Complications in Gynecologic Surgery

Complications in Gynecologic Surgery

PREVENTION, RECOGNITION, AND MANAGEMENT

Editors

James W. Orr, Jr., M.D.
Director
Division of Gynecologic Oncology
Watson Clinic
Lakeland, Florida

Hugh M. Shingleton, M.D.
J. Marion Sims Professor of Gynecology Emeritus
University of Alabama at Birmingham
National Vice President for Detection and Treatment
American Cancer Society
Atlanta, Georgia

with 19 contributors

J. B. Lippincott Company • PHILADELPHIA

Acquisitions Editor: Lisa McAllister
Sponsoring Editor: Emilie M. Linkins
Production Editor: Virginia Barishek
Indexer: Maria Coughlin
Interior Designer: William T. Donnelly
Cover Designer: Larry Pezzato
Production: P. M. Gordon Associates, Inc.
Compositor: Pine Tree Composition, Inc.
Prepress: Jay's Publishers Services, Inc.
Printer/Binder: Arcata Graphics/Kingsport

6   5   4   3   2   1

Library of Congress Cataloging-in-Publication Data

Complications in gynecologic surgery : prevention, recognition, and
    management / editors, James W. Orr, Jr., Hugh M. Shingleton ; with
      19 contributors.
        p.   cm.
    Includes bibliographical references and index.
    ISBN 0–397–51269–4
    1. Generative organs, Female—Surgery—Complications.   I. Orr,
James W.   II. Shingleton, Hugh M.
    [DNLM: 1. Genitalia, Female—Surgery.   2. Genital Diseases,
Female—surgery.   3. Intraoperative Complications.   WP 660 C7365
1994]
RG104.2.C66   1994
618.1′059—dc20
DNLM/DLC
for Library of Congress   93–41475
                                                               CIP

The authors and publisher have exerted every effort to ensure that drug selection
and dosage set forth in this text are in accord with current recommendations and
practice at the time of publication. However, in view of ongoing research,
changes in government regulations, and the constant flow of information relating
to drug therapy and drug reactions, the reader is urged to check the package insert
for each drug for any change in indications and dosage and for added warnings and
precautions. This is particularly important when the recommended agent is a new
or infrequently employed drug.

To Pamela Jo Orr
and Lucy Shingleton

Contributors

Kevin F. Browne, Jr., M.D.
Chairman of Research
Watson Clinic
Lakeland, Florida

Thomas W. Burke, M.D.
Associate Professor
Gynecologic Oncology
The University of Texas M. D. Anderson Cancer
   Center
Houston, Texas

Daniel L. Clarke-Pearson, M.D.
James Ingram Professor of Obstetrics and Gynecology
Duke University School of Medicine
Director, Division of Gynecologic Oncology
Duke University Medical Center
Durham, North Carolina

Benjamin E. Greer, M.D.
Professor
University of Washington School of Medicine
Director
Division of Gynecologic Oncology
University of Washington Medical Center
Seattle, Washington

David L. Hemsell, M.D.
Professor
Director, Division of Gynecology
University of Texas Southwestern Medical Center at
   Dallas
Director of Gynecology
Parkland Memorial Hospital
Dallas, Texas

Robert L. Holley, M.D.
Assistant Professor
Division of Medical and Surgical Gynecology
Department of Obstetrics and Gynecology
University of Alabama Medical Center
Birmingham, Alabama

Robert W. Holloway, M.D.
Division of Gynecologic Oncology
Watson Clinic
Lakeland, Florida

Walter B. Jones, M.D.
Associate Professor of Obstetrics and Gynecology
Cornell University Medical Center
Attending Surgeon, Department of Surgery
Gynecology Service
Memorial Hospital
New York, New York

Larry C. Kilgore, M.D.
Assistant Professor
Division of Gynecologic Oncology
University of Alabama at Birmingham
Birmingham, Alabama

Charles Levenback, M.D.
Assistant Professor
Gynecologic Oncology
The University of Texas M. D. Anderson Cancer
    Center
Houston, Texas

William J. Mann, Jr., M.D.
Gynecologic Oncologist and Director of Residency in
    Obstetrics and Gynecology
Riverside Regional Medical Center
Newport News, Virginia
Clinical Professor of Obstetrics and Gynecology
Medical College of Virginia
Richmond, Virginia

James W. Orr, Jr., M.D.
Director
Division of Gynecologic Oncology
Watson Clinic
Lakeland, Florida

Pamela Jo Orr, R.N., O.C.N.
Division of Gynecologic Oncology
Watson Clinic
Lakeland, Florida

Gustavo Rodriguez, M.D.
Assistant Professor
Duke University Medical School
Department of Obstetrics and Gynecology
Division of Gynecologic Oncology
Duke University Medical Center
Durham, North Carolina

Victoria L. Seewaldt, M.D.
Senior Fellow, Oncology
University of Washington
Department of Internal Medicine
Division of Oncology
University of Washington Medical Center
Seattle, Washington

Hugh M. Shingleton, M.D.
J. Marion Sims Professor of Gynecology Emeritus
University of Alabama at Birmingham
National Vice President for Detection and Treatment
American Cancer Society
Atlanta, Georgia

Barry S. Siller, M.D.
University of Alabama School of Medicine
University Hospital
Birmingham, Alabama

Peyton T. Taylor, Jr., M.D.
Richard N. and Louise R. Crockett Professor
Director, Division of Gynecologic Oncology
Clinical Director, Cancer Center
University of Virginia Health Sciences Center
University of Virginia Hospital
Charlottesville, Virginia

Ravinder Tikoo, M.D.
Gynecology Service
Department of Surgery
Memorial Sloan-Kettering Cancer Center
New York, New York

Preface

Each year, over four million surgical procedures of the reproductive tract are performed in this country. Fortunately, the vast majority of outcomes are good. When perioperative complications occur, however, early recognition and appropriate management can minimize their adverse effects. This book focuses on the prevention and management of problems encountered during pelvic surgery. Chapters, organized by organ system, stress both specific prophylaxis and management of complications related to individual procedures. The organ-specific complications of conventional and radical operative procedures are covered, both for malignant and nonmalignant diseases. Contributors representing all areas of the country have been selected for their expertise. The information presented is intended to assist physicians during their training or clinical practice and to provide an authoritative reference source. It is the editors' belief that this book provides the information necessary to recognize risks, prevent complications, and manage adverse outcomes to increase the safety of women undergoing surgery.

The editors specifically thank Sylvia Foltz and Josephine Taylor for their tireless efforts in the compilation of this text.

James W. Orr, Jr., M.D.
Hugh M. Shingleton, M.D.

Contents

Chapter 10

Hugh M. Shingleton and Barry S. Siller

Chapter 11

William J. Mann, Jr.

Complications in Gynecologic Surgery

Complications in Gynecologic Surgery: Prevention, Recognition, and Management,
edited by James W. Orr, Jr., and Hugh M. Shingleton.
J. B. Lippincott Company, Philadelphia, © 1994.

Chapter 1

Cardiovascular Complications

James W. Orr, Jr.
Kevin F. Browne, Jr.

The primary objective of reducing operative morbidity and mortality can best be achieved by incorporating an orderly method of perioperative risk assessment designed to detect an individual's coexisting physiologic or psychological abnormalities. This information allows the surgical team to utilize perioperative patient assessment and monitoring to optimize the patient's medical status and postoperative care. Even in optimal circumstances, perioperative complications occur, and it is imperative that surgeons not only understand surgical risks but react with appropriate or necessary therapeutic intervention when complications or unexpected events occur during the patient's postoperative convalescence.

Although risk reduction for the individual patient is important, the impact of risk stratification and risk reduction on a national scale becomes apparent when reviewing hospital discharge survey data.[1] Gynecologist-obstetricians annually perform over 4 million operative procedures in the United States. Cesarean section is the most frequently performed major surgical procedure (945,000 per year) in the United States, while hysterectomy (591,000 per year), and adnexal surgery (476,000 per year) are two of the five most frequently performed major surgical procedures. Recent technical innovations in diagnostic or therapeutic laparoscopic surgery offer a "minimally invasive" approach to many gynecologic surgical problems, and the frequency of

these procedures is increasing proportionately. Additionally, "short" anesthetics for uterine dilation and curettage (137,000 per year), hysteroscopy, or conization are frequently necessary. In fact, nearly 2% of women in the United States undergo reproductive tract surgery each year. Fortunately, most of these procedures are well tolerated by young and healthy women; however, significant complications and even mortality occur following gynecologic procedures (Table 1–1). Reducing an individual patient's surgical risk is paramount; improving outcome on a local, regional, or national level will likely effect a favorable reduction of health care expenditures.

Regardless of operative approach or technique, the majority of surgical procedures have in common the need for anesthesia. Modern anesthetic and monitoring techniques have evolved to safely produce the necessary relaxation and analgesia required for almost any surgical procedure, even in the elderly or in those with significant associated medical disease. Techniques of intraoperative monitoring have rapidly advanced, progressing from the "finger on the pulse" technique of the 1940s to invasive blood pressure monitoring in the 1970s and continuous oxygen saturation monitoring, pulmonary artery (PA) catheterization, pulse oximetry, and intraoperative transesophageal echocardiography in the 1980s.[2] Despite these innovations, anesthesia and the perioperative period should not be

TABLE 1–1. **Relative Complication and Mortality Rate, by Procedure**

	Complication Rate/1,000 Patients		
Surgical Procedure	*HEW* *(Ages 15–44)*	*Metropolitan Life* *(Ages 25–44)*	*Death Rate/* *1,000 Patients*
Dilation and curettage	8.86	1.09	0.10
Hysterectomy	4.77	7.00	0.25
Bilateral tubal ligation	3.97	—	0.04
Ovariectomy	2.77	1.10	0.30
Appendectomy	1.93	1.00	0.13

Modified from Houston MC: Preoperative medical consultation and evaluation of surgical risk. South Med J 80;1386–1397, 1987.

considered an isolated physiologic phenomenon. The psychological and physiologic stress of anesthesia and surgery is a tremendous assault on the reserves of any woman. Pain, apprehension, volume challenge, increased production and release of serum catecholamines, tachycardia, hypothermia, and hemorrhage may be well tolerated by women with normal cardiac and pulmonary function but may have catastrophic consequences in women with associated medical problems or limited cardiorespiratory reserve. In essence, surgery and anesthesia serve as a "stress test" of the cardiovascular and pulmonary system. Failure to evaluate associated risks preoperatively, or to develop a method of perioperative management to detect and treat cardiorespiratory complications, increases the potential of a poor surgical outcome, even with the best surgical technique.

Surgeons should continually strive for improvement in the quality of care in the delivery of surgical services. One potential method to improve perioperative outcome involves medical consultation, particularly when confronted with a high-risk surgical patient or a clinical situation in which surgical risks are difficult to define. In this setting, the internist's role should be to assist the surgeon in preventing and managing problems contributing to surgical morbidity and mortality. There is little need for or benefit from routine perioperative medical consultation in low-risk patients, as it rarely results in significant clinical recommendations but does increase costs by approximately $280 per patient.[3] However, pre- or perioperative medical consultation can offer a significant number of recommendations in those patients who are likely to undergo a medium- or high-risk surgical procedure and whose history, physical, or laboratory examination findings place them at high risk in the American Society of Anesthesiologists' (ASA) classification for perioperative complications.[3] Consultation for patients in high-risk categories may be appropriate, as higher ASA status is associated with increased acute and late perioperative mortality following elective and emergency surgery (Table 1–2). Even with consultation, it remains the surgeon's responsibility to understand the basis for medical recommendations and assist in their implementation when deemed appropriate, and to discuss or even reject specific recommendations if necessary.

The perioperative risks and management plans for surgical complications related to the reproductive, gastrointestinal, or urinary tract are stressed during residency and postresidency gynecologic training. Residents or physicians in practice are less likely to receive intensive training or education in the detection and management of perioperative cardiac or pulmonary complications. Additionally, the indications, results, and implications of new cardiovascular or pulmonary management schemes, drugs, or diagnostic studies are rarely published or reviewed in the gynecologic literature. This information void often makes it necessary to consult a nonsurgical subspecialist who may not completely comprehend the extent or necessity for operation. Additionally, specific subspecialists may focus their perioperative recommendation only on their organ of interest. These problems, as well as an increasing body of critical care knowledge and complex technology, a lack of economic incentive, and potential liability issues, have resulted in surgeons abdicating their traditional role of providing pre- and postoperative care in many situations, particularly in surgical intensive care units. One recent report suggested that surgeons relinquish their principal management role in intensive care units for surgical patients in 75% of hospitals.[4]

The primary goal of this chapter is to update the

TABLE 1–2. **Mortality Associated with American Society of Anesthesiologists (ASA) Physical Status Classification**

	ASA Class*				
	I	*II*	*III*	*IV*	*V*
48-Hour Mortality (%)					
(*n* = 68,388)					
Elective	0.07	0.24	1.4	7.5	8.1
Emergency	0.16	0.51	3.4	8.3	9.5
6-Week Mortality (%)					
(*n* = 856,000)					
Elective					
Low risk	0.03	0.31	1.9	5.6	20.0
Medium risk	0.02	1.7	7.2	17.2	31.4
High risk	2.2	5.4	14.6	20.5	42.4

Modified from Orr JW: Introduction to pelvic surgery: Pre- and postoperative care. In Gusberg SB: Female Genital Cancer. New York: Churchill Livingstone, 1988.
*ASA status: I—healthy, II—mild systemic disease, III—severe but not incapacitating disease, IV—incapacitating disease, V—moribund.

practicing gynecologist-obstetrician on pertinent issues as they relate to the identification and management of perioperative cardiac complications. Although the clinical interaction between cardiac and pulmonary risk factors is inseparable, they will be discussed individually for simplicity.

Cardiac Physiology

To understand surgical stress and risks, it is imperative that the surgeon have a basic understanding of cardiac physiology. Under normal conditions, the heart adjusts cardiac output (CO) to deliver an adequate amount of oxygenated blood and nutrients to satisfy total tissue metabolic requirements. When these metabolic needs are significantly increased during the perioperative interval, peripheral tissue requirements substantially increase CO, resulting in increased myocardial work.

Cardiac output is the amount of blood pumped to the peripheral circulation per minute and is the product of heart rate and stroke volume. Normal values are 5 to 6 L/min but with stress may increase to more than 10 L/min. Heart rate depends on the intrinsic rhythmicity of the sinoatrial node and is further affected by extrinsic neural or humoral factors. Stroke volume is primarily determined by *preload* (the volume of blood stretching the myocardial muscle *before* contraction) but is also affected by afterload and contractility of both healthy and diseased myocardium. *Preload,* or left ventricular

end-diastolic volume (LVEDV), is difficult to measure but can be approximated using echocardiography (precordial or transesophageal), ventriculography, or radionuclide scintigraphy. Left ventricular end-diastolic pressure (LVEDP), frequently measured clinically with a PA catheter, is used as an approximation of LVEDV. This relationship is not linear, particularly in the presence of myocardial ischemia or other conditions when ventricular relaxation (compliance) is abnormal. Important factors affecting *preload* include total blood volume, body position, intrathoracic pressure, intrapericardial pressure, venous tone, the pumping action of skeletal muscles, and atrial contribution to ventricular filling.

In 1895 Frank described the increased pressure generated by the myocardial muscle when the filling pressure was increased just prior to contraction. The presystolic or end-diastolic volume and filling pressure determine the magnitude of the all-or-none muscular response. These initial studies emphasized the dependence of the cardiac response on hemodynamic events immediately preceding electrical excitation. In 1914, Starling described the increased stroke volume produced when diastolic ventricular volume was increased or when venous return was augmented. Starling's conclusion that cardiac responsiveness was primarily related to presystolic muscle fiber length has been validated by nearly all investigators. The Frank-Starling curve (Fig. 1–1) represents a family of ventricular function curves demonstrating the relationship between

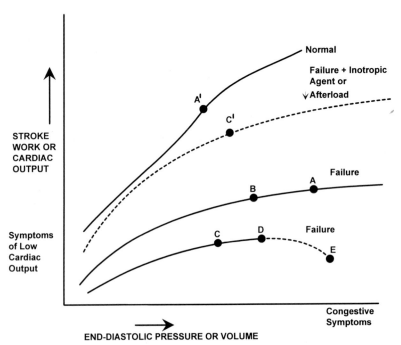

FIGURE 1–1. Ventricular function curves relating left ventricular filling pressure to ventricular performance expressed as cardiac output or stroke work. The filling pressure can be expressed as either the left ventricular end-diastolic pressure or volume. *Curve A*[1] indicates normal ventricular contractility. The normal left ventricle increases its stroke work as preload (often measured clinically as pulmonary capillary wedge pressure) increases, moving up the ascending limb of the curve until reserve is exhausted. In heart failure (*CDE*), the ventricular function curve is displaced downward and to the right. An increase in contractility, as after administration of norepinephrine or digitalis, displaces the curve to the left; i.e., a larger stroke output is accomplished at any given filling pressure (*BA*). Reduction in physical activity allows the failing heart to meet metabolic demands. Treatment of heart failure by a reduction in preload (i.e., with a diuretic or a vasodilator acting predominantly on the venous bed) causes a shift from point *A* to *B* on the same ventricular function curve. Administration of a positive inotropic agent or a vasodilator producing afterload reduction will shift the curve, resulting in improvement of the circulatory state in the direction shown by a shift from point *A* to *C*[1].

ventricular wall tension and diastolic fiber length or their physiologically measurable analogues. In any given circulatory state there is a consistent relationship between atrial pressure and stroke volume of the ipsilateral ventricle. At high filling pressures the curve flattens to a plateau. A descending line (decreasing ventricular volume with increasing effective filling pressure) usually does not occur in the normal heart but may occur in the presence of a compromised myocardium. The Frank-Starling effect is primarily responsible for the matching of CO and venous return and also ultimately the matching of right and left ventricular output. While important, preload and the contractile inotropic state of the myocardium cannot be considered theoretically independent determinants of myocardial performance.

Afterload is simplistically noted as the ventricular wall stress measured at end-systole and involves measurement of arterial input impedance. For the left ventricle, the sum of opposing forces (afterload or aortic input impedance) is composed of peripheral vascular resistance (friction), arterial capacitance (stiffness), the mass of the aortic column of blood, and blood viscosity. Left ventricular wall tension is thus an indicator of afterload but is not the same as afterload. Systemic vascular resistance (SVR) is the most commonly used clinical indicator of afterload; however, the measured mean pressure-flow phenomenon ignores the pulsatile component of ventricular ejection.

Contractility is an intrinsic property of the cardiac cell and is primarily determined by the availability of intracellular calcium (Ca^{2+}). Increasing intracellular Ca^{2+}, by facilitating entry into the cell or release by sarcoplasmic reticulum, increases the number of actin-myosin crossbridges. Ejection phase indices are clinically used as a measure of contractility and are commonly evaluated by non-invasive techniques. *Ejection fraction* (EF) is defined as the result of (stroke volume) ÷ (end-diastolic volume).

Blood pressure is often used as a surrogate for CO because it is easily measured and, in the absence of disease, frequently gives adequate clinical information. However, actual CO can be measured by several methods, including the Fick and dye dilution techniques, as well as by direct flowmeter techniques, including Doppler and aortic pulse contour measurement. If attention is given to injecting correct volumes, using a correct rate of delivery, or avoiding measurements during infusion of large intravascular volumes, thermodilution techniques using thermistors in PA catheters offer satisfactory results with a small standard deviation (4.6%) when performed in triplicate.[5] Measurements of CO, its derivatives (Fig. 1–2), and ventricular filling pressures allow construction of clinical ventricular function curves that assist in the detection of cardiovascular dysfunction and allow rational bedside intervention or prophylactic therapy.

The adequacy of CO and tissue perfusion can be inferred by measuring blood pressure, assessing tissue warmth or tissue color, or evaluating capillary refill time (normal, 2 to 3 sec). However, the important role of circulatory function relates to oxygen transport (TO_2), which is the product of CO × arterial oxygen content (CaO_2). Normal CaO_2 is primarily related to hemoglobin (Hb)-bound oxygen, with a lesser component from oxygen dissolved in plasma. Thus, CaO_2 is derived as:

$$CaO_2 = (1.39) \text{ (arterial } O_2 \text{ saturation)} + (0.003)(PaO_2),$$

where 1.39 is the oxygen-carrying capacity of Hb (mL/g) and 0.003 is the solubility of oxygen in plasma at 37° C (mL O_2/mL blood). Normal CaO_2 is

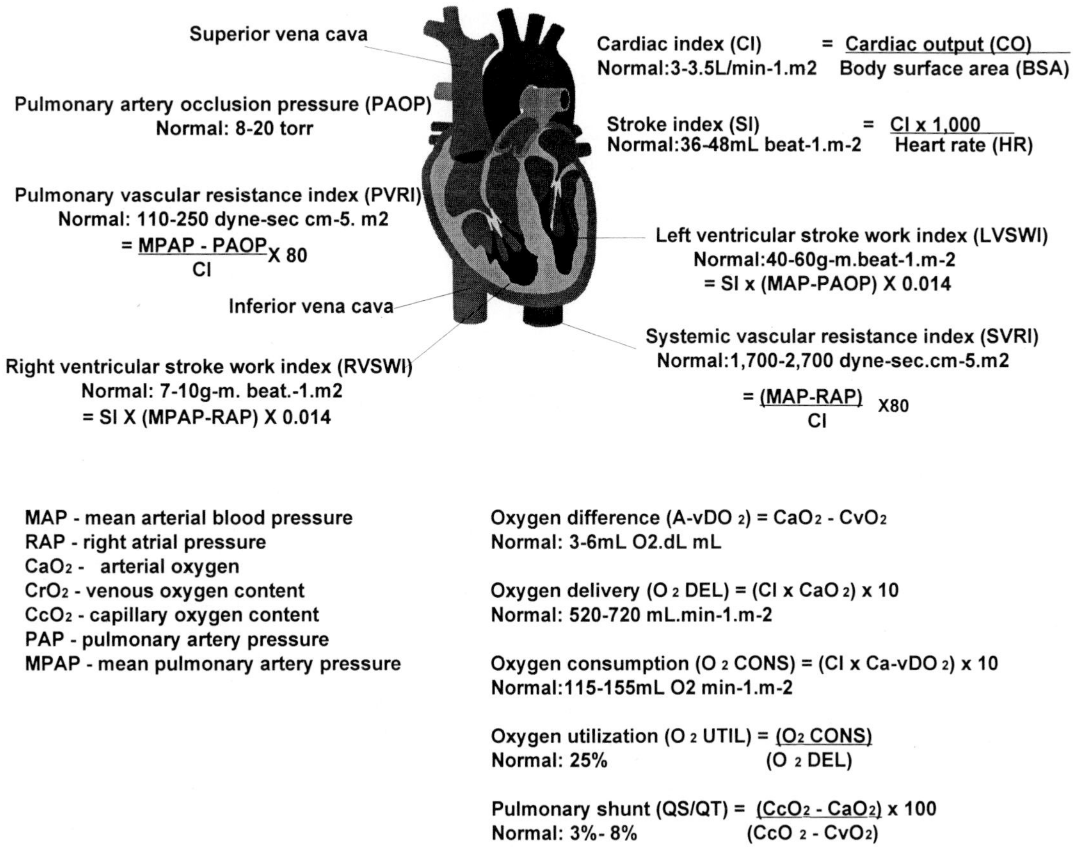

Superior vena cava

Pulmonary artery occlusion pressure (PAOP)
Normal: 8-20 torr

Pulmonary vascular resistance index (PVRI)
Normal: 110-250 dyne-sec cm-5. m2
$$= \frac{MPAP - PAOP}{CI} \times 80$$

Inferior vena cava

Right ventricular stroke work index (RVSWI)
Normal: 7-10g-m. beat.-1.m2
= SI X (MPAP-RAP) X 0.014

Cardiac index (CI) $= \dfrac{\text{Cardiac output (CO)}}{\text{Body surface area (BSA)}}$
Normal:3-3.5L/min-1.m2

Stroke index (SI) $= \dfrac{CI \times 1{,}000}{\text{Heart rate (HR)}}$
Normal:36-48mL beat-1.m-2

Left ventricular stroke work index (LVSWI)
Normal:40-60g-m.beat-1.m-2
= SI x (MAP-PAOP) X 0.014

Systemic vascular resistance index (SVRI)
Normal:1,700-2,700 dyne-sec.cm-5.m2
$$= \frac{(MAP-RAP)}{CI} \times 80$$

MAP - mean arterial blood pressure
RAP - right atrial pressure
CaO₂ - arterial oxygen
CrO₂ - venous oxygen content
CcO₂ - capillary oxygen content
PAP - pulmonary artery pressure
MPAP - mean pulmonary artery pressure

Oxygen difference (A-vDO $_2$) = CaO$_2$ - CvO$_2$
Normal: 3-6mL O2.dL mL

Oxygen delivery (O $_2$ DEL) = (CI x CaO $_2$) x 10
Normal: 520-720 mL.min-1.m-2

Oxygen consumption (O $_2$ CONS) = (CI x Ca-vDO $_2$) x 10
Normal:115-155mL O2 min-1.m-2

Oxygen utilization (O $_2$ UTIL) $= \dfrac{(O_2 \text{ CONS})}{(O_2 \text{ DEL})}$
Normal: 25%

Pulmonary shunt (QS/QT) $= \dfrac{(CcO_2 - CaO_2)}{(CcO_2 - CvO_2)} \times 100$
Normal: 3%- 8%

FIGURE 1–2. Important measurable and derived cardiac indices available with pulmonary artery catheter monitoring.

20 mL O_2/dL of blood, and with a normal CO, TO_2 is approximately 1 L/min.

The relationship between SaO_2, PaO_2, and CaO_2 is related to the oxyhemoglobin dissociation curve, and TO_2 can be dramatically affected by shifting this curve. In patients with a normal Hb, CaO_2 remains 20 mL O_2/dL when the PaO_2 is ≥50 mm Hg and SaO_2 is ≥90%, but diminishes rapidly below these levels.

Tissue oxygen consumption (VO_2) is the difference between oxygen transported and oxygen returned and is expressed by:

$$VO_2 = CO \ (C[a\text{-}v]O_2).$$

Thus, inadequate oxygen consumption can result from a decrease in CaO_2, CO, or tissue consumption of oxygen and can be favorably improved by manipulating any of these variables. CaO_2 is frequently reduced in the presence of anemia, in patients with decreased SaO_2, and in patients with abnormal hemoglobins (e.g., thalassemia). CO may be limited by cardiac decompensation or toxicity from drugs or metabolic products.

In some situations, critically ill postoperative patients shift from aerobic to anaerobic metabolism and develop lactic acidosis despite normal or elevated CO and CaO_2 levels. This failure of oxygen extraction is characterized by high (>50 mm Hg) mixed venous oxygen tension (PVO_2), high (>80%) mixed venous oxygen saturation (SVO_2), high (>181 mL O_2/mL) mixed venous oxygen content, and a small gradient (<5 mL O_2/mL) of arterial-venous content.[6]

Coronary Blood Supply

Both right and left coronary arteries originate at the root of the aorta. The right coronary artery (RCA) supplies the right atrium, ventricle, and, in most subjects, the inferior left ventricle. The left coronary artery (LCA) divides into the left anterior descending (LAD) and left circumflex (LCX) artery and supplies the left atrium and the remainder of the left ventricle. In humans, the sinus node is supplied by the RCA in 55% of people and the LCA in 45% of people. The RCA supplies the atrioventricular (AV) node in 90% of cases, while the AV node is supplied by the LCA in 10% of cases. The anterior papillary muscle is nearly always supplied by the LCA and the posterior papillary muscle is usually supplied by both coronary arteries. The majority of coronary blood flow returns to the right atrium via the coronary sinus; however, arterial sinusoidal as well as arterioluminal communication and thebesian vessels form an extensive plexus of subendocardial vasculature.[7]

Resting coronary blood flow is approximately 200 to 225 mL/min, comprising 4% to 5% of the total CO. The myocardium efficiently extracts approximately 65% of the available oxygen from arterial blood. Thus the only source of additional myocardial oxygenation during periods of increased demand is increased blood flow.

The normal coronary artery circulation demonstrates autoregulation, with blood pressure maintained within relatively narrow limits. Changes in coronary blood pressure are primarily related to vessel caliber changes in the coronary resistance vessels in response to altered myocardial metabolic demands. This regulation is specific, and maximum coronary dilation or constriction can be elicited within 15 to 20 seconds.[6]

The ratio of subendocardial to epicardial blood flow is approximately 1.25:1, and the majority of coronary artery blood flow to the left ventricle occurs during diastole as myocardial vessels are compressed during contraction impairing flow during systole.[6] The contraction-related pressure gradient is highest in the subendocardium and lowest in the epicardium, resulting in minimal or no blood flow through the left ventricular subendocardium during systole. Any elevation in heart rate decreases diastolic time and contribution to coronary artery flow as well as ventricular filling. An increase in heart rate from 50 to 70 beats/min is associated with a reduction in diastolic time from 70% to 50%. An increase from 70 to 90 beats/min further reduces diastolic time from 50% to 45%. This reduced blood flow places the subendocardium at the greatest risk of ischemia, particularly during episodes of severe hypotension and tachycardia.

Coronary artery perfusion pressure is defined as the aortic diastolic blood pressure minus LVEDP. Elevation of the latter can effectively decrease subendocardial blood flow at a level equivalent to a drop in diastolic blood pressure. In the presence of hemodynamically significant coronary artery disease (CAD), coronary artery perfusion pressure will decrease, and any elevation in LVEDP further jeopardizes subendocardial blood flow.

Coronary artery perfusion pressure is intimately related to coronary blood flow. The importance of this interaction becomes prominent when the perfusion pressure falls below 60 mm Hg. At or below this level, coronary arteries become maximally dilated and coronary flow becomes totally dependent on perfusion pressure.

Gynecologic surgeons are frequently confronted with patients "diagnosed" with CAD who are taking a variety of cardioactive medications that may require manipulation during the perioperative period. Currently, three classes of drugs—nitrates, β-blockers, and calcium channel blockers—are used clinically to improve coronary blood flow in patients with CAD (Fig. 1–3). Each drug class has a unique mechanism of activity, and combined administration of drugs of different classes produces synergistic effects.

Nitrates, the most commonly employed drugs for the treatment of CAD, have a primary effect of vasodilation, predominantly on the venous system but also directly on the coronary arterioles. Nitrates are the only one of the three groups of antianginal drugs that have no direct negative inotropic properties. Through a mechanism of action recently more fully understood, nitrates cause vascular smooth muscle vasodilation through nitric oxide receptors. The resultant dilation is associated with decreased blood return to the heart and a lowered preload, thereby reducing oxygen demand. Recent studies have also confirmed the presence of increased coronary blood flow secondary to arterial vasodilation. During the perioperative period, particularly in the presence of hypovolemia, the administration of nitrates can have a deleterious effect by creating systemic hypotension and a compensatory sinus tachycardia. Nitrates are most frequently administered intravenously (IV) in the patient with a rapidly changing hemodynamic status but also can be administered transcutaneously or orally.

β-blockers are highly effective drugs that suppress the β-sympathetic effect of circulating catecholamines and decrease heart rate and lower blood pressure. They are particularly useful in patients with stable constant threshold angina secondary to fixed obstructive coronary disease. β-blockers are most frequently employed during the perioperative period in those patients who had been receiving β-blockers preoperatively in an attempt to prevent rebound tachycardia. β-blockers may be administered IV to control hypertension and tachycardia associated with an increased sympathetic tone. Their use may adversely affect left ventricular function

MYOCARDIAL OXYGENATION

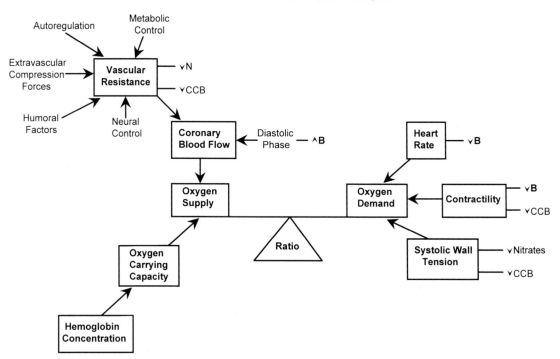

FIGURE 1–3. Factors affecting the balance of myocardial oxygen supply and demand. N, nitrates, CCB, calcium channel blockers; B, β-blockers.

and renal blood flow, and the perioperative initiation of these agents should be done cautiously and only after left ventricular function has been assessed.

Calcium channel blockers are potent vasodilatory agents that act directly on smooth muscle at the arterial level. Their use results in a significant increase in coronary blood flow and peripheral blood flow. Although as a class, calcium channel blockers should be considered to have negative inotropic effects, newer agents such as amlodipine and felodipine appear to have selective activity without significant negative inotropic effect. These agents are safe to use even in patients with mild to moderate congestive heart failure (CHF).

The patient receiving both IV β-blockers and calcium channel blockers should be continuously monitored. This is particularly true for patients who also receive digitalis in combination with two or three of these drugs. Digitalis can produce a high-degree AV block and severely depress sinus node function, resulting in hemodynamically destabilizing bradyarrhythmias. When administered orally in typical therapeutic doses, β-blockers plus calcium channel blockers are unlikely to produce substantial bradyarrhythmia.

Cardiac Alterations Specific to Pregnancy

Most of the 40% elevation in CO that occurs with pregnancy is devoted to the products of conception in direct support of the growing fetus. Increased cutaneous renal blood flow, which allows heat dissipation and excretion of specific metabolic products, also consumes a portion of the increased CO. Arteries, veins, capillaries, and many organs, especially the uterus, dilate, and blood volume increases by as much as 50%. Plasma volume expansion exceeds that of circulating red blood cell mass, contributing to the development of physiologic anemia.

As the metabolic demands of the fetus increase through pregnancy, so in theory should the maternal CO. However, maternal CO peaks at about the sixth gestational month, coinciding with the time that pregnant patients with cardiac disease often become symptomatic. From 6 months until term, CO may increase, decrease, or remain constant. In early pregnancy, stroke volume is responsible for the majority of the increment in CO. Later increases in CO follow heart rate and may become of critical significance in patients with limited cardiac reserve. The patient with obstructive valvular heart disease (e.g., mitral valve stenosis) in whom diastolic filling time limits performance is particularly at risk.[7]

Cardiac Effects of Anesthesia

Nearly all inhalational agents depress myocardial contractility, modify neural control of vascular tone, and are arrhythmogenic. Nitrous oxide and isoflurane increase heart rate but have minimal effect on actual CO, while the administration of halothane and enflurane can decrease cardiac output by 20% to 50%. Nitrous oxide has little to no effect on stroke volume; however, stroke volume is decreased by 40% to 60% by enflurane and by 20% to 40% by isoflurane and halothane.[8] Thiopental results in a 10% to 25% decrease in CO, and newer agents such as propofol also have a potentially significant negative inotropic effect. Some anesthetic techniques (balanced regimen of droperidol and fentanyl or nitrous oxide plus pancuronium bromide) produce little myocardial depression at the expense of increasing the time to reversal of the anesthetic.[9] Although all agents blunt coronary artery regulation, isoflurane is the most potent coronary artery dilator of epicardial vessels, and its use can result in coronary steal and decreased coronary perfusion pressure. These anesthetic-associated negative inotropic cardiac effects are usually well tolerated by the young, healthy woman undergoing transvaginal hysterectomy or repair; however, the same physiologic effects when coupled with coexisting disease are more likely to result in an adverse outcome in the obese, the elderly, those undergoing an extensive operative procedure, or women with coexisting CAD.

Because of the potential cardiac effects, it is the responsibility of both the pelvic surgeon and the anesthesiologist to evaluate associated cardiac risks so as to modify preoperative preparation, intraoperative technique, and methods of intra- or postoperative surveillance. The choice of anesthetic is influenced by specific preoperative findings (historical, laboratory, or radiologic) and by the surgeon's intraoperative and postoperative needs. Although anesthetic management may be modified (risk stratification) with input from the internist or cardiologist (Fig. 1–4), actual anesthetic management must be primarily decided by the anesthesiologist.

Prevention of Ischemia

Despite popular opinion, cardiac risks are not primarily dependent on the choice of regional versus general anesthesia[9] or on specific anesthetic agents, but rather on the anesthesiologist's techniques, skills, methods of monitoring, detection of specific problems, and appropriate intervention. Multiple studies have demonstrated no difference in peri-

ANESTHESIOLOGY

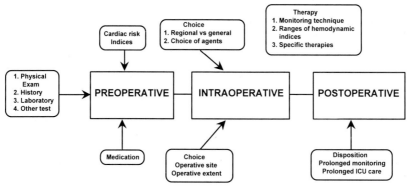

SURGICAL

FIGURE 1–4. Important factors related to the choice of anesthetic route and regimen.

operative myocardial infarction (MI) risks associated with regional or general anesthesia.[10] In patients with a history of prior MI, Rao et al. reported a 1.8% (12/659) reinfarction rate with general anesthesia and a 2.7% (2/74) reinfarction rate following regional anesthesia.[11] Additionally, there is no apparent difference in the incidence of perioperative arrhythmias between regional and general anesthesia. The only potential benefit of regional (subarachnoid, epidural) anesthesia is a possible decrease (10×) in the risk of developing postoperative CHF.[2]

Regardless of the individual risk stratification and the actual anesthetic technique, the anesthesiologist must maintain a positive effect on the cardiac oxygen supply and demand ratio and deliver anesthesia with a 50% or greater oxygen concentration in the inspired mixture. Avoiding hypoxia is a primary goal because hypoxia may contribute to 50% of all perioperative cardiac deaths.[12] Although some intubations remain difficult, the introduction of routine percutaneous oxygen saturation monitoring and the continuous measurement of intraoperative end-tidal CO_2 production has all but eliminated the risk of hypoxemia associated with improper placement of the endotracheal tube. Maintenance of adequate postoperative oxygenation is obviously important in preventing potential cardiac morbidity but may decrease infectious complications as well.[13]

Specific attention should be devoted to the detection or prevention of perioperative problems such as hypotension (which may be related to perioperative medications), sympathetic blockade, or existing intravascular volume depletion even in the absence of large volume blood loss. Hypotension

(systolic blood pressure < 90 mm Hg) reduces myocardial wall tension and oxygen demand; however, its adverse effects on coronary perfusion (oxygen supply) dominate. As many as 25% of perioperative ischemic events are associated with an episode of 20% or greater reduction in systolic blood pressure. At least five studies have demonstrated a causal relationship between hypotension and myocardial ischemia.[14] In those patients with a previous MI, reinfarction rates may increase by a factor of five if systolic hypotension (≥30% reduction) occurs for a 10-minute duration, particularly if associated with tachycardia. The risk of hypotension may be increased in specific patient subsets. As many as 38% of patients with gynecologic cancer enter the operating room with significant existing deficits in intravascular volume secondary to concurrent disease, concurrent use of medications such as diuretics, or even mechanical bowel preparation.[15] Additional blood loss in these patients clearly increases the incidence and severity of hypotension and its sequelae. In addition to evaluating preoperative volume status and minimizing blood loss, specific considerations to decrease the risk of postoperative hypotension might include the use of specific narcotics. Morphine is associated with hypotension secondary to vagally induced bradycardia, vasodilation, and splenic blood sequestration (secondary to histamine release). In specific situations it would be prudent to use fentanyl or other narcotics that do not release histamine and are associated with a lesser risk of hypotension. The recent introduction and use of injectable nonsteroidal anti-inflammatory agents has potentially decreased the need for high-dose narcotics.

The occurrence of hemodynamically significant perioperative or intraoperative hypertension (related to intubation or sympathetic stimulation) also significantly increases perioperative cardiac risks. Although fewer than 15% of intraoperative ischemic episodes are associated with hypertension, as many as 50% of perioperative ischemic episodes are associated with elevated blood pressure. In the nonfailing ventricle, associated increased diastolic pressures may raise coronary perfusion pressure; however, in the failing ventricle, the elevation in LVEDP (and intramyocardial wall tension) may exceed the elevation in systemic and coronary artery diastolic pressure, resulting in decreased coronary flow, increased static work, and myocardial ischemia.

Prevention of Arrhythmia

Postoperative tachycardia of 25% to 50% of the preoperative heart rate occurs in as many as 25% of patients and is associated with a decrease in oxygen supply (decreased diastolic filling and perfusion time) and an increased oxygen demand (increased ventricular work).[2] Although usually well tolerated, the adverse effects of an elevated heart rate on diastolic time can result in ventricular dysfunction. The use of short-acting β-blockers such as esmolol may be required. The initial approach to the management of tachycardia involves excluding other important physiologic events (hypovolemia, hypoxia) as a cause. Pharmacologic intervention should be considered only if no reversible factors are found. In the patient managed chemically with β-blockers preoperatively, tachycardia should be expected postoperatively unless these drugs are continued.

All anesthetics are considered arrhythmogenic; however, the incidence of perioperative arrhythmias depends greatly on inclusion criteria and methods of monitoring. It appears that the majority (72%) of perioperative arrhythmias occur during intubation or extubation.[16] Halothane is the most arrhythmogenic and enflurane the least arrhythmogenic inhalational agent.[17]

Alteration of thermoregulatory centers occurs during general anesthesia but not with regional anesthesia. These central changes, when combined with abdominal organ exposure, blood loss, rapid infusion of cool IV fluids, and prolonged operative times, often result in hypothermia. In fact, as many as 60% of patients are hypothermic (core temperature <36° C) on their return to the recovery room. Although the anesthesiologist assumes primary responsibility for maintaining normothermia in the cold operating room environment, the surgeon should be aware of associated adverse effects (Table 1–3).[18] Hypothermia-induced peripheral vasoconstriction may result in or contribute to hemodynamically significant hypertension, mask the presence of hypovolemia, and increase the risk of dysrhythmia, particularly if core temperatures are below 33° C. Associated postoperative shivering can increase oxygen consumption and postoperative oxygen demand by 300% to 800%.[18] Specific interventions to reduce the risks and sequelae of hypothermia can be undertaken by the entire surgical team. Room temperatures should be kept above 21° C until draping. Preparation solutions and large-volume infusions should be warmed. Recent information suggests that air warming systems may be the most efficient method to minimize the risk of intraoperative or postoperative hypothermia, and should be considered for use in women at greatest risk (the elderly, or those undergoing prolonged procedures).[18]

Although fever is not necessarily anesthetic related, its presence and the associated increase in heart rate and metabolic demands may have a deleterious effect in patients with borderline cardiovascular function. The evaluation and management of postoperative temperature elevation is discussed elsewhere. However, temperature suppression (after appropriate evaluation) can significantly decrease cardiac and metabolic demands. Care should be ex-

TABLE 1–3. **Effects of Hypothermia**

Cardiovascular
  Increased systemic vascular resistance (afterload)
  Increased blood viscosity
  Myocardial depression
  Arrhythmogenic
Respiratory
  Diminished response to hypoxemia
  Diminished response to hypercarbia
  Decreased CO_2 production
Neurologic
  Disorientation
  Confusion
Hematologic
  Increased viscosity
  Thrombocytopathy (impaired thromboxane synthesis)
  Thrombocytopenia
  Impaired coagulation
Renal
  Impaired sodium reabsorption
Metabolic
  Hyperglycemia

erted as neutrophil function is reportedly enhanced and macrophage oxidative metabolism is increased with temperature elevation. In fact, temperatures in the range of the usual fever may render host defenses more active and many pathogens more susceptible.[19]

Perioperative Vascular Access

Establishing adequate vascular access in the perioperative period is paramount in all patients but particularly in women with limited cardiorespiratory reserve or those undergoing extensive surgical procedures. Decisions regarding the need for monitoring and methods of volume replacement should be made before the procedure is begun.

Perioperative arterial cannulation may be necessary in patients who require continuous monitoring of arterial blood pressure or frequent measurement (more than three times daily) of arterial blood gases. Fortunately, the necessity for the latter indication has decreased dramatically with the routine use of percutaneous oximetry. Safe arterial access can be gained via the radial, axillary, femoral, or even dorsalis pedis route. The smallest-diameter catheter should be used, as patency is not related to catheter size. The most common complication of arterial access is thrombosis, which occurs in as many as 11% of radial arteries cannulized for 4 days and 29% for longer use. Fortunately, fewer than 1% of arterial thrombi require surgical intervention, but failure of pulse return or continued evidence of ischemia (for 6 hours) should prompt consultation.[20] Percutaneous insertion, replacement of the monitoring system every 48 hours, and catheter changes every 3 to 4 days are routinely recommended to minimize the risk of bacteremia. Arterial lines are responsible for 10% to 15% of hospital-acquired bacteremias. Cut-down placement should be avoided if possible because it increases the frequency of bacteremia ninefold when compared to percutaneous placement.[20]

Venous access must be established before the surgical procedure is begun to allow adequate drug administration as well as volume resuscitation. It must be remembered that catheter flow characteristics are primarily determined by the catheter's internal diameter and length and not by the actual catheter size. Thus, a 14-gauge, 2-inch-long catheter has a flow rate more than 1.5 times that of a 16-gauge catheter of the same length, which in turn has a flow rate double that of a 16-gauge, 12-inch-long catheter. Thus, long central venous catheters may not provide adequate access in those instances re-

quiring large volume resuscitation. The recent introduction of larger-gauge, shorter central lines has allowed central access to serve as a volume line. However, these larger catheters are subject to a potential risk of insertion or maintenance complications.

Sterile, centrally placed multilumen catheters can provide several IV routes with the risk and discomfort of a single access site. When compared to single-lumen catheters, multiple-lumen catheters cost more and have a larger outside catheter diameter. Additionally, multiple-lumen catheters have been associated with an increased risk of catheter sepsis (6×) when compared to single-lumen catheters, particularly if parenteral hyperalimentation is infused.[21] Regardless of lumen number, catheter infection is rare if the catheter is in place for 72 hours or less. Longer periods of use are associated with sepsis rates of 2% to 5%. The reported risk of infection varies widely, based in part on the investigator's definition of infection, selected patient population, number of breaks in aseptic technique, and catheter care routines.

In high-risk (septic or immunocompromised) patients, routine catheter care is important. Although routine catheter change at 3-day intervals has been recommended, one recent randomized prospective trial indicated that this practice did not prevent infection.[22] Although catheter change over guidewires decreased the risk of mechanical complication, it did not decrease the risk of bloodstream infection.[22]

A variety of complications have been reported following insertion and long-term use of central venous catheters. Insertion or mechanical complications are more closely related to the experience of the physician than to the route of access or the catheter type.[20] Cannulation failure rates are doubled when the catheter is placed by an inexperienced physician. Three unsuccessful insertion attempts at a single site should prompt attempts at another insertion site and perhaps by another operator.

Subclavian vein placement allows ready access to central circulation, provides a site that is well tolerated, and can be adequately secured to an immobile flat surface removed from body secretions. This site has the lowest infection risk of all possible sites. Mechanical complications range from 1% to 11% and are highest (15%) when the vein is accessed in the emergency setting. Cannulation of the jugular vein also permits access to the central venous circulation. Internal jugular cannulation is more likely to be successful than external jugular cannulation (91% vs. 76%); however, complications are higher (13% vs. 0%). The most common complication is inadvertent puncture of the carotid artery, which can result in hypovolemia, hemothorax, tracheal deviation, and airway compromise. Bedside ultrasound guidance can be of great benefit in placement of internal jugular catheters, particularly in difficult situations. Jugular insertion and neck movement are generally associated with a higher infection rate and lower stability than is subclavian access. In emergency or unusual situations, femoral or axillary access can be used.[20]

Another life-threatening complication, superior vena cava or cardiac perforation, may occur during insertion or as a result of later catheter movement or migration. The respective mortality from these complications approaches 67% and 100%. Immediate radiologic confirmation of catheter position and catheter immobilization potentially decreases these risks and is mandatory following every central venous line insertion.

Since its initial description in 1970, PA catheterization has become an integral part of perioperative or intensive care of high-risk surgical patients. Despite extensive clinical use, PA catheter placement has not been conclusively demonstrated to improve mortality rates, and its clinical utility in terms of the risk-benefit ratio is yet to be determined. A recent prospective study of 126 surgical patients that was undertaken to assess the clinical impact of PA catheterization in surgical intensive care units evaluated the accuracy of precatheterization predictions of PA wedge pressure, CO, and SVR. Results obtained after catheter insertion prompted a major change in therapy in 50% of patients, suggesting the value of obtaining hemodynamic variables with a PA catheter and improved accuracy of bedside evaluation.[23] Obviously, the important issue regarding PA catheter use does not relate to obtaining hemodynamic parameters but rather the therapeutic manipulations prompted or avoided because of these measurements.

In general, surgical patients do well, with overall mortalities much less than 2%; hence many surgeons are hesitant to depart from their organized perioperative routine until serious complications intervene. Unfortunately, by that time irreversible, potentially lethal cardiovascular changes may be present. Criteria for PA catheter placement include the necessity to make specific management decisions that are based on hemodynamic data obtained after insertion. Inadequate systemic and coronary perfusion can frequently be prevented or corrected by early aggressive therapy directed at attaining normal or supranormal values of hemodynamic pa-

rameters and results in decreased morbidity and mortality.[24]

Serious complications of PA catheterization are reported to occur in 5% of placements (Table 1–4). Most of these complications occur during insertion. Complications are substantially reduced when lines are placed by experienced physicians. Like any operation, PA catheter placement should not be considered a simple procedure but viewed with caution. Dysrhythmias occur in 50% of patients but are rarely hemodynamically significant or persistent.[20] Mechanical complications unique to PA catheterization include catheter knotting and PA rupture. The former should be suspected when difficulty in removing the catheter is encountered. Kinked or knotted catheters can be removed under fluoroscopic guidance, using angiographic techniques. Rupture of the PA related to prolonged balloon in-

TABLE 1–4. **Complications of Flow-Directed Pulmonary Artery Catheters**

Complication	Prevalence (%)
Central Venous Cannulation	
Arterial puncture/hematoma	8
Pneumothorax	2–4
Hydrothorax	2
Hemothorax, brachial plexus damage, air embolism, phrenic and recurrent laryngeal nerve damage, sheared catheter	(<1% each)
Passage of Catheter	
Arrhythmia	13–70; 1% serious
Right bundle-branch block	3
Cardiac perforation and tamponade	<1
Presence of Catheter in Circulation	
Infectious	
Frank infection	
Colonization/contamination	3–40
Sepsis	4–6
Thrombotic	
Thrombosis (evidence of)	60
Clinical thromboembolism	<1
Cardiac	
Endocardial damage	36
Valve damage	<1
Aseptic endocarditis at autopsy	21
Bacterial endocarditis	0–5
Pulmonary	
Pulmonary infarction	<1–7
Pulmonary artery rupture	<1% each
Mechanical	
Balloon rupture	1–5
Knotting	<1

flation, distal migration of the balloon followed by vigorous inflation, or disease of the PA segment is manifested by massive hemoptysis, occurs in one in 800 catheterizations, and carries a mortality rate of 80%.[20]

Perioperative Cardiac Morbidity

Clinical cardiovascular disease affects one in four Americans (65/239 million). Hypertension is the most prevalent (59.1 million), and CAD (6.7 million) causes the greatest morbidity and mortality (540,000 deaths annually). The associated annual mortality from CAD (1 million) accounts for one of every two deaths in the United States, exceeding the mortality from all other diseases combined. Significant annual cardiovascular morbidity includes 1.5 million MIs, 0.6 million strokes, and 0.4 million cases of CHF. Associated cardiac health care costs surpass $80 billion per year.[2]

Despite new or innovative medical or surgical therapy, cardiovascular disease will continue to be a perioperative problem because the prevalence of CAD increases with age. The population of the United States is aging rapidly; currently 25 million people (10%) are 65 years or older and nearly 3.0 million are older than 85 years of age. By the middle of the 21st century the population over 65 is expected to increase to nearly 70 million.[25] Although cardiovascular disease death rates have been reduced, the predominant influence of aging, which increases the overall incidence of cardiovascular disease, will offset this decreased mortality.

Perioperative cardiac morbidity, the leading cause of death after anesthesia and surgery, is generally defined as the occurrence of MI, unstable angina, CHF, serious dysrhythmia, or cardiac death during the intraoperative or immediate postoperative period (Table 1–5). Currently, fewer than 100 studies spanning 35 years allow review of outcome data for perioperative cardiac morbidity. Although none specifically address associated risks during gynecologic and obstetric procedures, the potential impact and adverse effects of cardiovascular disease in the gynecologic-obstetric surgical population cannot be ignored. Extrapolations from current data suggest that as many as 750,000 women are at risk for cardiac morbidity or mortality during gynecologic or obstetric procedures.[2] Approximately 125,000 have diagnosed CAD (classic angina, Q waves on preoperative ECG) and 290,000 have two or more major risk factors for cardiovascular disease. Although the usual obstetric patient population is young, at least 20% of the 591,000 women undergoing hysterectomy each year are elderly.[1] Specific procedures for vaginal repair, incontinence, or malignancy occur primarily in the older population. At least 75% of gynecologic surgical procedures are major intra-abdominal procedures, and a significant proportion are emergency procedures. Perioperative cardiac morbidity is increased with abdominal procedures and is dramatically increased (3×) in patients undergoing upper abdominal surgery, during procedures lasting more than 3 hours (3×), and in patients undergoing emergency procedures (5×).[2]

The occurrence of perioperative cardiac morbidity not only creates acute care problems but also serves as an important clinical marker. Patients who develop but survive perioperative cardiac complications remain at high risk for chronic cardiac problems. In effect, surgery and the emergence from anesthesia is a physiologic cardiac stress test, and patients who develop any evidence of perioperative ischemia are at a 2.2-fold increased risk for later cardiovascular problems. One recent study[25] reported that in patients with preexisting chronic disease, including CAD, a previous history of CHF, or vascular disease, or who sustained postoperative infarction/ischemia associated with unstable angina, there was a 28-fold increased risk for the subsequent development of cardiac complications over ensuing months. In fact, over 70% of all later adverse cardiac outcomes were preceded by evidence of perioperative myocardial ischemia. The majority (67%) of later events occurred within

TABLE 1–5. Perioperative Cardiac Morbidity

Outcome	Reported Incidence (%)
Myocardial ischemia	
Preoperative	24
Intraoperative	18–74
Postoperative	27–38
Myocardial infarction	
Population	0.1–0.7
Prior MI	1.9–7.7
Recent MI	1–15
Vascular surgery	0–37
Ventricular failure	
Intraoperative	4.8
Postoperative	3.6
Serious arrhythmia	
Intraoperative	0.9–36
Postoperative	14–40

Modified from Mangano DT: Perioperative cardiac morbidity. Anesthesiology 72:153–184, 1990.

the first postoperative year. This information clearly indicates that aggressive long-term cardiovascular follow-up and intervention should be the rule in individuals who develop perioperative cardiac morbidity.[25]

Myocardial Ischemia

Perioperative myocardial ischemia can be precipitated by an increase in myocardial oxygen demand associated with tachycardia, hypertension, anemia, stress, sympathomimetic drugs, or even discontinuation of antianginal medications. As many as one half of perioperative ischemic episodes are unrelated to these factors, however, which suggests a cause related to deficits in myocardial oxygen supply. The latter may be precipitated by hypotension, tachycardia, increased ventricular filling pressures, anemia, or hypoxemia. Acute coronary artery thrombosis precipitated by surgically induced platelet activation and aggregation and coronary artery spasm surely contributes to perioperative ischemia.

Intraoperative myocardial ischemia diagnosed by ECG or transesophageal echocardiography (TEE) occurs in 18% to 75% of patients with CAD undergoing noncardiac surgery.[2] ECG studies suggest that nonspecific ST-T-wave changes, of variable duration (1 to 258 minutes), most commonly occur in the lateral precordial leads (V_4, V_5). During cardiac surgery, segmental myocardial wall thickening and motion abnormalities detected by TEE are a more sensitive indicator of ischemia than ECG ST-T-wave changes. The relationship of TEE abnormalities to ECG changes have not been extensively investigated in noncardiac surgery, but most likely will apply equally as well.

Preliminary data suggest that the prevalence of postoperative myocardial ischemia may be higher than that of intraoperative or preoperative baseline ischemia. Postoperative ischemic episodes are frequently silent and most often occur during the initial 48 to 72 postoperative hours. Rarely, they may occur 7 days or more after surgery. Serial screening with ECG and cardiac enzyme levels indicates that 75% of ischemic episodes occur within 24 hours[26] and are frequently associated with an elevated heart rate. In addition to operative stress, five major preoperative factors (left ventricular hypertrophy on ECG, hypertension, diabetes, diagnosed CAD, and the use of digoxin) increase the risk of postoperative ischemia. The presence of one of these factors is associated with a 31% risk of postoperative ischemia. This risk increases to 46% if two risk factors are present and 77% if four risk factors are present.[27]

Myocardial Infarction

The mystique of perioperative MI is in part related to the silent nature of the process, which may be attributed to altered pain perception, residual anesthetic effect, administration of analgesics, or competing somatic stimuli such as incisional pain. While most symptomatic, transmural MIs can be detected by ECG, most perioperative MIs (≥6%) are silent and require the use of serial ECGs or the evaluation of cardiac enzymes for detection.[26] Many silent subendocardial MIs may require the use of more sensitive techniques such as radionuclide imaging for detection.

Although the pathophysiology of perioperative infarction remains unknown, it appears that events associated with a silent perioperative MI are not different from nonsurgically associated infarcts and represent a continuum of change involving atherosclerotic plaque rupture, intraluminal thrombosis, and coronary artery spasm. The perioperative period represents a high-flow state producing high shear stress. Additionally, the patient is in a procoagulant state. At the site of advanced atherosclerosis, plaque rupture with thrombosis can occur. Powerful biochemical mediators released from the aggregating platelets (including vasoactive thromboxane and serotonin), infiltrating leukocytes with subsequent release of free radicals and other chemo-attraction result in subsequent coronary artery stricture. Leukotrienes and abnormal arachidonic acid metabolites, including prostaglandins, and other pro-aggregates add to the propagation of intraluminal obstruction, constriction, and reduction of coronary artery blood flow.

The incidence of postoperative MI after noncardiac surgery is 0.15% in patients without a prior history of heart disease.[28] Following noncardiac surgery, a perioperative MI rate of 1.1% has been reported in patients with CAD and a nonfatal MI rate of 1.8% has been reported in patients over 40 years old, regardless of the presence or absence of CAD.[29] Reinfarction rates ranging from 5% to 8% have been reported in many patients with a history of prior MI, with reported risks increasing to 37% in patients who have had a recent (within 3 months) MI.[10,11] It appears that primary MI or reinfarction carries a higher mortality in the postoperative period than MI occurring in the absence of surgical stress; however, this information may be biased by the silent nature of perioperative MI.[15] The quoted proportionally high risk (37%) of perioperative reinfarction reported in patients with a prior recent (within 3 months) MI has recently been challenged by Rao et al., who reported an overall reinfarction risk of only 1.9%, increasing to 5.7% when the previous infarct was recent (Table 1–6).[11] This decreased risk has been reportedly related to preoperative identification, aggressive intraoperative monitoring, and extended postoperative stay in an intensive care unit. A critical review of the available literature does not confirm the actual benefit of these methods of care, however, additional studies have confirmed the lower risk of perioperative reinfarction.[10]

In the era of acute intervention for MI, previous data on the perioperative risk of reinfarction may no longer be valid in the evaluation of the vast majority of patients.[30] The ECG distinction of Q-wave from non-Q-wave infarcts may not be as clinically significant in the era of thrombolytic therapy. Currently, non-Q-wave infarcts are diagnosed from acute ST-T-wave changes on the ECG, with or without cardiac enzyme elevation. The risk of reinfarction is not significantly different regardless of whether the initial event was a Q-wave (transmural) or non-Q-wave infarct.[28] Patients with a complicated Q-wave infarct have a doubled mortality (19% vs. 10.2%) related to the acute event.[29] Individuals who survive a non-Q-wave infarct are at greater risk (15% vs. 5%) for reinfarction than those who survive a Q-wave infarction. Those patients who have not had a transmural infarct probably have high-risk "border" zones of myocardium supplied by either a very high-grade coronary stenosis or very unstable plaque with relatively low perfusion and remain at high risk for a subsequent infarct. The concurrent problem of hypertension significantly increases the risk of reinfarction in those patients surviving a non-Q-wave infarct.[31]

The potential impact of cardiac surveillance in the detection of acute perioperative MI is suggested by trials of early intervention in patients with nonsurgically related infarcts. These trials suggest that early, directed therapy (within 3 hours of MI) results in a 3% risk of cardiogenic shock, while delayed therapy (more than 3 hours) carries a higher risk (13%) of cardiogenic shock.[32] Appropriate surveillance allows early detection and appropriate institution of pharmacologic, catheter-based, and surgical intervention for an acute perioperative cardiac event.

Unstable Angina

The incidence of developing unstable angina (defined as a recent increase in frequency and duration of symptoms) postoperatively is unknown. However, the results of the Coronary Artery Surgery Study (CASS) following noncardiac surgery suggest that 8.7% of patients with known CAD develop postoperative chest pain.[33] This event occurs significantly less frequently in patients without CAD (4.5%) and in patients with a previous coronary artery bypass graft (CABG) (5.1%). Unfortunately, the incidence of perioperative angina is not representative of the overall risk of myocardial ischemia. Ischemic ST-T-wave changes occur in as many as 38% of perioperative studies. More than 85% of these ECG changes are silent.[2]

Congestive Heart Failure

The reported prevalence of perioperative CHF ranges from 2% in patients with no history of heart failure to more than 30% in patients with an S_3 gallop preoperatively (Table 1–7). The postoperative diagnosis of CHF is frequently difficult to make because pulmonary congestion may be precipitated not only by ventricular failure but also by decreased oncotic pressure, a pulmonary capillary leak due to preexisting disease, sepsis, or even transfusion-related problems.

In patients with CAD, isolated regional ischemia (i.e., papillary muscle dysfunction), global ischemia, or infarction may impair diastolic relaxation and systolic contraction, precipitating CHF. In addition, perioperative increases in afterload or preload (related to catecholamine release, temperature elevation, fluid shift, or respiratory changes) will mechanically affect both the diastolic and systolic myocardial function and potentially exacerbate the risk of CHF. The presence of cardiomyopathy or valvular heart disease significantly increases these risks.

Serious Dysrhythmias

Continuous perioperative and intraoperative ECG monitoring is necessary to detect the presence of dysrhythmia, to determine its severity, and to distinguish new operatively associated dysrhythmia from chronic arrhythmias. Although a number of studies have addressed the incidence of characteristic intraoperative dysrhythmias, few have used continuous recording techniques, and only one has studied the relationship of postoperative dysrhythmias to the preoperative baseline pattern. The reported incidence of intraoperative dysrhythmias ranges from 13% to 84%. The incidence of serious dysrhythmia (i.e., new, hemodynamically important multifocal premature ventricular contractions [PVCs], ventricular tachycardia, and ventricular fibrillation) has been reported to range between 4.9% and 6%.[15]

(*Text continued on p. 18.*)

TABLE 1-6. Perioperative Myocardial Infarction or Mortality in Patients with Previous Myocardial Infarction

Time from MI to Operation (mo)	Arkins, 1963	Topkins, 1959–1963		Fraser, 1960–1964	Tarhan, 1975–1976		Sapala, 1970–1974		Steen, 1980		von Knorring, 1981	
	Mort.	Reinf.	Mort.	Mort.	Reinf.	Mort.	Reinf.	Mort.	Reinf.	Mort.	Reinf.	Mort.
0–3	40% (11/27)	54.5% (12/22)	*	38% (19/38)	37% (3/8)	*	86% (6/7)	86% (6/7)	27% (2/18)	*	25% (4/16)	*
4–6	*		*	*	16% (3/19)	*			11% (2/18)			
7–12	*	25.0% (9/36)	*	*	5% (2/42)	*					18% (2/11)	*
13–18	*	22.4% (11/49)	*		4% (1/27)	*					11% (10/89)	*
19–24	*		*	*	4% (1/21)	*	5.7% (9/159)	1.9% (3/159)				
25–36		5.9% (3/51)	*	*					5.4% (30/544)			
>36		1.0% (5/493)	*	*	5% (11/232)	*						
Unknown		42.8% (3/7)	*		5.6% (7/73)	*					22% (9/41)	
Total no. of pts. with MI	*	6.5% (43/65)	4.7% (31/65)	*	6.6% (28/422)	3% (15/422)	9% (15/166)	5.4% (9/166)	6.1% (36/587)	4.2% (25/587)	15.9% (25/157)	4% (7/157)

16

TABLE 1-6. **Perioperative Myocardial Infarction or Mortality in Patients with Previous Myocardial Infarction** (continued)

Time from MI Operation (mo)	Goldman, 1975–1976		Eerola, 1970–1974		Schoeppel, 1980		Rao, 1973–1976		Rao, 1976–1982		Shah, 1990	
	Reinf.	Mort.	Reinf.	Mort.	Reinf.	Mort.	Reinf.	Mort.	Reinf.	Mort.	Reinf.	Mort.
0–3	4.5% (1/22)	23% (5/22)	8% (1/12)	8% (1/12)	0% (0/1)	0% (0/1)	30% (4/11)	*	5.8% (3/52)	*	4.3% (1.23)	*
4–6		5.9% (1/17)	5.9% (1/17)	0% (/1)	0% (0/8)	0% (0/8)	26% (8/31)	*	2.3% (2/36)	*	0% (0/18)	*
7–12	0% (0/13)						5% (6/127)	*	1.0% (1/104)	*	5.7% (10/174)	*
13–18		8% (1/133)			0% (0/10)	0% (0/10)	5% (6/114)	*	1.6% (4/258)	*		
19–24	3.3% (2/66)	3.3% (2/66)	4.9% (4/82)	12% (1/82)								
25–36					0% (0/26)	0% (0/26)	5% (4/81)	*	1.7% (4/235)	*		
>36												
Unknown											3.3%	
Total no. of pts. with MI		8.9% (9/109)			5.7% (3/35)	3.8% (2/53)	7.7% (28/364)	4.1% (15/364)	1.9% (14/733)	0.7% (5/733)		

*Not applicable.

17

TABLE 1–7. **Correlation of Preoperative Signs and Symptoms and Postoperative Cardiogenic Pulmonary Edema**

Sign or Symptom	% of Patients in Whom Cardiogenic Pulmonary Edema Developed
No history of congestive heart failure (CHF)	2
History of CHF: normal examination, normal chest roentgenogram	6
CHF detected on preoperative physical examination or chest roentgenogram	16
NYHA preoperative functional class for CHF	
I	3
II	7
III	6
IV	25
History of pulmonary edema	23
S$_3$ gallop	35
Jugular venous distention and clinical signs of CHF	30

Modified from Houston MC et al: Preoperative medical consultation and evaluation of surgical risk. South Med J 90:1391, 1987.

A 1992 report[34] on continuous Holter monitoring in the evaluation of patients with CAD or patients at risk for CAD indicated that asymptomatic ventricular arrhythmias occurred in 44% of patients, either preoperatively (21%), intraoperatively (16%), or postoperatively (36%). The apparent decrease in intraoperative risk as compared to former studies was noted by the authors to suggest less arrhythmogenicity of modern anesthetic techniques. Current anesthetic drugs blunt the response of the sympathetic nervous system, the hypothalamic-pituitary axis, and the renin-angiotensin pathway to stress. When compared to preoperative baseline, the arrhythmia severity increased 2% intraoperatively and 10% postoperatively. This risk was significantly increased in smokers (odds ratio = 4.1), those with a history of CHF (odds ratio = 4.1), and those with ECG evidence of myocardial ischemia (odds ratio = 2.2), suggesting the need to consider extended perioperative cardiac monitoring in specific high-risk populations. Importantly, the risk of postoperative MI was not increased in patients with preoperative arrhythmias. Other patient groups that should be considered at increased risk for the development of postoperative supraventricular tachyarrhythmias include elderly patients, those undergoing pulmonary surgery, patients with subcritical valvular stenosis, and patients with a prior history of supraventricular tachyarrhythmia. Although the data are limited and conflicting,[35] digitalis is commonly used in the hope of preventing the development of postoperative supraventricular tachycardia as well as to slow the rate of supraventricular tachycardia in pulmonary patients. Although low-dose β-blockers may be even more effective, their use may be associated with bronchospasm in patients with respiratory disease. Adenosine or verapamil may be useful while the underlying cause is sought and remedied.

Cardiac Death

Perioperative cardiac morbidity is a primary cause of death following anesthesia and noncardiac surgery, with as many as 50,000 patients per year sustaining a perioperative MI and 20,000 dying as a direct result.[2] Patients with no history of CAD are at lower risk of cardiac mortality than patients with CAD (0.5% vs. 2.4%).[33] For patients over 40 (with or without CAD) Goldman and Braunwald reported a cardiac death rate of 1.9%.[36] This mortality rate associated with perioperative MI ranges from 36% to 70% and is highest if associated with reinfarction.[15] Mortality rates associated with other perioperative cardiac events remain unknown.

The occurrence of perioperative cardiac arrest is devastating. The ability to resuscitate the patient successfully strongly relates to coexisting disease. In one recent retrospective report, the records of 114 cancer patients suffering cardiopulmonary arrest during a 3-year period at Memorial Sloan-Kettering Hospital and Cancer Center were evaluated. Although 65.7% of these patients were initially successfully resuscitated, only 12 (10.5%) were discharged alive from the hospital. Median survival after discharge was 150 days. Univariate and multivariate analysis suggested that the only variable predicting the likelihood of a patient being discharged alive after arrest was the performance status at the time of admission to the hospital. A patient spending more than 50% of the time in bed at the time of admission had only a 2.3% chance of being discharged alive after a cardiopulmonary event.[37] In other critical care situations, initial successful resuscitation is common (44%); however, few (5%) are ultimately discharged, and the majority (75%) of these patients survive less than 1 year. Significant disability is common in survivors.[38] This information should not direct therapy, but it does emphasize the necessity and benefits of prevention.

Cardiac arrest can occur during or after *any* surgical procedure. Even the conceptual "minimally invasive" laparoscopy procedure is associated with a risk of cardiovascular collapse (1/2,500). Any cause, including air emboli and hypercapnia associated with the Trendelenburg position and elevated intra-abdominal pressures, can contribute.[39]

Cardiac Risk Assessment

More than 40 years ago reports appeared suggesting an increased risk of potentially lethal postoperative MIs in patients with CAD.[40] Since that time numerous clinical risk indices, including those devised by the American Society of Anesthesiologists (ASA scale), Dripps (1961), Goldman (1977), and Detsky (1986), have attempted to stratify preoperative surgical risks.[36] Unfortunately, despite the magnitude of morbidity and mortality associated with perioperative cardiac morbidity, the optimal risk assessment scheme remains undefined.

As expected, clinical or historical preoperative risk factors as well as classic and dynamic intraoperative predictors (Table 1–8) have been the primary focus of investigations attempting to identify those patients at highest risk for perioperative cardiac morbidity. Only recently have the results of sophisticated laboratory evaluation been incorporated. Although no reports specifically address cardiac risks associated with reproductive tract procedures, extrapolation from other subspecialty evaluations allows some basis for developing a rational preoperative evaluation, as well as appropriate methods of perioperative cardiac surveillance.

Historical Factors

Age

The incidence of CAD increases with age. By the year 2000, the proportion of the American population between 65 and 69 years of age will remain essentially the same as it is today, but the number of people aged 80 years or older is expected to increase by 66%.[41] At present, the U.S. population includes about 2.6 million persons who are 85 years or older, and this segment of the population, now 1% of the total, is projected to be the fastest-growing segment in the coming decade, doubling by the year 2000 and increasing to 5% by the year 2050.[42]

TABLE 1–8. **Predictors of Cardiac Risk**

Historical Predictors
    Age
    Previous MI
    Angina
    Left ventricular dysfunction
    Hypertension
    Diabetes
    Dysrhythmia
    Peripheral vascular disease
    Valvular heart disease
    Previous CABG or PTCA
    Risk indices

Intraoperative Predictors
Classical
    Anesthetic choice
    Surgical site
    Duration of surgery
    "Emergency" surgery
    Hypertension
    Hypotension
    Tachycardia
    Ventricular dysfunction
    Myocardial ischemia
    Dysrhythmias

Dynamic
    Hypertension
    Hypotension
    Tachycardia
    Myocardial Ischemia
    ST-T-wave changes
    TEE-demonstrated wall motion/thickening
    Pulmonary artery monitoring
    Cardiokymographic detection
    Biochemical markers
    Ventricular dysfunction
    Arrhythmias

Current life expectancy at age 60 is 20 years, at age 70 it is 13 years, and at age 80 it is 7 years. Currently, in patients 65 years or older, 7 of 15 hospital diagnoses and 12 of 15 prescriptions are for cardiac or pulmonary problems.[43]

Although there is no absolute age-related effect on cardiac systolic performance, age is associated with a depressed cardiac response to different forms of stress such as exercise or catecholamines and impaired relaxation. Left ventricular wall thickness increases by 25% with age.[43] This suggests that age itself may not be as important as coexisting medical problems (Table 1–9). In one prospective study of 288 older (>65 years) general surgical patients, significant coexisting preoperative medical problems were present in 80%. Respiratory disease was present in 29%, 14% gave a history of previous CHF, 9% had symptoms of angina,

TABLE 1–9. **Preoperative Risk Factors and Postoperative Cardiovascular Complications in the Elderly**

Preoperative Risk Factor	Postoperative CVS Complications: Increase in Relative Risk			Comments
	Myocardial Infarction	*Cardiac Death*	*All CVS Complications*	
Age over 70	↑ 2–4×	↑2–12×	↑2–3×	Age effect much less when patients with known heart disease excluded
Emergency admission		↑4× in cardiac surgery	↑2×	
Myocardial infarction within 3 months	↑ 5–8×	↑5–8×		Studies included middle-aged and elderly
Myocardial infarction 3–6 months previously	↑ 2–4×	↑2–4×		
Stable angina, controlled heart failure		↑1.5–2×	↑2–3×	
Acute heart failure	(?)↑2×	↑10–15×		Potentially treatable risk factor
Dyspnea on moderate exercise	↑2–4×	↑2–4×	↑2–4×	
Sex, obesity, smoking, diabetes, systolic BP	←————— No proven correlation with adverse CVS outcome in elderly —————→			

Modified from Seymour DG: Aspects of surgery in the elderly: Preoperative medical assessment. B J Hosp Med 37: 102–112, 1987.

5% had been treated for a stroke, and 9% had an impaired mental score. Three or more preoperative medical problems were detected in 30% of patients.[41,44] The same problems are true of women with endometrial cancer[45] as well as other gynecologic disease.[46] Additionally, there is a statistical association between age and nonelective admission. Emergency admission in the elderly population is strongly associated with a poor surgical outcome.[44] Another study evaluating 304 general surgical patients 80 years old or older reported an overall surgical mortality rate of 14%; it was twice as high (19.9%) in patients admitted under emergency conditions than in patients undergoing elective procedures (8.9%). The majority (79%) of patients were discharged; however, 7% required postoperative care in a skilled nursing facility. When compared to standard life tables, survival rates were equal to that of all 80-year-old patients, and the authors concluded that health care resources devoted to the elderly should be directed toward early intervention for surgical problems such as carcinoma before complications develop or emergency procedures are necessary.[41]

In a study by Orr et al.,[45] major perioperative morbidity was reported to occur in 22% of 101 patients over 70 years of age with gynecologic disease. Older women have operative mortality rates of 1.3%, with 1-year survival rates of 86%. Many elderly women (at least 29%) require perioperative intensive care admission or intensive cardiovascular monitoring.[45]

The elderly may require a more intensive preoperative cardiac evaluation, particularly if other diseases (e.g., arthritis) limit the ability to accurately assess important historical factors. One report evaluating hemodynamic parameters demonstrated poor cardiopulmonary reserve in a group of 75 elderly patients. In this subgroup of patients scheduled to undergo vascular surgery, information obtained from preoperative PA catheterization indicated that only 25 patients (33%) had normal left ventricular function. In this specific study, incremental changes in preload were necessary in 20 patients (26.7%) to improve myocardial function. Thirty patients (40%) had abnormal left ventricular function and required pharmacologic modulation including preload adjustment, inotropic support, or afterload reduction. These therapeutic changes, all completed within 3 days, resulted in improved left ventricular function in 93% of patients. This short surgical delay had no measurable adverse effect on eventual outcome.[47] This type of information clearly indicates the necessity of careful preoperative assessment of the elderly to detect important potential coexisting disease that may further increase perioperative cardiac morbidity.

Even perioperative mortality rates following CABG in patients over 65 years of age (range, 1.6%–19%) is increased threefold (5%) in most centers, compared to rates in younger patients (1.5%). Cardiovascular morbidity associated with CABG may also be higher in elderly patients.[48]

Age alone does not appear to play a significant role in the primary success rate of percutaneous transluminal coronary angioplasty (PTCA) with satisfactory outcomes in the same range as younger patients. In some opinions, PTCA is the preferred treatment in elderly patients with localized CAD (defined as a single- or two-vessel disease) and relatively normal left ventricular function.[48]

Previous Myocardial Infarct

Patients with a prior MI and CAD are at greater risk for reinfarction than patients without CAD (5%–8% vs. 0.1%–0.7%). Surgically related reinfarction mortality rates are reported to be 5% to 70%.[16] Classic teaching indicated that the risk of postoperative reinfarction was highest shortly (within 6 weeks) after previous MI and decreased toward normal after 6 months. Although previous data suggested a time-related decreased risk, recent data from the CASS trials and other studies have failed to confirm that a previous infarct (regardless of duration) carried a markedly increased risk of perioperative cardiac morbidity or mortality. Rao et al. reported that an intensive perioperative care regimen was associated with an apparent reduction of reinfarction to 5.7% for patients than 3 months post MI and a further decrease to 2.3% between 3 and 6 months.[11]

Although modern anesthetic techniques and monitoring apparently decrease the risk of reinfarction, patients usually do not return to full physical activity until at least 6 weeks following an acute MI, and it would appear prudent to delay all but the most necessary procedures during this interval. Myocardial function may be significantly depressed during the initial interval as the myocardial scar remodels and fibrosis develops.[30]

The beneficial impact of prior CABG surgery on subsequent perioperative mortality is well documented. Mahar[49] compared the surgical outcome of 49 patients with angiographic CAD and 99 patients who had undergone previous bypass surgery. Five percent of the initial group suffered perioperative infarcts compared to none of the patients who had

previously undergone bypass surgery. The CASS study[33] evaluated 1,600 patients undergoing major noncardiac surgery. Perioperative cardiac mortality was extremely low (0.5%; 2/399 patients) in patients without significant CAD and not significantly different from that in patients with CAD post CABG (0.9%, 7/743; $p = 0.42$). Patients with significant CAD who had not undergone a bypass operation had a perioperative cardiac mortality of 2.4% (11/458; $p < 0.009$). When considering the role of presurgical CABG after MI or in a patient with angina, one must remember that the mortality associated with CABG is 2.3%, increasing to 2.9% in those with a lower EF (<50%) and to 7.9% in patients more than 70 years old.[50]

In the CASS study, CABG-related operative mortality was less (1.9%) for men than women (1.9% vs. 4.5%; $p < 0.001$). The overall crude in-hospital mortality rate (4.3%) for isolated CABG varied greatly among centers and increased with age, female sex, small body surface area, greater comorbidity, reoperation, poor cardiac function (as indicated by lower EF), increased LVEDP, and emergency or urgent procedures.[51] Recently, a contemporary surgical series provided compelling evidence that the excessive operative mortality in women following CABG could be completely explained by the referral for surgery later in the course of the disease, when CHF was an important part of the clinical presentation.[52]

The initial literature on coronary angioplasty suggested that this procedure had a history similar to that of CABG surgery, with initial comparative reports suggesting that women were older and had more advanced clinical disease than men at the time of referral for angioplasty. More recent reports no longer note a sex-related difference in actual outcomes, and most studies seem to indicate that if angioplasty is successful, female sex may be associated with a more favorable long-term clinical and angiographic outcome.[52] At present, prospective data comparing the perioperative mortality in men and women after PTCA are not available. Recent retrospective data suggest a significant decrease in perioperative cardiac risks.[53]

Angina

Angina is usually associated with angiographically significant coronary artery stenosis (>70%). Although 90% of older women (>60 years) with classic angina have significant coronary artery stenosis, fewer than 65% of those with atypical angina have significant stenosis.

Although a history of stable angina significantly increases the risk of MI and sudden death in ambulatory patients with CAD, its predictive role remains controversial in noncardiac surgical patients. Goldman and Braunwald's classic study found stable angina to be a "conspicuously insignificant" predictor of perioperative cardiac mortality.[36] However, it must be remembered that 75% of all perioperative ischemic episodes are silent, suggesting the bias or hazard in assessing cardiac risks by symptoms alone. More recent data suggest that angina is a significant risk factor in the development of perioperative ischemia; however, quantitative analysis is lacking.[30,54]

In a population of patients without chest pain the likelihood of significant CAD is small. Pooled data from 23,996 autopsies and 4,952 coronary arteriograms indicated that women aged 40 to 49 without chest pain have a 1% likelihood of CAD. For women with nonanginal chest pain, this likelihood doubles to 3%. CAD is present in 13% of women with atypical angina and 55% of women with typical angina.[55] In women aged 50 to 59 years, 3.2% of asymptomatic women have CAD and 8.5% of women with nonanginal chest pain have significant CAD.[55]

Congestive Heart Failure

To a physiologist, heart failure is defined as the inability of the heart to pump blood at a rate commensurate with the requirements of the metabolizing tissues, irrespective of high, normal, or low CO.[56] Clinical manifestations of heart failure may be chronic or acute, depending on the rapidity with which ventricular decompensation occurs and whether or not enough time is allowed for compensatory mechanisms to partially alleviate the consequences of reduced CO.

CHF is the leading diagnosis in hospitalized patients aged 65 years or older. Radiologic or clinical evidence of CHF correlates with a poor prognosis in patients with CAD and is an important predictor of acute and chronic cardiac mortality in the patient with an acute MI. The overall 5-year survival of patients with clinically apparent CHF is 50% or less.[2] In those patients with EF of ≤30%, the 1-year cumulative mortality approaches 30%. A 2-year mortality of 78% is reported in patients with an elevated filling pressure (>25 mm Hg) and a depressed stroke work index (<20 g/m²), differing significantly from the 10% 2-year mortality in patients with compensated left ventricular dysfunction.

Although preoperative CHF is a predictor of perioperative cardiac morbidity, the value of specific signs is controversial. One older report suggested that patients with a relevant history but no clinical signs were three times more likely to develop CHF than controls without such a history, even in the absence of clinical symptoms.[57] Perioperative CHF is increased 17-fold in those with a previous history. It is now apparent that more than 50% of patients who develop perioperative pulmonary edema have no antecedent history.[58] Clinical signs of left ventricular dysfunction dramatically increase risk (8×) when compared to controls. The more apparent the heart failure, the greater is the likelihood of developing a life-threatening perioperative cardiac event.[59]

Goldman and Braunwald suggested that the presence of a third heart sound (S_3) and clinical jugular venous distention were predictive but cardiomegaly was not.[36] Foster, reporting for the CASS study,[33] reported that S_3 and orthopnea were univariate predictors, but only the left ventricular wall motion score was predictive in a multivariate analysis. A number of studies have evaluated preoperative EF and suggest that a value <40% is predictive of perioperative CHF, MI, or reinfarction.

One recent report suggests that hypertensive patients with preoperative cardiac disease (previous MI, valvular disease, or CHF) have a high risk (17%) of developing postoperative CHF when compared to controls (1%) without known cardiac disease. Diabetics with cardiac disease are at a particularly high risk when compared to nondiabetics (12% vs. 2%). Additionally, patients who experience an intraoperative decrease or increase of 40 mm Hg in mean arterial pressure compared to preoperative baseline values are also at increased risk. In a report by Charlson et al., the risk of postoperative CHF was not necessarily related to volume overload. The risk of CHF was highest among those patients with less than 500 mL/hr of net intake.[58]

The risk of developing perioperative CHF follows a bimodal pattern, with the initial risk occurring on the day of surgery, often associated with aggressive fluid resuscitation and the potential myocardial depressant effects of anesthesia. While intraoperative volume administration may not be important, a simple and predictive perioperative measurement of cardiac morbidity and mortality involves the evaluation of changes in body weight (Table 1–10).[60] The second peak in incidence occurs on day 3, when sequestered third space fluid is resorbed into the intravascular space. In one recent report, all of the 15 episodes of postoperative CHF developed within the first 3 postoperative days—

TABLE 1–10. **Postoperative Fluid Overload**

	Weight Gain* (as % of Body Weight)		
	<10%	*1%–20%*	*>20%*
Mortality[†]	10.3	18.8	100
Vasopressor (days)[‡]	3.6 ± 1	8.7 ± 5	26 ± 12

Modified from Lowell JA: Postoperative fluid overload: Not a benign problem. Crit Care Med 18:728–733, 1990.
*APACHE II—not different.
[†]$p < 0.0008$.
[‡]$p < 0.04$.
< 15% received adequate perioperative caloric intake nutrition.

six on the day of surgery, one on the first postoperative day, and six on the second postoperative day.[58] This bimodal risk pattern makes it appropriate that intensive clinical or hemodynamic monitoring be continued for at least 72 hours postoperatively in patients at risk.

Evaluation of the perioperative patient presenting with symptoms of heart failure demands a careful history, physical examination, and appropriate studies to explain the underlying cause. Prior to surgery, there should exist an understanding of the potential pathophysiologic basis for the development of cardiac decompensation. During the entire perioperative period, surveillance for any acute precipitating events is required. Objective assessment of cardiac performance should be ongoing and may require the use of a PA catheter throughout the perioperative period.

The clinical diagnosis of heart failure as well as the majority of the underlying structural causes can be determined by ECG, chest radiography, PA catheterization, and/or echocardiography. A concerted effort to determine the underlying structural cause is important not only to exclude potentially correctable lesions but to avoid inappropriate therapy (e.g., pericardial effusion or constriction). CAD is by far the most common cause of heart failure. In most cases, heart failure is precipitated by volume shifts and perioperative stress on a ventricle with limited myocardial reserve. A vicious, potentially lethal loop ensues of myocardial stress creating coronary ischemia, which produces greater myocardial stress. This results in rapidly downward-spiraling cardiac decompensation. Although MI is not required for this scenario, mortality increases significantly if infarction occurs. Patients with decreased myocardial reserve from causes other than CAD

may also develop pulmonary edema. Left ventricular function depressed as a result of cardiomyopathy can result in pulmonary edema. The two syndromes can often be differentiated with the use of echocardiography to evaluate for the presence of segmental versus global wall motion abnormalities. PA catheter monitoring with appropriate pharmacologic therapy (Table 1–11) can frequently diminish the risk of the development of pulmonary edema and interrupt the cycle of dysfunction before pulmonary edema develops.

Diminished CO in patients with pump failure is often associated with a fall in blood pressure. SVR (ventricular afterload) may increase in an effort to maintain coronary and cranial blood flow and can lead to further depression of cardiac performance. The widespread successful use of vasodilators in

TABLE 1–11. **Recommended Dosages of Specific Agents in Congestive Heart Failure**

Drug	Dosage
Diuretics	
Furosemide	IV: 40 mg; maximum: 1 g/d PO: 40 mg/d in 1 or 2 doses, titrated to clinical response
Ethacrynic acid	IV: 50–100 mg PO: 50–400 mg/d
Bumetanide	IV: 0.5–1.0 mg; maximum: 10 mg/d PO: 1–10 mg/d
Metolazone	PO: 2.5–10.0 mg/d
Spironolactone	PO: 200 mg/d in divided doses
Inotropic Agents	
Digoxin	IV: For rapid digitalization, 0.75–1.0 mg; maintenance: 0.25–0.50 mg/d PO: Maintenance: 0.25 mg/d
Dopamine	IV: 2–5 µg/kg/min
Dobutamine	IV: 5 µg/kg/min, titrated to hemodynamic response; maximum: 20 µg/kg/min
Amrinone	IV: Bolus of 0.75 mg/kg/min, followed by infusion of 5–10 µg/kg/min
Vasodilators	
Nitroprusside	IV: 0.5–10.0 µg/kg/min, titrated to hemodynamic response
Nitroglycerin	IV: 10–15 µg/min, titrated up to 200 µg/min
Hydralazine	IV: 10–25 mg; maximum: 200 mg/d
Captopril	PO: 6.5–50.0 mg 3×/d
Enalapril	PO: 2.5–15.0 mg 2×/d
Lisinopril	PO: 5–20 mg 1×/d

Reproduced by permission from Jafri SM, Goldstein S: Choosing the best therapy for congestive heart failure. J Crit Illness 5:1259–1270, 1990.

the treatment of heart failure has highlighted the impact of an elevated SVR in regulating the performance of a diseased left ventricle, which is more sensitive than a normal ventricle to changes in peripheral vascular resistance. Increased venous return has little effect because the diseased left ventricle is operating at the apex of a depressed ventricular function curve.

Increased adrenergic activity to improve contractility and elevate heart rate is an important compensatory mechanism to support cardiac function. Sympathetic stimulation is augmented in heart failure, which contributes to increased peripheral resistance to raise blood pressure in the face of falling CO. There appears to be progressive depletion of myocardial norepinephrine stores that usually parallels the climbing left ventricular function curve, resulting in the loss of an important mechanism to increase inotropic support. Although a substantial amount of evidence supports a role for the β-adrenergic system in sustaining inotropic activity in the failing myocardium, the mechanism itself may be self-limiting because of progressive reduction in myocardial norepinephrine stores and, more important, decreased sensitivity (down-regulation) in the β-adrenergic receptor pathway. In the failing heart, β-adrenergic receptor density is decreased in direct relationship to decreasing ventricular function.

The renin-angiotensin-aldosterone system is also activated in patients with heart failure to support cardiac function by increasing preload and blood pressure through saltwater retention. Unfortunately, the potent vasoconstrictor effects of angiotensin may contribute to an excessive increase in SVR. Stimulation of aldosterone promotes saltwater retention, which results in interstitial edema and possibly increased sodium content of the vascular walls. The associated decreased vascular compliance when combined with extrinsic compression from interstitial edema potentially heightens vascular tone.

Recently a group of locally active neurohormones have been described that participate in controlling peripheral vasoconstriction. Endothelin, a hormone that causes intense vasoconstriction, is released by the endothelium in CHF and is at least partially responsible for the rise in SVR seen in this clinical state. Endothelial-derived relaxing factor (EDRF) or nitric oxide is also a locally acting vasodilator. Less EDRF is released in the presence of CHF.[61]

Once the diagnosis of ventricular failure is established, treatment involves improving CO and systemic perfusion (Table 1–12). The popularity of

TABLE 1–12. **Treatment of Heart Failure**

Clinical Finding	Treatment Approach
Decreased contractility	Digitalis glycosides or other intropic agents
Increased preload	Salt restriction
	Diuretics
	Venodilators
	Mechanical removal of fluid
	Phlebotomy
	Thoracentesis
	Paracentesis
	Dialysis
Low cardiac output and high vascular resistance	Arteriolar vasodilators
	Intra-aortic balloon pump
Rapid heart rate (atrial fibrillation or sinus tachycardia)	Improve left ventricular performance
	Increase atrioventricular block (digitalis)

digoxin in the treatment of patients with heart failure in sinus rhythm has waxed and waned over the years. Recent well-controlled trials support its use.[62] A large National Heart, Lung and Blood Institute trial is ongoing. This drug occupies a prominent place in the management of CHF and certain rhythm disturbances, particularly those of a chronic nature. The major indications for its use are in the treatment of CHF related to depressed contractility, and in the treatment of supraventricular dysrhythmia, including atrial fibrillation, flutter, and supraventricular tachycardias. There is little benefit to digoxin use in patients with obstructive valvular heart disease or diastolic dysfunction.

A number of other inotropic drugs, clinically available or investigative, play a prominent role in the management of CHF. Dopamine stimulates myocardial contractility by direct activity on the β_1-adrenergic receptors of the myocardium and indirectly by leaching norepinephrine from the sympathetic nerve terminals. Dobutamine, a synthetic sympathomimetic, has high affinity for the α_1 and β_1 receptors and a weak affinity for α_2 and β_2 receptors, and increases contractility without producing tachycardia or increasing peripheral vascular resistance. This drug does not alter renal blood flow but causes a redistribution of CO in favor of coronary and skeletal muscle beds over the mesentery or renal vascular beds. Dopexamine, a potent β-adrenergic stimulant with additional dopamine$_1$ and dopamine$_2$ receptor activity, causes a marked reduction in SVR and a moderate increase in CO and myocardial contractility.[63]

Inodilators are the newest drugs for the treatment of CHF and the low-output syndrome during the perioperative period.[63,64] Phosphodiesterase inhibitors include amrinone, milrinone, enoximone, and piroximone. The effectiveness of amrinone in patients with low-output syndrome, particularly after cardiac surgery, has been demonstrated by a number of investigators. Amrinone is a biperidin that acts through inhibition of phosphodiesterase and augments myocardial contractility, resulting in smooth muscle relaxation. It increases CO and reduces filling pressure and SVR in patients with CHF, with minimal change in heart rate. Amrinone produces a very modest inotropic effect and moderate vasodilation. Significantly, heart rate and mean arterial pressure are not affected. Amrinone promotes diastolic relaxation (lusitropism). Peak response occurs within 5 minutes after an IV dose is administered.[64] The joint administration of amrinone with dobutamine or dopamine may augment myocardial contractility more than administration of either agent alone. In addition, amrinone may be especially useful in patients on large doses of catecholamines who have "down-regulated" their β receptors. Amrinone may have an adverse effect on platelets.

Following inotropes, diuretics are the most commonly used drugs in the treatment of acute and chronic heart failure. Diuretics primarily reduce venous return, although venous dilation (decreased preload) has been proposed as an additional beneficial mechanism of action following the acute administration of potent diuretics such as furosemide.[64] The overall hemodynamic effect is a reduction in ventricular filling pressure not necessarily associated with improved CO. In fact, CO may initially decline following diuretic administration in some patients with acute heart failure.

The introduction of vasodilators has been a major advance in the treatment of severe heart failure. Left ventricular afterload reduction improves CO and reduces pulmonary venous pressure and myocardial oxygen demand. Useful direct smooth muscle relaxants include nitrates and nitroprusside. Nitrates are primarily venous dilators but produce arterial dilation at high concentrations. They are particularly effective in women with CHF associated with high ventricular filling pressures and low CO. Sodium nitroprusside relaxes both arterial and venous smooth muscle, producing a balanced arterial and venous dilation, and has no direct cardiac inotropic activity. Nitroprusside must be administered IV, and the hemodynamic effects should be carefully monitored to assess the effectiveness of afterload reduction and avoid excessive systemic hypotension. Flosequinan, a phosphodiesterase inhibitor, is now approved for treating moderate CHF. It can be considered hemodynamically equivalent to nitroprusside.

Hydralazine, administered orally or IV, is a predominantly arterial vasodilator that increases CO, reduces left ventricular filling pressure, reduces systemic arterial pressure, and increases heart rate in patients with pump failure. Unfortunately, overall myocardial demand increases with this agent alone.

Specific α-adrenergic antagonists including phentolamine or prazosin are sometimes useful in the treatment of patients with CHF. Phentolamine, an α-adrenergic blocking agent, was the first vasodilator used to augment CO in patients with heart failure. It dilates arterioles and veins and releases cardiac norepinephrine, exerting a mild positive inotropic effect. Prazosin is a potent α-adrenergic receptor antagonist possessing direct smooth muscle relaxant properties derived from phosphodiesterase inhibition. Long-term tachyphylaxis has been shown for this drug in CHF.

Captopril, the first oral angiotensin-converting enzyme (ACE) inhibitor, acts by blocking the converting enzyme that catalyzes conversion of inactive angiotensin I and angiotensin II. Its use has been associated with improved CO and reduction of pulmonary vascular pressures in severe heart failure conditions refractory to Lanoxin (digoxin) and diuretic therapy. Improvement in mortality has been shown for patients with moderate and severe CHF.[65] Oxygen supplementation with positive pressure may decrease the need for acute intubation and ventilation in the treatment of severe cardiogenic edema.[66]

Hypertension

Hypertension affects more than 60 million Americans and at least 20% of surgical patients.[2] As early as 1929, Sprague (in Heuser) reported hypertension to be an important risk factor during anesthesia and surgery with perioperative mortality rates of 30%.[67]

Blood pressure is controlled within narrow limits in healthy, resting, awake humans; however, data obtained from continuous monitoring indicate that wide fluctuation occurs, with systolic pressures ranging from 60 mm Hg during sleep to 200 mm Hg with excitement.[68] Regulation involves a complex, integrated neural mechanism that includes the sympathetic (increases heart rate, contractility, systemic vascular resistance) and parasympathetic systems. The principal sensors are the aortic and carotid pressor receptors. Integration of information processors occurs in the central nervous system, with the heart and vascular compartments being the effectors. Humoral regulation is provided by the renin-angiotensin system, atrial natriuretic factor, and a number of vasoactive peptides. Anesthetics affect nearly all aspects of these control mechanisms, making blood pressure regulation less precise during the perioperative period. Additionally, a number of other perioperative factors (Table 1–13) may elicit hypertensive responses and require evaluation and intervention during perioperative care, particularly if hypertension occurs de novo during the perioperative interval.[67,68]

Classically, hypertension has been divided into essential and secondary causes. Essential hypertension accounts for approximately 85% of all hypertension cases and, while no definite cause can be identified, hereditary factors, salt intake, alterations in the renin-angiotensin system, and disturbances in sympathetic nervous system control have been correlated with incidence. With the exception of pregnancy-induced hypertension, secondary hypertension is rarely discovered during the care of the obstetric or gynecologic patient. Definable causes (acute or chronic) include connective tissue disorders, endocrine diseases (hyperaldosteronism, pheochromocytoma), renal artery stenosis, and other causes, including aortic coarctation.

Increased SVR is the primary hemodynamic characteristic of women with essential hypertension. Recent data implicate locally produced and locally acting neurohormones such as endothelin and EDRF as potentially pathogenic. The smaller nutrient arterioles and capillaries undergo rarefaction (reduction in number), resulting in a reduced surface area for exchange. These changes place specific end organs (kidney, brain) at risk for ischemia.

Chronic hypertension results in concentric ven-

tricular hypertrophy secondary to pressure overload. Increased contractility results in increased myocardial oxygen demand. Elevated intracavitary pressure and myocardial wall tension results in reduced myocardial blood flow and oxygen delivery, particularly in the subendocardium. This combination severely compromises the myocardial oxygen supply/demand ratio and explains the increased incidence and severity of myocardial ischemia and failure in hypertensive women. The close association between CAD and hypertension suggests that the management and not just the measurement of blood pressure during anesthesia and the perioperative period should be undertaken in a similar manner to that for patients with CAD.

Despite controversies regarding study design, the majority of trials evaluating antihypertensive therapy have demonstrated significant reductions in vascular morbidity and mortality, particularly in patients with severe diastolic elevations. Although controversy exists as to the desired "limit" of elevation, current data suggest no significant increase in associated perioperative morbidity if the diastolic pressure is less than 110 mm Hg.[15] However, the overall incidence of hypertension in the general population, the associated risk of perioperative hypertension, and the role of hypotension in perioperative cardiac morbidity make it imperative that the practicing pelvic surgeon be aware of the risks, the role and methods of intervention, and other aspects in the management of the hypertensive patient.

Currently several options exist as to the most appropriate drug therapy for hypertension. To simplify these issues, the perioperative management might be classified into three areas: routine, urgent, or emergency treatment of hypertension. The latter two demand immediate attention and close surveillance if they occur pre- or postoperatively. Although other causes should be excluded, epidemiologic studies indicate that 5% to 10% of patients with essential hypertension will experience an acceleration of their disease or transition to malignant hypertension at some time during the course of their disease.[36] Additionally, the asymptomatic state of hypertension probably encourages patients to become noncompliant because they do not feel sick. This problem is exaggerated if one considers the cost to patients of drug treatment ($100–$200/mo) and the wide array of potential side effects, including sexual dysfunction (β-blockers), sleep disturbances, easy fatigability, and exercise intolerance (α- and β-blocker). Reflex tachycardia and sodium retention (vasodilators), headaches, dizziness, flushing (calcium antagonists), and rash,

TABLE 1–13. **Perioperative Hypertension**

Stimuli

Hypoxemia
Hypercapnia
Acidosis
Direct laryngoscopy
Pain
Peritoneal stimulation
Hypothermia (shivering)
Hypovolemia
Subsequent to induced hypotension (rebound)

Modified from Heuser D: Acute blood pressure increase during the perioperative period. Am J Cardiol 63:26c–31c, 1989.

distorted taste, and cough (ACE inhibitors) all contribute to poor patient compliance, with the possibility of a precipitous rise in blood pressure.

In newly diagnosed patients, antihypertensive therapy should be instituted before elective procedures are undertaken. Untreated patients are likely to have excessively high initial values of SVR with a more pronounced level of hypotension (and associated myocardial and cerebral hypoperfusion) related to the anesthesia-associated decrease in CO.[67] Normotensive and adequately treated hypertensive patients maintain a more constant SVR during the perioperative period.[69] Associated intraoperative hypotension in hypertensive women may increase perioperative cardiac morbidity by a factor of 8.

A number of regimens are available for the medical treatment of hypertension. Urgent or emergency treatment is usually initiated with rapid-acting drug therapy (Table 1–14).

VASODILATORS. Sodium nitroprusside, a potent arterial and moderate venous dilator, initiated at 0.1 to 0.5 mg/kg/min, is a direct, rapid-acting approach to the treatment of emergency or urgent hypertension. Onset of action occurs within 2 minutes and offset less than 5 minutes after the infusion is terminated. Cyanide and thiocyanate toxicity, clinically manifested by headaches, nausea, vomiting, tremulousness, and confusion, is rare but can occur after 48 to 72 hours of continuous therapy. The infusion is light sensitive and must be covered during administration. If continuous infusions are necessary for 24 hours or longer, serum thiocyanate levels should be monitored daily. The risk of toxicity is increased in women with renal insufficiency and those requiring long-term administration.

Diazoxide, a potent peripheral arterial vasodilator, has immediate activity (within 5 minutes) and a peak effect within 30 minutes following IV administration. Initially this drug was thought to be effective only in bolus dosing (secondary to protein binding). Minibolus and continuous infusion strategies are efficacious[70] and decrease the risk of serious prolonged hypotension. Its protein binding may

TABLE 1–14. **Antihypertensive Effects**

Class	HR	CO	SVR	PCWP	Myocardial Oxygen Balance	Renal Blood Flow	Total Cerebral Blood Flow	Dose
Vasodilators								
Nitroprusside	↑	↑	↓	↓	↑	↑	↑	IV infusion: 0.3 mg/kg/min
Diazoxide	↑	↑	↓	↑	↓	↑	–	IV bolus: 300 mg IV minibolus: 1–3 mg/kg IV infusion: 15 mg/min
Hydralazine	↑	↑	↓	↑	↓	↑	↓	IM: 10 mg IV: 10 mg IV infusion: 02 mg/min
Minoxidil	↑	↑	↓	↑	↓	↑	↑	PO: 5 mg
Sympatholytics								
Labetalol	↓	↓	↓	↑	↑	–	↓	IV: 1–2 mg/kg IV minibolus: 20 mg IV infusion: 0.5 mg/min
Trimethaphan	↓	↓	↓	↓	↑	↓	–	IV: 0.3–0.5 mg/min
Clonidine	↓	–	↓	–	–	–	↓	PO: 0.2 mg
Prazosin	–	↑	↓	↓	–	–	–	PO: 5.0 mg
Calcium Antagonists								
Nifedipine	↑	↑	↓	↓	↑	↑	↑	PO/bite-swallow: 10 mg
Nicardipine	↑	↑	↓	↓	↑	↑	↑	IV infusion: 2–15 mg/hr
ACE Inhibitors								
Captopril	–	↑	↓	↓	↑	↑	↑	PO: 12.5 mg SL: 6.25 mg
Enalapril	–	↑	↓	↓	↑	↑	↑	IV bolus: 1.25 mg

Abbreviations: HR, heart rate; CO, cardiac output; SVR, systemic vascular resistance; PCWP, pulmonary capillary wedge pressure.

displace other protein-bound drugs (warfarin, theophylline) and may inhibit islet cell function and insulin secretion, resulting in hyperglycemia. Finally, injectable diazoxide is extremely alkaline (pH = 11.6), and extravasation is associated with superficial thrombophlebitis, cellulitis, and sometimes tissue necrosis.

With the exception of the treatment for pregnancy-induced hypertension, hydralazine, a direct-acting arterial vasodilator, is rarely used. IV administration results in a moderately rapid onset of activity (10–30 minutes) with a maximal effect 10 to 40 minutes later. The immediate side effects related to hydralazine vasodilation are well tolerated, but reflex tachycardia and increased myocardial oxygen consumption may exacerbate angina in patients with CAD.

Minoxidil is a potent oral vasodilator that has an action onset of 30 to 60 minutes, a maximum effect at 2 to 4 hours, and a long duration (12–72 hours) of activity. Its use is mainly reserved for severe, refractory patients.

SYMPATHOLYTICS. Labetalol, a unique antihypertensive, exerts α_1-blockade ($\leq 50\%$ of phentolamine) and noncardioselective β-blockade (equal to propranolol). The predominant effect is that of reduced SVR (α-blockade). Heart rate and CO remain unchanged. Onset of activity occurs 5 minutes after IV administration and maximal activity is reached within 10 minutes. Antihypertensive effects continue for 3 to 6 hours. This latter duration is increased to 12 hours following oral administration. Unfortunately, side effects related to β-blockade make this drug relatively contraindicated in patients with CHF, bradydysrhythmias, and bronchospastic pulmonary disease. Severe hypotension may be lessened when IV infusions are initiated at 0.5 mg/min and titrated to achieve the desired antihypertensive effect.

Trimethaphan depletes norepinephrine from the sympathetic ganglia, reducing heart rate, CO, and SVR. Its rapid action (1–5 minutes) and short duration (10 minutes) requires infusion administration. As with sodium nitroprusside, constant arterial pressure monitoring and the use of an infusion pump are necessary. Significant postural hypotension is common. Unfortunately, trimethaphan depletes neurotransmitter release in cholinergic ganglia, resulting in adynamic ileus and acute urine retention, both undesirable during postoperative recovery.

The central α_2-agonist clonidine acts to decrease SVR within 30 minutes following a 0.2-mg oral dose with a duration of activity of 8 to 18 hours.[71] In emergency situations, an initial dose of 0.2 mg with a continued oral loading of 0.1 mg/hr allows 0.6 mg to be given within 6 hours of the initial treatment. Drowsiness is common (60%), and dry mouth occurs in 44% of patients. Although these symptoms usually decrease in intensity during the ensuing 4 weeks, the appearance and troublesomeness of these symptoms during the postoperative interval make them less than optimal. The feared acute discontinuation syndrome of rebound hypertension occurs infrequently.

Methyldopa, a central α_2-agonist less potent than clonidine, is used in the treatment of pregnancy-induced hypertension and occasionally when weaning patients from prolonged sodium nitroprusside infusions. As with clonidine, somnolence and neurologic drowsiness frequently occur.

CALCIUM CHANNEL BLOCKERS. A host of neurogenic and hormonal mechanisms regulate blood pressure through a final common pathway at the level of vascular smooth muscle. Calcium appears to be a primary link between the electrical activity of excitation and the mechanical activity of contraction. Calcium channels play an integral role in the development of vessel wall tension and blood pressure control. Calcium transport involves at least three potential sites for ion flux: the voltage-dependent channel, a receptor-operated channel, and the sodium/calcium exchange. During the past decade a number of chemically and pharmacologically diverse calcium channel blockers have been developed (Table 1–15). The papaverine-like compounds (verapamil), the dihydropyridine compounds (nifedipine, isradipine, nicardipine, nimoipine, nitrendipine) and the benzothiazepine, diltiazem, all inhibit the calcium flux through the voltage-dependent gate but have differing activities. All available calcium channel blockers decrease myocardial contractility to some extent.[72] Verapamil and its related compounds are highly effective in those calcium channels that open and close rapidly (i.e., the sinus and AV nodes) and are most effective in managing supraventricular tachyarrhythmias. The dihydropyridines exert their primary effects on the peripheral smooth muscle. As a class, calcium antagonists are effective in controlling blood pressure, result in regression of left ventricular mass, have no adverse effects on total serum cholesterol, and have no significant effects on blood glucose or insulin responses.

Nifedipine is the antagonist most commonly used in the management of severe hypertension. Its

TABLE 1–15. **Calcium Antagonists**

Parameter	Nifedipine	Diltiazem	Verapamil	Nicardipine
Conduction				
Sinoatrial node	↑	↓	↓↓	↑
Atrioventricular node	↑	↓	↓↓	↑
Heart rate				
Acute	↑	↓	↑	↑
Chronic	–	↓	↑↑	↑
Myocardial contractility	↓	↓	↓↓	↓
Cardiac output	↑	↓	↓	↑
Coronary blood flow	↑	↑	↑	↑
Systemic vascular resistance	↓↓	↓	↓↓	↓↓
Sodium retention	↑	↑	↑	↑
Dose:	30–180 mg/d tid	180–360 mg/d tid	240–480 mg/d tid	60–120 mg/d tid

reduction in SVR is not accompanied by a significant negative inotropic or chronotropic effect. Oral administration, sublingual administration, and "bite" swallows have all been evaluated. Buccal absorption is erratic and minimal; however, the bite swallow dose of 10 mg begins to have antihypertensive effects within 20 minutes and achieves maximal effect at 60 minutes, with a duration of action of approximately 3 hours. Administration of an oral dose at 6- to 8-hour intervals may result in peripheral edema, associated depressed sodium excretion, and enhanced fluid transudation secondary to vasodilation.

Nicardipine, a dihydropyridine calcium channel blocker with potent vasodilator effects, is not associated with the degree of myocardial depression seen with other calcium channel blockers. It may also have positive inotropic activity and is a potent coronary vasodilator that augments coronary blood flow in patients with CAD.

IV nicardipine (1–15 mg/hr infusions) results in a rapid decrease in SVR, increases coronary blood flow (without inducing a coronary steal), and has a significantly less negative inotropic effect than nifedipine. Symptoms related to systemic vasodilation (flushing, palpitations) are well tolerated, and the risk of thrombophlebitis is decreased by reducing infusion concentrations to ≤0.1 mg/mL and limiting the infusion to less than 15 hours.[72]

It would appear that urgent and emergency perioperative hypertension can be treated successfully with Ca^{2+} antagonists, and that long-term oral administration of sustained-release preparations gives equal results as treatment with diuretics, β-blockers, or other combinations.[73]

β-BLOCKERS. β-blockers are not considered primary agents in urgent or emergency perioperative hypertensive episodes. The acute effects of these drugs result in a reduction in CO. However, they may be useful as adjunctive therapy in patients with coronary insufficiency or tachyarrhythmias.

In general, β-blockers decrease cardiac automaticity, slow conduction velocity, decrease heart rate, reduce myocardial contractility, stroke volume, and CO, and are contraindicated in patients with bradydysrhythmias, advanced AV block, or CHF. $β_2$-blockade results in potential bronchospasm and may mask the systemic manifestations of hypoglycemia (tachycardia, diaphoresis).

The primary perioperative β-blocker used is ultra-short-acting esmolol, a cardioselective β-blocker that has proved useful in the management of perioperative hypertension as well as ventricular and supraventricular tachyarrhythmias. Its duration of action is less than 30 minutes.

ACE INHIBITORS. ACE inhibitors block the peripheral conversion of angiotensin I to angiotensin II, directly reducing SVR and indirectly lessening preload by decreasing angiotensin II stimulation of aldosterone.

Although well tolerated, severe hypotension with initial dosing may occur, particularly in patients with intravascular volume depletion. This side effect may be particularly important before radical or ultraradical procedures in which as many as 38% of patients enter the operating room with significant existing volume deficits. The use of ACE inhibitors and the associated reduction in aldosterone may result in hyperkalemia and metabolic acidosis, particularly in the elderly. In the presence of prerenal volume deficits, ACE inhibition of angiotensin II may worsen prerenal azotemia or may even result in acute renal insufficiency. Other potential side effects, including taste disturbances and agranulocytosis, make these agents less than optimal for the treatment of perioperative hypertension.

Captopril (12.5 mg PO or 6.25 mg sublingually) is the most commonly administered ACE inhibitor. Oral and sublingual administration are accompanied by different onset times (<60 minutes vs. <5 minutes), different times to maximal effect (60 minutes vs. 15 minutes), and different durations of action (6 hours vs. 3 hours). Enalapril, a recently released IV-administered ACE inhibitor, has been used in those unable to receive oral medication.

Regardless of the agent chosen, drug therapy, when instituted, should be simplified. Outpatient compliance on a t.i.d. medication regimen is 59% but increases to 83.6% compliance when medications are prescribed on a once daily regimen. This 42% improvement can only benefit the patient.[73] Additionally, prescribing errors can and do occur in an in-patient setting. The evaluation of medication orders written in a tertiary teaching center during 1 year found 905 errors (out of 28,941 prescribing orders), which were detected and averted. At least 522 (57.5%) were rated as having the potential for adverse consequences. The overall detected medication error rate was 3.3/1,000 written orders, with a significant error rate of 1.8/1,000 written orders. The error rate is greatest (4.1/1,000 orders) between 12:00 P.M. and 3:59 P.M. The obstetrics and gynecology service (3.54/1,000 orders) has a relatively high rate of errors when compared to other services.[74]

In a patient with hypertension, the pelvic surgeon should focus on and evaluate the effect of hypertension on target end organs, including the heart, kidney, and central nervous system. The surgeon must be aware of the association between hypertension, peripheral vascular disease, and diabetes, as well as the role of specific antihypertensive drugs, their routes of administration, their potential interactions, and their side effects.

Although uncontrolled studies previously suggested that continuation of any hypertensive agent would increase the risk of perioperative hypoten-

sion, substantial subsequent data indicate that patients whose hypertension is well controlled do as well or better if their medications are continued up to the time of the operative procedure. Uncontrolled hypertension places patients at higher risk for labile blood pressures and hypertensive episodes during surgery, especially just after extubation.[36]

Periods of preoperative and postoperative fasting strain the ability to maintain scheduled perioperative drug treatment. In fact, 15% (256/1,746) of single prescriptions scheduled to be given on the day of surgery or first postoperative day were not administered. As expected, analgesics were not omitted, and when these drugs were excluded from evaluation the proportion of prescriptions that were not administered increased to 29%. Nearly one third (38/95) of omitted drugs had been prescribed for cardiovascular disease or respiratory disease (34/103).[75]

As previously noted, hypertension is the leading cause of ischemic heart disease, and the severity of hypertension correlates directly with atherosclerotic changes.[2] Hypertension doubles the risk of angina and MI, and progressive CAD is worsened in the presence of hypertension. Unfortunately, alterations in blood volume and SVR increase the perioperative risks of hypotension and its sequelae. Recent information suggests this risk of intraoperative hypotension to be significantly increased in patients whose perioperative mean arterial pressure equaled or exceeded 110 mm Hg, those with walking distance of less than 400 meters, or those who had a plasma volume of less than 3,000 cc.[76] Additionally, patients undergoing intra-abdominal procedures or prolonged operations (>2 hours) were at increased risk of perioperative cardiac morbidity. It would appear that the level of change (i.e., instability) and not necessarily the degree of change (i.e., 40 mm Hg vs. 20 mm Hg) is significant. While the majority (62%) of patients had an arterial pressure decrease (>20 mm Hg), the postoperative risks were doubled, related to the duration of this decrease.[76] Interestingly, this 20 to 30 mm Hg change closely corresponds to the effects of coronary and renal autoregulation.

Arrhythmias

As previously mentioned, major ventricular arrhythmias occur in 44% of patients with known CAD or risk factors for CAD who are evaluated with continuous perioperative ECG monitoring.[44] Perioperative arrhythmias were more common in smokers (odds ratio = 4.1), those with a history of

CARDIOVASCULAR COMPLICATIONS **31**

CHF (odds ratio = 4.1), and those with ECG evidence of myocardial ischemia (odds ratio = 2.2). Perioperative nonfatal infarction and cardiac death were not increased in patients with documented cardiac arrhythmias.

Although dysrhythmias are common, particularly in the critically ill, they are usually benign in patients without coexisting heart disease. Conduction system disease or premature ventricular or premature atrial contractions may serve as markers for underlying cardiac disease, and their presence in association with CAD or left ventricular dysfunction is more ominous. Their occurrence with acute MI correlates with poor outcome, and the combination of ventricular arrhythmias and hypokalemia in patients with acute myocardial ischemia increases the risk of ventricular fibrillation.[2] While four studies have assessed the importance of perioperative arrhythmia, current data suggest that frequent PVCs or other nonsinus rhythms on preoperative ECG are independent predictors of perioperative cardiac morbidity. To the contrary, the presence of bifascicular, trifascicular (complete or incomplete) bundle-branch block, right bundle-branch block, or left anterior hemiblock in the absence of other conditions such as acute MI does not apparently increase the risk of PCM.

Almost no clinical patient subset is free from cardiac arrhythmias. Atrial tachycardia is the most common arrhythmia noted in the general population. Chronic atrial fibrillation of more than 3 weeks' duration is present in 1.7% of the general population. It occurs with a variety of conditions, including systemic hypertension, CAD, lung disease, and valvular heart disease. In the absence of a known recognizable cause, it is called lone atrial fibrillation.[77] CAD is present in 50% to 60% of patients with atrial fibrillation, and hypertension is present in 40% to 60%. Hyperthyroidism occurs in approximately 2.5%.[78] Critically ill patients with atrial tachyarrhythmias, nodal rhythm, ventricular bradycardia, and rapid ventricular rhythms have a significantly higher mortality than patients without arrhythmias. The relative risk of dying in those clinical groups was increased by a factor of 1.16, 1.27, 2.20, and 1.47, respectively.[79]

In one series of patients undergoing cardiac surgery, 4% of patients developed new supraventricular tachyarrhythmias postoperatively. Within this group, 46% of patients had acute cardiac conditions, 31% had major infection, 29% had preexisting hypotension, 26% had anemia, 23% had metabolic disorders, 23% had received new parenteral drugs that could be implicated, and 20% were hypoxic.[80] Therefore, tachyarrhythmias following surgery should be considered a manifestation of bleeding, infection, acid–base electrolyte imbalance, and/or iatrogenic disease. New postoperative supraventricular tachyarrhythmias should prompt a search for remedial medical problems.

Atrial fibrillation is often a manifestation of atrial enlargement, and any supraventricular rhythm other than sinus appears to be a risk factor for the development of perioperative complications. Depending on its cause, duration, and hemodynamic significance, as well as on the symptomatic state of the patient, the goal of treating atrial fibrillation is either control of ventricular rate or termination of fibrillation. Digoxin has been proposed as treatment for a rapid ventricular response, for terminating recent-onset atrial fibrillation, for maintaining sinus rhythm, and prophylactically in patients with paroxysmal atrial fibrillation to prevent excessive tachycardia during the paroxysm. Studies now suggest that in patients with atrial fibrillation, digoxin is a poor choice for controlling heart rate during exertion, has little or no effect in terminating arrhythmia, and may occasionally aggravate paroxysmal atrial tachycardia.[35]

In the patient presenting with new-onset atrial fibrillation and a rapid ventricular response, a careful clinical assessment is needed to determine the presence of concomitant CHF and to assess the degree of urgency for control of ventricular rate. Oral or IV digitalization is still appropriate for the hemodynamically stable patient for whom there is no urgency. Digoxin will be less effective or ineffective if there is associated fever, thyrotoxicosis, hypoxia, acute blood loss, or any other condition in which sympathetic tone is elevated. In the absence of CHF, digoxin does not act as an antiarrhythmic drug in the atrium. In a double-blind, randomized, placebo-controlled study of digoxin in recent-onset atrial fibrillation not associated with CHF, no benefit was found for digoxin compared to placebo for reversion of arrhythmia to sinus rhythm. This observation is supported by electrophysiologic evidence that digoxin shortens the refractory period of the atrial myocardium and could potentially increase the fibrillary rate and at least theoretically lessen the possibility of reversion to sinus rhythm.[35]

Although all patients with atrial fibrillation are at increased risk for systemic embolization, emboli are more often associated with atrial fibrillation in rheumatic heart disease. In the Framingham study, stroke occurred at a rate 17.56 times the expected rate in patients with rheumatic heart disease with atrial fibrillation, compared to 5.6 times the expected rate in other patients with atrial fibrillation.[77]

There is general agreement among physicians that patients with atrial fibrillation and mitral valve disease should be treated with long-term anticoagulation.[77] Both left ventricular and left atrial anatomy are significant predictors of thromboembolisms in patients with nonvalvular atrial fibrillation. Standard echocardiography may contribute to the risk stratification, differentiating the one third of patients without clinical risk factors who are at increased risk for stroke from the remainder who may not need antithrombotic prophylaxis.[81]

In the Stroke Prevention in Atrial Fibrillation trial, the presence of three independent clinical predictors—recent CHF, a history of hypertension, and previous thromboembolism—defined patients with rates of thromboembolism of 2.5% per year (no risk factors) to 7.2% per year (one risk factor) and 17.6% per year (two or three risk factors). Nondiabetic patients without these risk factors, composing 38% of the cohort, had a low risk for thromboembolism (1.4% per year). Patients without clinical risk factors who were under 60 years of age had *no* thromboembolic phenomena.[81]

Prospective trials indicate that the rate of stroke in patients with nonvalvular atrial fibrillation is substantial, about 5% per year. More important, they have convincing documentation that low-dose warfarin therapy reduces stroke rates with minimal risk for significant hemorrhage in properly chosen patients with nonvalvular atrial fibrillation.[78]

The presence of PVCs should serve as a clinical clue to the possible presence of cardiac pathology. If a careful history, physical examination, and indicated imaging studies confirm the absence of underlying cardiac disease, no further evaluation or treatment is necessary. Patients who have PVCs but no evidence of underlying heart disease on detailed examination have an apparently normal cardiac prognosis, and PVCs in the absence of underlying heart disease should not be considered a risk factor for cardiac complications with noncardiac surgery. The extent of diagnostic testing necessary to determine the presence or absence of underlying heart disease varies with the clinical setting. The history, including a specific review of coronary risk factors and a detailed review of exercise capacity, coupled with careful physical examination remains the most valuable element of the comprehensive assessment. In patients in whom careful history and physical examination do not suggest underlying possible cardiac disease, no further diagnostic testing may be required. Further testing is advisable only if

deemed necessary to clarify particular aspects of the history and physical examination.[82] The lack of ECG complexity further negates the need for treatment. Electrolyte and metabolic abnormalities clearly underlie lethal ventricular arrhythmias in a wide variety of clinical situations and should be routinely considered as a potential cause and evaluated in patients with ventricular arrhythmias, particularly those patients with hypertension and CHF who are receiving thiazide and loop diuretics.[83] The presence of perioperative arrhythmias is frequently associated with electrolyte disturbances, particularly hypokalemia. Concentrated potassium chloride (200 mEq/L) infusions at a rate of 20 mEq/hr via central or peripheral vein to correct hypokalemia (evaluated in 1,351 infusions) resulted in a mean increment in the serum potassium level of 0.25 mmol/L per 20-mEq infusion. No temporally related life-threatening arrhythmias were noted; there were ten instances of mild hyperkalemia.[84] This schedule has been confirmed in another select group of hypokalemic patients in whom a potassium infusion of 20 to 40 mmol was safely delivered over 1 hour and effectively increased serum potassium levels in a dose-dependent and predictable fashion, independent of the patients' underlying renal function or associated diuretic administration.[85] Although arrhythmias may be associated with hypokalemia, the presence of hypokalemia per se is not associated with an adverse anesthetic cardiac outcome.[86]

While PVCs may signal underlying heart disease, the use of antiarrhythmic drugs to suppress PVCs in certain instances may actually be harmful. In patients with chronic obstructive pulmonary disease, ventricular ectopy may be caused by underlying disturbances or by pharmacologic therapy. For most patients with structurally normal hearts and for those with mitral valve prolapse without murmur, reassurance and avoidance of substances that can increase ventricular ectopy are the only treatment necessary. If perioperative treatment is deemed necessary, a prophylactic bolus of lidocaine (3 mg/kg) followed by a continuous infusion of 1 to 4 mg/min can be used but is not well tolerated by the elderly, those with renal dysfunction, or those with severe CHF. If antiarrhythmic drug therapy has been initiated previously, it should be continued up to and resumed immediately after the operative procedure.

Patients with complete heart block must augment stroke volume in response to the demands for increased CO. Unfortunately, many of these patients cannot increase myocardial contractility. Anesthetic-associated myocardial depression and peripheral vasodilation may create perioperative problems. Furthermore, anesthesia may further depress myocardial automaticity and myocardial conduction, and may alter ventricular rate in order to meet the increased demands placed on the cardiovascular system by anesthesia. A permanent or temporary pacemaker should be inserted before general anesthesia even in asymptomatic, untreated patients with complete heart block. A significant fraction of patients with chronic bifascicular block develop complete heart block following MI. Progression from bifascicular to complete lethal heart block has not been documented during the perioperative period in patients without a previous history of third-degree heart block. In this regard, patients with chronic asymptomatic bifascicular block do not need routine preoperative prophylactic pacemaker placement but are best managed with continuous ECG monitoring and continuous evaluation by a physician skilled in the placement of a pacemaker, should one be needed. The risk of complete heart block is estimated to be less than 1%, and the block is rarely lethal.[59] Therefore, we do not recommend prophylactic pacemaker placement for patients with first-degree AV block or Type I second-degree AV block (Wenckebach), although a pacemaker should always be available in the operating room for emergency placement. In patients who have bifascicular block *and* either Mobitz Type II second-degree AV block or a history of unexplained syncope or transient third-degree AV block, or symptomatic sick sinus syndrome, the risk of developing complete heart block is much higher and a temporary pacemaker should be placed preoperatively.[87,88]

Additional indications (Table 1–16) for temporary perioperative pacing include inadequate medical control of supraventricular dysrhythmias or severe bradycardia associated with drug therapy or drug toxicity.

Patients with existing permanent pacemakers should be carefully evaluated during the preoperative and intraoperative period to ensure proper pacemaker function. Demand pacemakers are sensitive to electrocautery-induced electromagnetic interference, which can result in failure to pace. This potentially hazardous interaction can be reduced by placing the indifferent pole of the cautery as far as possible from the lead and pulse generator. In this clinical situation, intraoperative electrocautery should be used in brief bursts rather than continuously. A magnet to convert the pacemaker from the demand to the fixed mode should be readily avail-

TABLE 1–16. Guidelines for Pacemaker Implantation

Complete heart block (permanent or intermittent) occurring with:
  Symptomatic bradycardia
  Congestive heart failure
  Arrhythmia requiring drugs that suppress escape rhythm
  Documented asystole ≥3 sec or escape rate <40 beats/min
Second-degree AV block with symptomatic bradycardia
Bifascicular block with intermittent complete heart block and symptomatic bradycardia
Symptomatic bifascicular block with intermittent type II second-degree AV block
Sinus node dysfunction with documented symptomatic bradycardia
Persistent, advanced second-degree AV block or complete heart block

Modified from Collins JJ, et al: Guidelines for permanent cardiac pacemaker implantation. Circulation 70:331, 1984.

able in the operating room. Finally, cautery may interfere with ECG monitoring, rendering it temporarily uninterpretable. Direct arterial pressure should be monitored when cautery is being used in patients with permanent pacemakers.[89]

Valvular Heart Disease

The risk of developing perioperative cardiac morbidity depends primarily on the functional state of the heart, including the presence of ventricular dysfunction, dysrhythmias, pulmonary hypertension, or CAD. Therefore, patients with valvular disease who exhibit little or no limitation of physical activity tolerate surgical procedures well and require little more than careful perioperative evaluation and prophylaxis for infective endocarditis. Those with more severe impairment of cardiac reserve (i.e., those in New York Heart Association [NYHA] functional class III or IV) tolerate noncardiac operations poorly, and their prognosis for surviving major surgery is distinctly worse.

The normal area of the aortic valve is 3 cm². Signs and symptoms of aortic stenosis consistently occur when valvular area falls below 1.0 cm². Patients with aortic stenosis and good left ventricular function who do not have a significant pressure gradient across the aortic valve are not at significant risk for perioperative cardiac morbidity. Significant aortic stenosis is associated with a 14-fold increase in the risk for perioperative cardiac morbidity.[36] Preoperative aortic valve replacement or valvuloplasty should be considered in symptomatic patients or in asymptomatic patients with documented significant aortic valvular stenosis. General anesthesia is preferable to regional anesthesia in patients with aortic stenosis because the latter may produce hypotension and tachycardia, which are not well tolerated. Mitral valve prolapse is present in 5% to 17% of otherwise healthy women. Hereditary transmission through an autosomal dominant pattern with reduced expressivity in humans has been proposed. Mitral valve prolapse is associated with thoracic skeletal abnormalities, migraines, anxiety attacks, neurosis, autonomic dysfunction, von Willebrand's syndrome, and polycystic kidney disease.[89,90] In general, women with mitral valve prolapse without mitral regurgitation are not at significant risk for perioperative cardiac morbidity.

Mitral stenosis or insufficiency is associated with an increased risk of CHF with a 15% incidence of associated left ventricular dysfunction.[91] Atrial contraction is important for adequate ventricular filling early in the course of mitral stenosis, but as left atrial size increases, the most important factor in adequate ventricular filling becomes the duration of diastole. Thus, in patients with mitral stenosis, CO can be dramatically decreased if atrial fibrillation or any supraventricular tachycardia intervenes.

Patients with symptomatic, critical aortic, or mitral valve stenosis are prone to sudden death or acute pulmonary edema during the perioperative period. The risk is particularly increased if cardiac demands are suddenly increased or if atrial fibrillation and a rapid ventricular rate are precipitated by anesthesia or operation. Corrective valve surgery should be considered before an elective operative procedure in patients with severe stenotic or regurgitant valve disease. Women undergoing emergency noncardiac operations should benefit from intraoperative hemodynamic monitoring, afterload reduction, and preload augmentation. Balloon valvuloplasty may relieve severe valvular obstruction in those situations where open surgery for valve replacement is deemed undesirable.

Prosthetic Heart Valves

Many patients with mechanical prosthetic heart valves receive long-term anticoagulants to prevent or decrease the risk of thromboembolic complications. This risk is higher in those with prosthetic mitral valves (5%) than in those with a prosthetic aortic valve (2%). Oral anticoagulants can be temporarily discontinued during the perioperative period with minimal risk of thrombosis. In 159 patients with prosthetic mitral valves who underwent 189 noncardiac procedures, warfarin was discontinued 2.9 days preoperatively and resumed 2.7 days postoperatively, with no thromboembolic complications.[92] Using a similar approach, there were no thromboembolic complications in 25 of 27 noncardiac operations in patients with prosthetic aortic valves.[92] Katholi reported that two of 38 patients sustained fatal embolic events when anticoagulants were discontinued 3 to 5 days preoperatively and resumed 3 to 5 days postoperatively.[93] In patients with prosthetic valves and who are at high risk, we prefer to discontinue oral anticoagulation 2 to 3 days preoperatively to allow the prothrombin time to recover to approximately 2 to 3 seconds above control. At that time, supplemental intravenous heparin is started; the heparin is discontinued 6 hours before the operation and restarted 36 to 48 hours postoperatively. Oral anticoagulation is resumed and heparin is discontinued when the prothrombin time is within therapeutic range.

Endocarditis Prophylaxis

Patients with significant valvular heart disease as well as those with prosthetic heart valves should receive prophylactic antibiotics when undergoing contaminated surgical procedures.[94] Bacteremia commonly occurs after daily events such as teeth brushing (20%–24%) or use of an oral irrigation device (20%–24%), as well as after specific procedures, including dental extraction (30%–80%), barium enema (11%), transurethral prostate resection (10%–57%), upper gastric endoscopy (8%), and nasotracheal intubation (16%).[89] Nearly all gynecologic, gastrointestinal, or genitourinary operations can be complicated by either gram-positive or gram-negative bacteria and require specific antimicrobial prophylaxis in this clinical subset of patients.

The role and benefit of antibiotic prophylaxis before noncardiac operations in patients with mitral valve prolapse remains controversial. Most studies suggest that patients with mitral valve prolapse who have the clinical murmur of mitral regurgitation are at a substantially higher risk than patients who do not have this murmur. Cost-benefit analysis argues against routine prophylaxis in patients with mitral valve prolapse without a murmur.

Cholesterol

Hypercholesterolemia, familial or nonfamilial, is predictive of cardiovascular mortality, but insufficient data are available to determine the risk of perioperative cardiac morbidity. Treatment may reduce the risk of future cardiac events but probably plays little role in perioperative cardiac morbidity.

Cigarette Smoking

Nicotine has dose-related effects on the cardiovascular system, causing systemic vasoconstriction as well as an increase in the heart rate, systolic blood pressure, and other aspects of cardiopulmonary function (Table 1–17). Smoking abstinence is followed by a 20 beat/min decrease in heart rate as well as a decrease in blood pressure and serum catecholamine levels.

Smoking also acutely increases oxygen demand, increases coronary vascular resistance, and increases carboxyhemoglobin levels. Chronic nicotine abuse is associated with vasoconstriction, enhanced platelet aggregation, loss of endothelial integrity, and an increased risk of accelerated atherosclerosis. These adverse cardiovascular effects of smoking may theoretically contribute to perioperative cardiac morbidity, and short-term abstinence from smoking may be beneficial. However, only a single report has evaluated the effects of cigarette smoking on perioperative cardiac morbidity,[33] and the authors could find no measurable adverse effects.

Diabetes

Among hypertensive and diabetic patients undergoing elective noncardiac surgery, preoperative status and intraoperative changes in mean arterial pressure are predictive of postoperative ischemic complications. In one report, 30 diabetic patients (12%) developed postoperative ischemia, infarction, or cardiac death. Of diabetic patients with a previous MI or cardiomegaly, 24% had an ischemic postoperative event, while only 7% of diabetics without either preexisting condition sustained ischemic complications. No other preoperative characteristics, including the presence of angina, predicted ischemic cardiac risk. Diabetics are at risk for sequelae of intraoperative hypotension, with ischemic cardiac complications occurring in 19% of patients with a ≥ 20 mm Hg decrease in intraoperative mean arterial pressure lasting 60 minutes or more.[95] Appropriate cardiac evaluation of the diabetic woman may decrease the potential for perioperative cardiac morbidity.

Estimation of Cardiac Risks

There are numerous potentially pertinent preoperative evaluable cardiac factors that can be investigated during a preoperative consultation. Attempts to classify and correlate preoperative condition and postoperative morbidity were initially reported in 1963 by the American Society of Anesthesiologists using their ASA scale.[96] Although the ASA classification correlates with the risk of preoperative mortality following specific procedures, many surgeons consider it subjective, nonspecific, imprecise, and vague.

Before 1977, univariate analysis of individual clinical variables was routinely used to predict the risk of perioperative cardiac events. Goldman and Braunwald, evaluating results of 1,001 noncardiac operations, published the first multivariate approach and described a cardiac risk index that included variables from the history, physical examination, and laboratory evaluation.[36] In their initial report, specific factors (Table 1–18) were correlated with increased cardiac risk, but importantly, this categorization indicated the presence of a number of apparent "non-risk" cardiac variables. Notably unimportant cardiac risk factors included smoking, glucose intolerance, hyperlipidemia, hypertension, peripheral vascular disease, class I or II angina, and a history of remote MI. This initial report suggested that a direct linear relationship existed between the Goldman score, life-threatening complications, and postoperative mortality. This risk increased from 0.2% in those patients with scores less than 5 to 56% for patients with scores greater than 26. Unfortunately, this index was de-

TABLE 1–17. **Smoking Effects on Cardiopulmonary Function**

Cardiovascular
↑ HR
↑ BP (systolic/diastolic)
↑ Myocardiocyte CA^{2+} regulation
↑ Hematocrit
↓ O_2 delivery/utilization

Respiratory
↑ Mucous secretion
↓ Mucociliary clearance
↑ Small airway activity
Altered surfactant activity

Immune
↑ IgE
↑ WBC
↓ Chemotaxis

TABLE 1–18A. Cardiac Risk Factors

Factor	Points
History	
• Age > 70	5
• MI (<6 mos)	10
Physical	
• S_3, JVD	11
• Aortic stenosis	3
ECG	
• Arrhythmia	7
• PVC (>5/min)	7
General	
• $Pao_2 < 60$, $Paco_2 > 50$ mm Hg	3
• $K^+ < 3$, Cr > 3.0	
• Abnormal LFTs	
• Bed confined	
Operation	
• Abdominal/thoracic	3
• Emergency	4
Total	**53**

rived from a group of unselected general surgical patients above the age of 40 and may actually underestimate the risk of perioperative cardiac morbidity after specific surgical procedures. A review of Goldman and Braunwald's report suggests that 31 (59%) of 53 of the possible cardiac risk points can be altered. However, it remains to be documented that correction of any of these factors would reverse associated operative risk.[12] Specific unalterable preoperative factors that correlate with perioperative cardiac morbidity include advanced age, emergency operation, cardiomegaly, a history of CHF, angina, an abnormal ST segment on the ECG, and an abnormal QRS complex on the ECG.[89,90]

TABLE 1–18B. Risk Categorization

Goldman Score	Life-Threatening Complication (%)*	Mortality (%)
< 5	0.7	0.2
6–12	5.0	2.0
13–25	11.0	2.0
> 26	22.0	56.0

Modified from Goldman L, Caldera DL, Nussbaum SR, et al: Multifactorial index of cardiac risk in noncardiac surgical procedures. N Engl J Med 297:845, 1977.
*Myocardial infarction, failure, ventricular tachycardia.

This classic study was a "hypothesis-generating" report and subsequently a number of investigators have published "hypothesis testing" reports (Table 1–19). More recent reports[97] have modified Goldman's index by adding clinically relevant features such as anginal classification, history of remote MI, the presence of unstable angina, suspected critical aortic stenosis, and alveolar pulmonary edema. These latter studies support the predictive ability of a multifactorial index but caution against "ruling out" significant cardiac risk in patients undergoing extensive, high-risk surgical procedures. They have also suggested the potential benefit of information obtained from additional noninvasive cardiac studies. The hypothesis-testing studies also suggested that "cardiac risk" indices be used with caution unless each institution or physician has defined specific patient subsets in which the information obtained from these indices would be of benefit. Obviously, the impact of a surgical procedure on cardiovascular morbidity can be stratified by dividing operations into those that are likely to increase perioperative ischemia and those that do not increase the risk of ischemia. At best, the use of indices for predicting cardiac complications should serve as an aid and not replace good judgment during preoperative evaluation.[98]

Attempts to further define perioperative risk have involved the use of the acute physiology and chronic health evaluation (APACHE) score, which classifies patients according to severity of disease. An APACHE score represents the sum of 34 physiologic variables, recently reduced to 12 physiologic variables that are most predictive of mortality of patients in an intensive care setting (Table 1–20). Age points and chronic health points are added to this physiologic score, which is now referred to as the APACHE II score. The APACHE II score is not ideal for evaluation of the patient scheduled for elective surgery because the scores are generated from data relevant to patients in intensive care units. Although the APACHE II score is an easily determined objective tool, its use has not yet been predictive of the risks of perioperative cardiac morbidity, with the exception of one report indicating its predictive value in those undergoing major upper abdominal surgery.[96]

Recommendations

Preoperative cardiac evaluation should begin before hospitalization or surgery. The patient's visit to the surgeon's office represents the one consistent

TABLE 1–19. **Major Complication* Rates Analyzed with the Multifactorial Cardiac Risk Index**

	Series and Patient Type					
	Goldman 1977 Unselected Major Noncardiac Surgery, ≥ 40 yrs old	*Zeldin 1984* Unselected Noncardiac Surgery, ≥ 40 yrs old	*Detsky 1986* Preoperative Medical Consultations	*Jeffrey 1983* Abdominal Aortic Aneurysm Surgery	Pooled	Pooled Likelihood Ratio (Sensitivity/ 1-Specificity)
Overall complication rate	58/1,001 (6%)	35/1,140 (3%)	17/268 (10%)	11/99 (11%)	131/2,508 (5.2%)	
Complication rate by class						
Class I (0–5 pts.)	5/537 (1%)	4/590 (1%)	8/13 (6%)	4/56 (7%)	21/1,317 (1.6%)	0.29
Class II (6–12 pts.)	21/316 (7%)	13/453 (3%)	6/88 (7%)	4/35 (11%)	44/889 (5%)	0.94
Class III (13–15 pts.)	18/130 (14%)	11/74 (15%)	9/45 (20%)	3/8 (38%)		3.4
Class IV (≥ 26 pts.)	14/18 (78%)	7/23 (30%)	4/4 (100%)			22.7

Modified from Goldman L, Braunwald E: General anesthesia and noncardiac surgery in patients with heart disease. In Braunwald E (ed): Heart Disease. Philadelphia, WB Saunders, 1992.
*Documented myocardial infarction, cardiogenic pulmonary edema, ventricular tachycardia, or cardiac death.

point in the preoperative process where potential problems can be identified in a time frame suitable to schedule appropriate studies, seek medical consultation, and alert the anesthesiologist. The early detection and treatment of pathologic variations in essential body systems has always been a primary goal of physicians. If the surgeon assumes only the role of a technician, the patient may appear in the holding unit on the day of surgery with less than desirable evaluation or preparation. Failure to adequately evaluate associated medical problems can

result in surgical delay, potential confrontation, expedited evaluations, and potentially increased surgical risk for the individual patient.

Anesthetic or perioperative management of a patient may be altered by discovery of a specific laboratory test abnormality that cannot be identified by careful history or physical examination. In general, abnormalities suggesting a condition that poses a significant risk of perioperative morbidity that can be modified by preoperative treatment are uncommon. Specific laboratory results may assist in ensuring that a patient's preoperative condition is optimal. When added to a carefully obtained history and thorough physical examination, the value of any routine screening preoperative laboratory study is dubious. It is well documented that screening studies frequently fail to uncover new pathologic conditions, offer little improvement in patient care or outcome, and are inefficient in screening for asymptomatic disease. Even if abnormal, the actual values or recommendations are frequently not recorded or acted on (30%–95%) regardless of the medical setting (university or community).[90] It is clear that routine preoperative screening increases costs. Blue Cross/Blue Shield estimates that in 1984, more than $30 billion was spent in the U.S. health care system for preoperative evaluations.[99]

A carefully obtained medical history is paramount and allows for selective additional evalua-

TABLE 1–20. **Apache II**

Temperature
Age
Mean blood pressure
Heart rate
Respiratory rate
Oxygenation
Arterial pH
Serum sodium
Serum potassium
Serum creatinine
Hematocrit
White cell count
Glasgow Coma Score

tion. We believe that patients can assist in providing information regarding current or past medical problems, procedures, or medications. Every patient is asked to complete a detailed medical questionnaire at her first or preoperative visit and annually thereafter. This information is carefully evaluated and the patient's medical data base is increased during the history and physical examination. Even the simplest historical factors may require evaluation. If a patient is unable to walk two blocks at a normal pace because of claudication, the historical presence of Canadian Cardiovascular Society (CCS) class III angina cannot be ascertained[100] and additional cardiac evaluation may be indicated, depending on the extent of planned surgery. Additionally, subtle symptoms suggesting peripheral vascular disease may be elicited and guide additional preoperative evaluation. Of note, peripheral vascular disease is a significant risk factor for the development of ischemic heart disease that may be difficult to detect on physical examination and may not be manifested in an abnormal ECG. In a report on 500 patients with peripheral vascular disease, a normal ECG, and no prior history of MI, additional cardiac evaluation revealed a high incidence of significant (at least 70%) coronary artery stenosis.[89]

Obviously, relevant findings on the physical examination should prompt additional evaluation. Each patient should undergo a thorough multisystem examination, with the alert physician adding additional indicated preoperative studies based on physical findings. For instance, the existence of asymptomatic carotid bruits does not predict the site or influence the risk of perioperative stroke but does predict mortality from ischemic heart disease.[89] Thus, the presence of carotid bruit may alert the physician to the need for additional cardiologic evaluation.

Laboratory Studies

Numerous studies have failed to document the efficacy of routine preoperative laboratory biochemical screening studies.[90] Korvin et al.,[101] reviewing the results of routine admission biochemical tests in 1,000 patients, were unable to find any laboratory result that produced a diagnosis that was unequivocally beneficial to any patient. Olsen et al.[102] performed a controlled prospective trial evaluating the benefits of multiphasic laboratory screening in 1,500 patients and could not detect any difference in morbidity between controls and those who underwent the screening studies.[102] Durbridge et al.,[103] comparing 1,500 patients randomly assigned to

screening or nonscreening admission laboratory tests, reported no benefit in length of hospitalization or patient outcome from the additional 8,363 laboratory investigations performed for the group that underwent screening tests.[103]

The ultimate benefit of routine laboratory screening is questionable even in the elderly, a group of patients at much higher risk of surgical morbidity and mortality. Domoto et al.[104] examined the yield and benefit of a battery of 19 screening laboratory tests (3,093 total screening tests) performed in 70 functionally intact elderly patients whose average age was 82.6 years. Although "new" abnormal results occurred frequently, only 0.1% of all results led to a change in patient management, none of which, the authors concluded, benefited any patient in an important way.

Results obtained from routine laboratory screening rarely alter the timing of the surgical procedure. In one study abnormal laboratory results changed the preoperative clinical course (surgical postponement) in 28 (1.5%) of 1,924 patients evaluated. However, only three (0.16%) had laboratory screening abnormalities not explained or suggested by historical factors or findings from physical examination. Thus, the history and physical examination findings dictated appropriate laboratory testing in over 99% of the 1,924 patients evaluated.[105]

It appears that routine screening laboratory studies contribute little to the preoperative evaluation of asymptomatic patients; however, selective laboratory evaluation is paramount in patients with cardiovascular disease, and specific tests should be directed by the history and physical examination findings, current medication, surgical indications, and extent of operative procedure. Although a "cookbook" approach is not advocated, it is clear that selective laboratory testing is more likely to benefit patients and to be cost-effective.

Electrocardiography

A prospective study of the value of preoperative ECGs has not been reported and would be challenging to design. However, the utility of a normal ECG may be underestimated. A preoperative ECG can be useful in three ways: (1) to screen for abnormalities that are known to increase the risks associated with anesthesia and require a change in plans, (2) to provide a baseline recording of rhythm and morphologic features in case of significant cardiovascular complications, and (3) to provide information that would be of value in the future management of the patient.[106]

It has been amply demonstrated that screening

preoperative ECGs obtained in a population of relatively healthy adults yield very few specific end points, including recent unsuspected MI, serious arrhythmias, or serious metabolic abnormalities. In a recent study reported by Gold et al., 26 (3.3%) of the 782 patients studied had abnormalities that resulted in the cancellation of surgery.[107] Of the 12 patients with adverse cardiovascular outcomes, eight had ECG abnormalities that should have occasioned concern in giving an anesthetic and four of the eight patients were between the ages of 40 and 59.[107] Six of the 12 are said to have benefited from the baseline ECG, but only one of them was under the age of 60. Nine of the 12 patients who experienced adverse cardiovascular outcomes had worrisome preoperative ECG changes that would have been further investigated or would have influenced future management. Four of the nine were under the age of 60. Thus, a cookbook approach cannot be advocated, and clinical judgment remains important in determining who would benefit from a preoperative ECG.[107]

Specific ECG abnormalities with the potential to alter anesthesia management include atrial flutter or fibrillation, first-, second-, or third-degree AV block, ST-segment changes suggesting myocardial ischemia or recent pulmonary embolism, new or frequent premature ventricular and atrial contractions, left or right ventricular hypertrophy, short PR interval, Wolf-Parkinson-White syndrome, MI, a prolonged QT segment, and peaked T waves. The prevalence of ECG abnormalities has usually been determined by studies of hospitalized patients and epidemiologic surveys in healthy people. Pooled data indicate that the prevalence of abnormal preoperative ECGs exceeds 10% at 40 years of age and 25% by the age of 60. As expected, those studies evaluating ECG abnormalities in asymptomatic patients report a lower prevalence of significant abnormalities. Rabkin and Horne[108] examined the records of 165 patients having a new, "surgically" significant ECG abnormality (i.e., a change from previous ECG that represented a condition possibly affecting perioperative management or outcome). In only two (1.2%) instances was the anesthetic or surgical plan altered by the discovery of an abnormal ECG not predicted by history or examination. One of these patients had atrial fibrillation that should have been detected on examination. In this report, the benefits of a screening preoperative ECG were unproven, and individual case management was nearly always determined by historical factors or physical findings. McKee and Scott reported no significant abnormalities during preoperative evaluation of 116 individuals less than 60

years old and without cardiac symptoms.[109] Only two (1.6%) abnormalities were found in the 163 patients older than 60 years of age. Moorman et al.[110] reported that only one (0.4%) of 275 asymptomatic patients under the age of 45 years and seven (1.4%) of 500 asymptomatic patients over the age of 45 had preoperative ECG abnormalities. In another study, Blery et al.[111] indicated that only 0.6% of 2,256 asymptomatic patients under age 40 had an abnormal ECG. That report suggested that in the absence of a pertinent cardiovascular history, symptoms, or physical findings, the need for routine screening preoperative ECG begins at age 40 unless patients are undergoing extensive, high-stress procedures.

Preoperative ECG abnormalities occur in as many as 24% of ambulatory patients[112] and 70% of patients with CAD.[2] One recent retrospective study of 325 ambulatory surgical patients suggested that one in four patients had an abnormal ECG. The incidence of an abnormal ECG was 14% in patients under 40 years of age and 33% in those older than 40. All potentially serious ECG abnormalities such as PVCs, atrial arrhythmias, ischemia, or infarction occurred in patients over age 50 or in those with a prior history of cardiac disease.[112]

The rate of detection of an unsuspected MI in younger patients (<35 years) by screening ECG is approximately 1/1,000.[2] Nonspecific ST-T-wave changes are common (65%–90%), with left ventricular hypertrophy (10%–20%), and Q waves (0.5%–8%) occurring less frequently. Approximately 40% of abnormal preoperative ECG findings are new, occurring within the preceding 24 months.[2] New abnormalities on subsequent ECGs (25%–50%) occur as frequently as the sum of all abnormalities occurring on previous ECGs. Thus, one would be justified in obtaining screening ECGs before elective surgery in all patients over 40, even in those who recently had an ECG. Goldberger and O'Konski believe that the most important potential benefit of the preoperative ECG is in the detection of previously unrecognized myocardial ischemia.[113] This risk increases with increasing age; however, even in the highest risk group (those over 75 years of age), the estimated incidence of unrecognized Q-wave infarction within the preceding 6 months is relatively small (<0.05%). They concluded that the risk of obtaining a preoperative ECG and subsequent physician reactions probably exceed its benefit if patients are asymptomatic, do not have important risk factors for CAD, and, if female, are under age 55.[90]

Unfortunately, the data on the predictive value of an abnormal ECG are controversial. Goldman and

Braunwald[36] suggested that the presence of Q-wave changes, ST-T-wave changes, or a bundle-branch block was not predictive; however, other reports[114] have indicated that ischemic ST-T-wave changes or intraventricular conduction delays were the abnormalities occurring most frequently in patients with adverse cardiac outcomes. Clearly, any preoperative ECG abnormality requires explanation or additional evaluation prior to anesthesia induction.

Chest Radiography

The detection of tracheal deviation, mediastinal masses, pulmonary nodules, aortic aneurysm, pulmonary edema, pneumonia, atelectasis, new fractures of the vertebrae or clavicles, or cardiomegaly is important prior to proceeding with anesthesia and surgery. Clinical data also suggest that a tortuous or calcified aorta is predictive of perioperative cardiac morbidity.[36] Unfortunately, when compared to a history and physical examination, a screening chest roentgenogram in an asymptomatic woman contributes little to the detection of acute or chronic heart disease that would mandate a change in anesthetic technique. The risk of chest radiography probably exceeds possible benefits in the asymptomatic patient less than 60 years old. This analysis, of course, is predicated on maximizing benefit to society in general, because one cannot predict in advance which patients will benefit and which will be harmed.

Although rarely contributing to a cardiac evaluation in the asymptomatic patient, preoperative chest radiographs may be abnormal in as many as 19% of patients. Findings, including cardiomegaly (6%), COPD (4%), pneumonia (1%), and interstitial changes (1%), are less likely to be present in patients through 40 years old (9%) than in those older than 40 (27%). The majority (91%) of chest radiographs suggesting COPD, chronic heart failure, cardiomegaly, or pneumonia are obtained in patients older than 50. Unfortunately, the positive predictive value of an abnormal chest x-ray is only 8%.[112]

Tape and Mushlin[115] evaluated the effect on clinical management of preoperative chest radiographs in 341 patients. Only nine (2.6%) patients admitted for vascular surgery had abnormal films. Three (0.9%) patients (all symptomatic), two with CHF and one with pulmonary fibrosis, potentially benefited from radiologic findings. All three patients were known by history to have significant disease prior to its demonstration on a chest radiograph. No asymptomatic patient benefited. Unfortunately, six (1.8%) patients were subjected to additional evaluation and a potentially detrimental clinical outcome. Two were given incorrect diagnoses of tuberculosis, with subsequent therapy initiated in one; two had false positive diagnoses of pulmonary nodules, and two had false normal chest radiograph readings.

Roizen[90] retrospectively evaluated the potential adverse effects of screening chest radiography in 606 patients. An additional 368 extra chest radiographs were ordered without specific indication. Among those patients the discovery of only one (0.3%) abnormality (an elevated hemidiaphragm probably related to phrenic nerve palsy) resulted in improved care for that patient. On the other hand, the existence of three (0.8%) abnormal chest radiographs was responsible for three unrevealing sets of invasive tests, including one thoracotomy. These additional procedures did not result in the discovery of new disease and caused significant morbidity, including one pneumothorax and 4 months of disability for those three patients.

It is clear that routine screening chest radiographs are rarely revealing and not recommended for women less than 50 years old. Preoperative chest radiographs should be obtained based on historical or physical findings, influenced by surgical indication (i.e., malignancy) as well as the potential extent of radicality of the actual surgical procedure.

Cardiac Evaluation

Inability to exercise is probably the best clinical predictor of the risk of perioperative cardiac morbidity, and patients with normal exercise tolerance rarely need further preoperative cardiac testing. There is little need for additional cardiac evaluation if the diagnosis of CAD would have no impact on perioperative care. Additional cardiac studies are indicated and are of the most clinical benefit in patients whose risk of CAD is in the moderate range (30%–40%). Exercise ECG probably remains the initial diagnostic test of choice because this study is easy to perform, adds minimal expense, and carries predictive value for future coronary events (Table 1–21).

The evaluation of the patient with a poor or questionable exercise test result presents a difficult diagnostic challenge. Recognizing the limitations of ECG stress testing in patients with impaired exercise tolerance related to abnormal joint mobility, dementia, muscle weakness, claudication, or exertional angina is important. In these patients, an assessment of resting LVEF can be quite helpful in determining the risk of perioperative CHF. New

TABLE 1–21. **Screening Exercise Electrocardiography in the Coronary Primary Prevention Trial**

For Silent Ischemia:	
Sensitivity	37%
Specificity	79%
Pos. predictive value	3%
Neg. predictive value	98%

Modified from Siscovick DS, et al: Sensitivity of exercise electrocardiography for acute cardiac events during moderate and strenuous physical activity. Arch Intern Med 151:325–330, 1991.

pharmacologic stress testing using either radionuclide-labeled pharmaceuticals or echocardiography to detect new regional or global wall motion abnormalities has changed the thought process for the evaluation of those patients with suspected ischemic heart disease who are unable to exercise. Although long-term prospective studies are not available to determine the ability of these methods to predict future cardiac events, it is clear that their ability to demonstrate hemodynamically significant coronary stenosis is excellent. With the widespread availability of these studies, the surgeon should feel that patients who are unable to exercise can be adequately risk stratified.

Prior Myocardial Infarct

The patient with a recent Q-wave or non-Q-wave MI who has not returned to full exercise capacity is at high risk for developing preoperative myocardial ischemia and should undergo further preoperative cardiologic evaluation. If abdominal surgical intervention is contemplated, coronary angiography should be considered the initial diagnostic test of choice. Although the risks of reinfarction probably decrease as the interval (6 weeks) from the time of the acute MI increases, these patients should still be considered at significant risk. A determination of LVEF should be considered in all of the patients. Despite previous CABG, thrombolytic therapy, or PTCA, the majority of these patients should undergo radionuclide stress or pharmacologic testing and/or coronary angiography.

One recent report evaluated 275 patients with a prior MI who underwent noncardiac surgery. The choice of anesthetic technique had no effect on the incidence and outcome of perioperative MI. The reinfarction rate was 5% and mortality was 23%. Importantly, reinfarction occurred in 12 (92%) of

13 patients during the first 48 postoperative hours. An additional 21.5% of patients suffered serious nonlethal complications, suggesting that even though the risk of reinfarction has been reduced, patients with a prior MI remain at high risk for other postoperative complications.[10]

In this specific subset as well as in other patients at risk for postoperative myocardial ischemia, surveillance for reinfarction should routinely include serial ECGs and serial determination of cardiac enzymes on postoperative days 1 and 2 because the highest risk occurs immediately perioperatively. The sensitivity of this method of surveillance is 98%; however, false positive rates are relatively high (23%) and frequently require additional evaluation.[26]

Angina

Unstable angina, defined as the new onset of or a recent increase in frequency and duration of ischemic symptoms, is associated with a considerably higher long-term risk of cardiac morbidity. In a recent report by Shah et al.[10] evaluating 688 patients with cardiac risks, seven (28%) of 25 patients with unstable angina who underwent noncardiac surgery developed a perioperative MI or suffered cardiac death.[10] The risk of perioperative MI or cardiac death was 11.4% in those with chronic stable angina and 3% in those without chest pain. This information suggests that patients with unstable angina pose a prohibitive perioperative risk and that noncardiac operations should be performed only in emergency situations. Cardiologic evaluation and additional studies are mandatory. The development of a perioperative MI in this patient subgroup is difficult to manage because thrombolytic therapy may be contraindicated and emergency PTCA or CABG carries additional morbidity. Radionuclide or pharmacologic studies and/or coronary angiography are the initial preoperative studies of choice. In an emergency situation, intensive mechanical management including the perioperative use of an intra-aortic balloon pump as a bridge until a more definite cardiac treatment can be implemented may be necessary to reduce the risk of cardiac ischemia.[30]

Hypertension

Hypertensive patients have a higher prevalence of silent MI than the general population. However, a history of hypertension is not necessarily associated with an increased risk for perioperative cardiac morbidity. Perioperative hemodynamic fluctuations can be correlated with cardiac morbidity and are less frequent in treated than in untreated hypertensive patients.[91] Preoperative evaluation of the hypertensive patient should focus on radiographic, ECG, and echocardiographic evidence of left ventricular hypertrophy, which often signifies long-standing, poorly controlled disease. Echocardiographic evidence of ventricular hypertrophy may occur with no change in ECG voltage. If present, left ventricular hypertrophy alone increases the risk of developing an imbalance in myocardial oxygen supply and demand and ischemia, even in the absence of significant CAD. For example, ECG-demonstrated left ventricular hypertrophy is associated with a significantly higher incidence of postoperative myocardial ischemia (20/26 patients; 77%) than is found in hypertensive patients without left ventricular hypertrophy (57/137; 42%).[30] Additional preoperative cardiac evaluation including appropriate stress testing should be considered based on historical, clinical, or radiologic findings or in those patients undergoing extensive surgical procedures.

Diabetes Mellitus

Diabetes accelerates the development of arteriosclerosis and is a recognized risk factor for CAD. Diabetics have a high rate of silent myocardial ischemia and infarction, and the absence of cardiac symptoms probably correlates with autonomic dysfunction rather than with altered pain perception. Depending on the extent of surgical procedure, these patients should be considered for additional cardiac evaluation. An ECG should be obtained in all diabetics, with additional studies based on clinical findings. In view of the frequency of coronary disease, some authors have suggested that patients with a long history of diabetes should be considered for further diagnostic testing regardless of anginal history.[30]

Abnormal ECG

A change in the ECG from the preoperative tracing is always concerning and should be interpreted as evidence of ischemia until proven otherwise. It must be remembered that the classic ECG changes of an evolving MI are present in only approximately 66% of patients.[2] When evaluating an ECG with ST-segment elevation, it is important to exclude other nonischemic causes, including acute cor pulmonale, hyperkalemia, cerebrovascular accidents, left ventricular hypertrophy, left bundle-branch block, hypertrophic cardiomyopathy, hypo-

thermia, invasion of the heart by neoplastic tissue, and early repolarization.[116]

Pathologic Q waves in the preoperative ECG represent an important danger sign. However, Q waves shorter than 0.04 second in duration and less than 25% of the height of the R wave usually represent septal depolarization and may be part of a "perfectly normal" ECG. Although Q waves assist in determining a previous MI, noninfarction-associated Q waves may be present in patients with myocarditis, neuromuscular disorders, cardiac amyloidosis, postpartum cardiomyopathy, scleroderma, sarcoidosis, and hypertrophic cardiomyopathy.[116]

In patients with an abnormal baseline ECG, stress thallium imaging offers a sensitive method of detecting ischemia. If a stress thallium image is abnormal, discussion with a cardiologist is essential to determine the necessity of further evaluation as well as the role of preoperative cardiac catheterization and medical management.[30]

Congestive Heart Failure

Radiographic cardiomegaly suggests a significantly low EF (<40 %) in over 70% of patients with CAD. However, some studies suggest that cardiomegaly is not predictive of the risk of developing perioperative cardiac morbidity.[36]

Results from the CASS study indicate that patients with an EF of 35% or less have a 5-year survival of 54% with medical treatment, vs. a 5-year survival of 68% after CABG. In patient subgroups with EFs of 25% or less, the 5-year survival is 43% with medical treatment vs. 63% with CABG. An added benefit to coronary revascularization is improvement in myocardial function and clinical status after surgery.[117]

It appears that a minimal cardiac evaluation in patients with CHF includes ECG, measurement of ventricular EF, and stress or pharmacologic radionuclide imaging to assess and allow optimization of cardiac function. Stress echocardiography can substitute for radionuclide studies in some patients.

Special Cardiac Studies

A number of special procedures are available for cardiac evaluation (Table 1–22). Pharmacologic radionuclide studies such as dipyridamole–thallium stress testing, dipyridamole–technetium sestamibi stress testing, and adenosine–thallium stress testing use pharmacologic vasodilators combined with thallium or technetium imaging to assess left ven-

TABLE 1–22. **Cardiac Evaluation Techniques**

Technique	Advantages	Disadvantages
Exercise electrocardiography Low-level (predischarge following MI)	Safe, noninvasive; provides information about exercise tolerance, blood pressure response, heart rate response, exercise-induced angina, ischemia, and arrhythmias; will substantiate clinical impressions.	High-risk patients often unable to exercise; trend toward early discharge after uncomplicated infarction makes test difficult to obtain; low cutoff reduces potential for evaluating exercise capacity.
Symptom-limited (3–6 weeks)	Same advantages of low-level testing, plus evaluation of exercise capacity.	Lacks sensitivity of other tests for identifying severe coronary disease.
Coronary angiography	Direct visualization of affected vessels; will establish need for revascularization; exercise not required.	Invasive; expensive; associated risk greater, especially in elderly; does not evaluate physiologic significance of lesions.
Thallium 201 scintigraphy	Noninvasive; may be performed with or without exercise	Strict quality control required to ensure accuracy of results; severely ischemic areas may reperfuse slowly; image may be attenuated by breast tissue, high diaphragm, or large ventricular blood pool; expensive.
With pharmacologic vasodilators	Assists in identifying areas of jeopardized myocardium; helpful in patients who cannot exercise.	Can potentiate hypotension, cause gastrointestinal distress.
Radionuclide ventriculography	Allows evaluation of changes in segmental ventricular wall motion; less susceptible to operator error.	Exercise required; information not as direct as that from ^{201}Tl scintigraphy; data on test as a "risk stratifier" are limited.
Two-dimensional exercise echocardiography	Demonstrates changes in contractility in response to exercise.	Accuracy of results operator dependent; imaging may be inadequate in some patients; exercise required.

Modified from Krone R: What is the role of exercise testing after MI? J Crit Illness 5:1143–1157, 1990.

tricular regional blood flow. These studies do not require exercise but carry limitations related to known side effects of both dipyridamole and adenosine. Relative contraindications include bronchial asthma, COPD, theophylline use, and high-degree cardiac conduction abnormalities. Many centers rely on pharmacologic echocardiographic evaluations, in which echocardiographic images of the left ventricle are obtained at rest, during and after infusion of either dobutamine or amrinone. New regional wall motion abnormalities have been demonstrated to correlate with areas of ischemic myocardium. This technique suffers from the limitation of requiring a good echocardiographic window to allow sufficient imaging. Compared with other methods, it is as sensitive and slightly less specific in detecting myocardial ischemia.[118]

Continuous Monitoring

Continuous Holter monitoring of intermediate-risk patients can assist in the detection of asymptomatic myocardial ischemia. In a review of 176 asymptomatic vascular surgery patients, evidence of preoperative ischemia on continuous Holter monitoring was an independent predictor of perioperative cardiac morbidity.[90] The overall sensitivity of continuous monitoring for the prediction of perioperative cardiac morbidity was 92% and the specificity was 88%. This technique had a positive predictive value of 38% and a negative predictive value of 99%.[90]

Currently, the American Heart Association does not recognize ambulatory ECG as a preoperative diagnostic test for CAD.[30]

Exercise Stress Testing

Exercise stress testing is a readily available, simple, relatively inexpensive, well-standardized technique for screening for CAD. It is highly predictive of subsequent cardiac outcome in patients who start with normal ST segments and exhibit exercise-related ST-segment depression of >2.5 mm. These changes must occur within the first 3 minutes of testing, be sustained into the recovery period, or be associated with subnormal blood pressure elevation. Non-ECG responses that predict severe CAD include low achieved heart rate (<120 beats/min), unexplained systolic hypotension (decrease >10 mm Hg), elevated diastolic blood pressure (to >110 mm Hg), and the inability to exercise for 10 minutes.[90] Exercise stress testing is less predictive in patients with excellent exercise tolerance, particularly in patients undergoing low-risk surgical procedures. Associated disorders producing physiologic exercise limitation include obesity, hypertension, peripheral vascular disease, CAD, cardiomyopathy, valvular heart disease, vascular disease, obstructive lung disease, interstitial lung disease, carboxyhemoglobinemia, metabolic disorders, musculoskeletal disorders, and behavioral disorders. Its predictive value is lower in women; in patients with resting ECG abnormalities, including myocardial hypertrophy, conduction defects, a preexcitation pattern, or digitalis effect; in patients with limited exercise capacity (<85% of predicted maximal heart rate); and in patients taking cardioactive drugs, especially β-blockers and digitalis.[100,120,121] It must be remembered that patients with reduced exercise capacity may have a cardiovascular, ventilatory, or musculoskeletal limitation. Specific evaluation is necessary as the clinical history may be misleading. In fact, reduced exercise capacity even in patients who were previously asbestos workers is frequently (37%) related to cardiac etiologies.[121]

Although the risk of perioperative MI may be increased 20-fold in patients with a positive exercise stress test, its test sensitivity does not justify its use for routine surveillance, and exercise stress testing is of relatively little value in the screening of healthy asymptomatic patients. Although a positive exercise stress test may be present in 27% of those patients with a negative cardiac history and a normal ECG, only 26% of these patients (7% of those with a positive exercise stress test) are at risk for developing a perioperative MI.[2] As previously noted, the ability to exercise remains an important predictor of perioperative cardiac morbidity. Cutler et al.[122] found no risk of perioperative cardiac mortality or infarction in patients without ECG changes who could exercise to 75% of their maximal predicted heart rate. However, 4.3% of patients with characteristic ischemic changes developed nonfatal perioperative MIs. The development of ischemic changes occurring at less than 75% predicted maximal heart rate defined a very high-risk group of patients with a 25.9% risk of perioperative infarction and a 18.5% risk of cardiac mortality.

Current consensus suggests that exercise stress testing should be the initial test for evaluating those women with a moderate probability of CAD, particularly if the diagnosis of CAD would alter the timing or choice of the surgical procedure or alter intraoperative or perioperative surveillance care. It remains the initial study for assessing cardiac risk in patients with symptomatic peripheral vascular disease who can exercise or those women with stable angina.[59]

Gated Blood Pool Scanning

Pasternak et al.[123] utilized radionuclides to evaluate resting LVEF in patients undergoing aortic aneurysm repair. The risk of infarction increased in a linear fashion to 80% in patients with EFs below 36%. Although these patients were not chosen with specific selective criteria, this observation suggested that RNA evaluation was superior in predicting the risk of perioperative cardiac morbidity when compared to historical studies evaluating the predictive value of ECG in patients with CAD.[124] More recent studies have confirmed the predictive value of LVEF determined by resting gated pool blood studies and suggest that an LVEF below 35% is associated with a significant (75%) risk of perioperative ischemia following vascular procedures.[100]

Although considered of some value, RNA studies have been replaced by other methods of evaluation.

Precordial Echocardiography

Current state-of-the-art noninvasive techniques using refined two-dimensional echocardiography for assessment of anatomy and function, combined with the evaluation of physiology and hemodynamics using color flow imaging with Doppler echocardiography at rest and during exercise, have revolutionized the diagnosis and management of cardiovascular diseases. The relatively inexpensive application of these noninvasive techniques to patients with possible coronary heart disease allows identification of the proximal segments of the coronary arteries, detection of the presence and extent of prior MI (scar, resting abnormal wall motion, aneurysm), papillary muscle dysfunction, thrombus formation, and the presence of ischemia and its effects on ventricular systolic (regional and global) and diastolic function. In addition, Doppler and color flow imaging information can assist in determining the presence of mitral regurgitation, as well as other valvular abnormalities and pulmonary and right ventricular pressures. A complete evaluation utilizes dynamic (treadmill or bicycle), isometrics (handgrip, cold pressor), or pharmacologic (adenosine, dobutamine, dipyridamole) stress testing in conjunction with ECG and blood pressure monitoring, evaluation of myocardial wall motion, or myocardial perfusion imaging. Although the exact prognostic value of echocardiography is unknown, the diagnosis of preoperative ventricular dysfunction or wall motion abnormalities predicts the risk of perioperative dysfunction.[2] A regional ventricular wall motion abnormality and the inability to exercise for 2 minutes to a heart rate of more than 99 beats/min are independently predictive of a perioperative cardiac event.[28]

Hemodynamically significant CAD is essentially excluded with echocardiographic documentation of normal global and regional left ventricular function at rest and maximal exercise. Altered ventricular function during physical or pharmacologic stress may also occur in some older (>60 years) patients free of CAD or in patients with atrial fibrillation, left bundle-branch block, hypertension, valvular abnormalities, or intrinsic myocardial disease.

An objective measure of left ventricular function can be obtained from echocardiographic evaluation of resting LVEF. Although the predictive utility of the resting LVEF is controversial, the resting LVEF provides a baseline assessment of myocardial function that is most useful in patients with documented CAD, particularly those with poor or questionable exercise tolerance.[90]

The overall sensitivity of exercise echocardiography is approximately 80% and is higher in those patients with multivessel CAD. The overall specificity of exercise echocardiography approaches 95%. Stress echocardiographic imaging is more sensitive and specific than the standard treadmill ECG, and clinical results approximate the predictive value of radionuclide scintigraphy (thallium 201) with the advantages of less expense, no time delay, no radiation exposure, and beat-to-beat analysis of EF instead of averaging counts over 2 to 3 minutes.[125] Dipyridamole echocardiography also may be highly sensitive, and dobutamine echocardiography may be beneficial in predicting perioperative risks.

Transesophageal Echocardiography

Two-dimensional transesophageal electrocardiography is a complex, expensive, but potentially revealing cardiovascular monitoring tool. A typical TEE transducer (42 mm long, 13 mm wide, 11 mm thick) is mounted on the tip of a 9-mm-diameter gastroscope and uses intermittent pulses of ultrasound at 2.5 to 5 million cps. Thirty cross-sectional images per second are displayed in real time on a monitor screen and can be recorded on video tape for later review.[126]

Esophagitis, esophageal ulceration, or esophageal stricture and an uncorrected bleeding disorder are relative contraindications to TEE. The presence of a large hiatal hernia has been found to cause suboptimal transgastric imaging.[127]

TEE facilitates rapid assessment of ventricular volumes, EF, ventricular contractility, and ventricular filling, which is usually obtained indirectly from the Swan-Ganz catheter. It has remarkable sensitivity in detecting regional wall abnormalities, which have been reported to be more sensitive than ECG in detecting myocardial ischemia.[2,128]

The predictive value of awake TEE evaluation prior to noncardiac surgery has not been studied. It appears that following coronary occlusion and initiation of myocardial ischemia, the myocardial wall thickens and wall motion abnormalities develop that often precede ECG changes. TEE-demonstrated segmental wall motion and thickening abnormalities are more sensitive in the diagnosis of ischemia than is ECG, even 12-lead ECG. In one report of high-risk patients, segmental wall abnormalities occurred in 24 (48%) of 50 patients. All patients (12%) with ECG changes had characteristic TEE changes. In contrast, 12 of 24 patients with TEE changes had no ECG changes.[2] As many as 61% of TEE wall motion abnormalities occurred without significant change in heart rate, systolic arterial pressure, or PA pressure.[2,128] In one recent study of patients at risk for CAD, the use of intraoperative TEE and 12-lead ECG added little to the incremental predictive value of developing perioperative ischemia when compared to preoperative clinical data and routine two-lead intraoperative ECG monitoring.[129]

Radionuclide Imaging

The application of noninvasive nuclear medicine imaging techniques to the preoperative evaluation of patients at risk for or with known CAD offers important diagnostic, pathophysiologic, and prognostic information that can potentially modify patient management. Two factors regulate myocardial thallium uptake: viability of the myocardial tissue and the magnitude of regional myocardial perfusion. Ischemic but not infarcted regions are eventually perfused with thallium. Thallium washout from an ischemic region is delayed relative to washout from normally perfused regions because of the exercise-induced regional hypoperfusion.

Regional myocardial perfusion imaging using thallium 201, initially reported in 1985, is usually coupled with exercise or pharmacologic stress (dipyridamole, adenosine, dobutamine, or amrinone) to maximize coronary blood flow. Immediate postexercise images are compared to redistribution images obtained 3 to 4 hours later. The hallmark of myocardial ischemia is delayed uptake and washout. Therefore, quantitative discrimination of fixed and reversible thallium defects can distinguish scar from ischemia. Defects that persist on delayed imaging (fixed defects) were previously thought to represent an area of "old" infarction; however, fixed defects on standard delayed imaging (3 hours) may also occur in the presence of viable myocardium supplied by a severely stenotic vessel; this condition has been termed hibernating myocardium.

In scintigraphic studies, ^{201}Tl redistribution is defined as the total or partial resolution of initial postexercise defects when assessed by repeat imaging 2.5 to 4 hours after tracer administration. Thallium 201 rapidly washes out of normal myocardial zones and exhibits late accumulation or slower washout in the ischemic segment perfused by the stenotic vessel. Perfusion defects demonstrated by ^{201}Tl through myocardial perfusion imaging representing ischemia may now be distinguished from scar by the demonstration of delayed ^{201}Tl redistribution or enhanced uptake after reinjection of a second dose of [201]Tl. Redistribution on serial imaging is also observed when inhomogeneity of myocardial blood flow is produced by IV infusion of dipyridamole.[130]

Exercise thallium scintigraphy is a sensitive, noninvasive method for diagnosing CAD, especially in patients with abnormal resting ECGs or inadequate stress tests (Table 1–23). Results may define the perioperative prognosis of patients with known or suspected CAD. The sensitivity of exercise thallium scintigraphy when compared with angiography in the diagnosis of CAD ranges from 68% to 96%. Specificity ranges from 65% to 100%, averaging out to 87%. The sensitivity of thallium scintigraphy for detecting one-vessel disease is 78%; it is 89% for two-vessel disease, 92% for

TABLE 1–23. **Sensitivity and Specificity of Thallium Scintigraphy in Patients with Inconclusive Electrocardiographic Stress Tests**

[201]Tl Sensitivity/Specificity	No.	(%)
*ECG inadequate**		
[201]Tl sensitivity	72/92	(78%)
[201]Tl specificity	56/66	(85%)
ECG uninterpretable[†]		
[201]Tl sensitivity	32/43	(74%)
[201]Tl specificity	33/37	(89%)

Modified with permission from Kotler TS, et al: Exercise thallium-201 scintigraphy in the diagnosis and prognosis of coronary artery disease. Ann Intern Med 113:684–702, 1990.
*<85% of age-adjusted maximum predicted heart rate without exercise-induced ST-segment abnormalities.
[†]Abnormal resting electrocardiogram.

three-vessel disease, and 84% for any vessel disease. The specificity of thallium studies for the detection of any vessel disease was 87% in 10,000 studied patients (Table 1–24).[131] Stenosis of the left circumflex coronary artery is less easily detected than lesions of the right and left anterior descending arteries.

A normal maximum exercise thallium study is associated with a very low risk (0.5% per year) of cardiac events in the ensuing 4 years.[132] In patients unable to adequately exercise, IV dipyridamole–thallium imaging has been found to be an alternative means of stress testing. IV administration of dipyridamole causes coronary artery vasodilation, which results in increased blood flow to the myocardium supplied by nonstenotic vessels but limited perfusion of regions supplied by the diminished flow in stenotic vessels. This heterogeneity of blood flow is reflected in the heterogeneous uptake

TABLE 1–24. **Sensitivity and Specificity of Thallium Scintigraphy by Visual Assessment***

[201]Tl Sensitivity/Specificity	No.	(%)
Sensitivity		
One-vessel disease	193/247	(78%)
Two-vessel disease	224/275	(89%)
Three-vessel disease	303/328	(92%)
Any vessel disease	1,175/2,118	(84%)
Specificity (any vessel disease)	990/1,140	(87%)

Modified with permission from Kotler TS, et al: Exercise thallium-201 scintigraphy in the diagnosis and prognosis of coronary artery disease. Ann Intern Med 113:684–702, 1990.

of thallium, producing a reversible redistribution defect in the immediate images that resolves on the delayed images. A reversible defect on dipyridamole–thallium imaging suggests a significant risk of potential cardiac morbidity with a positive predictive value of 33%. Although the specificity of an abnormal scan is low, a scan without a redistribution defect is extremely reassuring, with a negative predictive value above 98%.[28] Stress thallium imaging under near maximal coronary blood flow is more sensitive than resting imaging and is capable of detecting perfusion heterogeneity with stenosis of 50%.[2] Exercise thallium scintigraphy reportedly has a 90% sensitivity in patients with multivessel disease and 60% in those with single-vessel disease.[131]

The administration of dipyridamole results in maximal coronary artery vasodilation equivalent to that produced by exercise without affecting oxygen consumption or producing tachycardia. The first test was introduced by Albo and co-workers in 1978 and found to be safe and minimally invasive. Compared to angiography, it reliably identifies significant stenosis with a sensitivity of approximately 90% and a specificity of approximately 70%. Aminophylline, an adenosine antagonist, can be administered to reverse dipyridamole-associated side effects, including systemic hypertension, chest pain, ST-segment depression, and nausea.[133]

Dipyridamole–thallium imaging is highly sensitive (89%–100%), relatively specific (53%–80%), and superior in risk stratification when compared to historical predictors or exercise stress testing. The risk of false positives decreases and the positive predictive value increases when reperfusion criteria include multiple dysfunctional segments or when high-risk subsets (prior MI, angina, CHF, diabetes) are investigated. The role of pharmacologic stress testing with the coronary artery vasodilator adenosine is under evaluation, and this agent may replace dipyridamole in patients who cannot exercise.[30] Adenosine is better tolerated, uses the same pharmacologic pathway as dipyridamole, and has a much shorter half-life.

Beller, evaluating patients with a prior history of angina and MI, reported that ^{201}Tl redistribution during preoperative dipyridamole–thallium scanning was better than any other clinical variable in predicting perioperative cardiac death, infarction, unstable angina, and pulmonary edema.[134]

Dipyridamole–thallium scanning was performed in 68 consecutive patients judged clinically to be at low risk for perioperative cardiac complications who presented for elective aortic surgery. Forty-two patients had a history of previous MI, stable angina, or abnormal ECG findings (group I). Twenty-six had no history of these findings (group II). In group I, 34 of 42 patients had positive results on dipyridamole–thallium scanning, and 15 of these patients were found to have critical CAD on subsequent cardiac catheterization. Nine underwent immediate CABG and in six others the CAD was treated medically and the vascular operation was canceled. The remaining 27 patients in group I underwent elective operations, but six (22%) of the 27 sustained postoperative cardiac complications. None of the group II patients were found to have critical CAD, and all patients underwent an aortic operation without cardiac complication.[135]

Beller[134] has reported that women may have a false positive test, thought to be secondary to attenuation from overlying breast. Reversible or fixed perfusion defects of the left ventricular septum may occur in patients with left bundle-branch block in the absence of significant CAD. False positive scans may occur as a result of attenuation artifacts, most commonly caused by overlying breast tissue or by a high left hemidiaphragm.

It appears that the sensitivity of ^{201}Tl–dipyridamole imaging for CAD is comparable to the sensitivity of ^{201}Tl exercise scintigraphy. It is sometimes difficult to differentiate between ischemia and scar, but this test may be used to differentiate the presence of residual myocardial viability in patients with regional wall abnormalities.[134]

Thallium redistribution abnormalities are also predictive of patients destined to develop TEE-demonstrable regional wall motion abnormalities during noncardiac surgery. A group of 360 patients underwent preoperative cardiac risk assessment that used 23 clinical parameters, seven multivariate clinical scoring systems, and quantitative dipyridamole–thallium imaging to predict postoperative or long-term MI and cardiac death following noncardiac surgery. There were 30 postoperative and an additional 13 cumulative long-term cardiac events after an average follow-up of 15 months. Clinical findings were not useful in predicting the outcome of individual parameters. The postoperative or long-term cardiac event rates were 1% and 3.5% respectively in patients with normal scans or fixed perfusion defects, and 17.5% and 22% in patients with reversible defects on ^{201}Tl imaging. Preoperative cardiac risk assessment should identify three patient subgroups: those with significant CAD, those with coronary stenosis who can safely undergo noncardiac surgery with anti-ischemic medication, and a small group of high-risk coronary patients who required preoperative coronary angiography. Most of these patients had some form of revascularization. These authors found that the quantitative perfusion indices, which reflect the amount of potentially ischemic myocardium, correlated strongly with both the preoperative and long-term outcome; and using quantitative indices it is possible to convert a test initially designed to screen for CAD into a true, simple, noninvasive risk stratification procedure.[136]

Patients with a positive preoperative nuclear imaging test that demonstrates a large or reversible defect should undergo coronary artery catheterization if noncardiac surgical intervention is considered.

Two new labeled myocardial perfusion agents, ^{99m}Tc-sestamibi and ^{99m}Tc-teboroxime, are now available for routine clinical applications. Both agents allow assessment of EF by first-pass techniques at rest or during exercise testing as well as evaluating myocardial perfusion. ^{99m}Tc-sestamibi has a long myocardial residence time as well as an adequate myocardial extraction, providing images of higher count density and superior quality compared to thallium. ^{99m}Tc-teboroxime has excellent myocardial uptake characteristics but is cleared very rapidly from the myocardium. Pharmacologic stress test studies may be more rapidly assessed using one of these two new perfusion agents.[137]

Positron Emission Tomography

Positron emission tomography (PET) and single-photon emission tomography are currently being investigated. Cardiac PET has evolved rapidly from a relatively esoteric research tool into clinical applications, providing unique, quantitative information on myocardial perfusion, metabolism, and cell membrane function. Currently these techniques are being applied only in patients in whom coronary revascularization is being considered.[138]

Magnetic resonance imaging/spectroscopy is a noninvasive test that can demonstrate subtle myocardial events, but its role in perioperative evaluation remains to be determined.

Cardiac Catheterization

Cardiac catheterization remains the reference standard for preoperative evaluation of patients with cardiac disease. EF, wall motion abnormalities, end-diastolic volume, and change in end-diastolic pressure are predictive of perioperative ventricular dysfunction. These studies also suggest that preoperative CABG significantly decreases mortality

both early (1.5% vs. 12%) and late (12% vs. 26%). Unfortunately, CABG-related mortality is twice as high in women. Short-term complications from angioplasty are also increased in women when evaluating mortality (1.7% vs. 0.3%), need for CABG (30% vs. 24%), or necessary emergency surgery.[139]

Angioplasty offers a less invasive approach to revascularization with very little recovery time. Although complications in women are higher than in men (mortality of 1.7% vs. 0.3%), and the need for emergency CABG is higher in women, they remain relatively infrequent.[52]

References

1. Graves EJ: National hospital discharge survey: Annual summary, 1990. Vital Health Stat 13(112), 1992.
2. Mangano DT: Perioperative cardiac morbidity. Anesthesiology 72:153–184, 1990.
3. Gluck R, Munoz E, Wise L: Preoperative and postoperative medical evaluation of surgical patients. Am J Surg 155:730, 1988.
4. Trask AL, Faber DR: The intensive care unit: Who's in charge? Arch Surg 125:1105–1108, 1990.
5. Moore FA, Haenel JB, Moore EE: Alternatives to Swan-Ganz cardiac output monitoring. Surg Clin North Am 71(4):699–721, 1991.
6. Ardehali A, Ports TA: Myocardial oxygen supply and demand. Chest 98:699–705, 1990.
7. Caton D: Pregnancy: Essential physiologic concerns. In Civetta JM, Taylor RW, Kirby RR (eds): Critical Care, 2nd ed, chap 64. Philadelphia: JB Lippincott, 1992.
8. Layon AJ, Bernards WC, Kirby RR: Fluids and electrolytes in the critically ill. In Civetta JM, Taylor RW, Kirby RR (eds): Critical Care, 2nd ed, chap 35. Philadelphia: JB Lippincott, 1992.
9. Sklaroff HJ: Preoperative evaluation of the patient with cardiac disease. Mt Sinai J Med 58:48–57, 1991.
10. Shah KB, Kleinman BS, Sami H, et al: Reevaluation of perioperative myocardial infarction in patients with prior myocardial infarction undergoing noncardiac operations. Anesth Analg 71:231–235, 1990.
11. Rao TL, Jacobs KH, Ei-Etr AA: Reinfarction following anesthesia in patients with myocardial infarction. Anesthesia 59:499–505, 1983.
12. Kroenke MK: Preoperative evaluation. The assessment and management of surgical risk. J Gen Intern Med 2:257–269, 1987.
13. Orr JW Jr: Infectious disease in the oncology patient. Contemp OBGYN 36(11):101–110, 1991.
14. Kotler JA, Stewart JM, Kurzon JD: Pharmacologic myocardial perfusion stress tests: Adenosine thallium stress test. J Fl Med Assoc 79:31–36, 1992.
15. Orr JW Jr: Intraoperative and postoperative care. In Copeland LC (ed): Textbook of Gynecology. Philadelphia: WB Saunders, 1992.
16. Bertrand CA: Disturbances of cardiac rhythm during anesthesia and surgery. JAMA 216:1615–1617, 1971.
17. Layon AJ, Segal E: Anesthesia: Physiology and post-anesthesia problems. In Civetta JM, Taylor RW, Kirby RR (eds): Critical Care, 2nd ed, chap 42. Philadelphia: JB Lippincott, 1992.

18. Entrup MH, Davis FG: Perioperative complications of anesthesia. Surg Clin North Am 71:1151–1173, 1991.
19. Styrt B, Sugarman B: Antipyresis and fever. Arch Intern Med 150:1589–1597, 1990.
20. Purdue GE, Hunt JL: Placement and complications of monitoring catheters. Surg Clin North Am 71:723–731, 1991.
21. Clark-Christoff N, Watters VA, et al: Use of triple-lumen catheters for administration of total parenteral nutrition. J Parenter Enter Nutr 16:403–407, 1992.
22. Cobb DK, High KP, Sawyer RG, et al: A controlled trial of scheduled replacement of central venous and pulmonary artery catheters. N Engl J Med 327:1062–1068, 1992.
23. Celoria G, Steingrub JS, Vickers-Lahti M, et al: Clinical assessment of hemodynamic values in two surgical intensive care units. Arch Surg 125:1036–1039, 1990.
24. Shoemaker WC, Kram HB, Appel PL, Fleming AW: The efficacy of central venous and pulmonary artery catheters and therapy based upon them in reducing mortality and morbidity. Arch Surg 125:1332–1338, 1990.
25. Mangano DT, Browner WS, et al: Long term cardiac prognosis following noncardiac surgery. JAMA 268:233–239, 1992.
26. Charlson ME, Mackenzie CR, Ales K, et al: Surveillance for postoperative myocardial infarction after noncardiac operations. Surg Gynecol Obstet 167:407–414, 1988.
27. Hollenberg M, Mangano DT, Browner WS, et al: Predictors of postoperative myocardial ischemia in patients undergoing noncardiac surgery. JAMA 268:240, 1992.
28. Freeman WK, Gibbons RJ, Shub C: Preoperative assessment of cardiac patients undergoing noncardiac surgical procedures. Mayo Clin Proc 64:1105–1117, 1989.
29. Racine N: Acute myocardial infarction: Contemporary management strategies. In Civetta JM, Taylor RW, Kirby RR (eds): Critical Care, 2nd ed, chap 84. Philadelphia: JB Lippincott, 1992.
30. Fleischer LA, Barash PG: Preoperative cardiac evaluation for noncardiac surgery: A functional approach. Anesth Analg 74:586–598, 1992.
31. Berger CJ, Murabito JM, Evans JC, et al: Prognosis after first myocardial infarction. JAMA 268:1545–1551, 1992.
32. Lee L, Bates BR, Pitt B, et al: Percutaneous transluminal coronary angioplasty improves survival in acute myocardial infarction complicated by cardiogenic shock. Circulation 78:1345, 1988.
33. Foster ED, David KB, et al: Risk of noncardiac operation in patients with defined coronary disease: The Coronary Artery Surgery Study (CASS) registry experience. Ann Thorac Surg 41:42–50, 1986.
34. O'Kelly B, Browner WS, et al: Ventricular arrhythmias in patients undergoing noncardiac surgery. JAMA 268:217, 1992.
35. Falk RH, Leavitt JI: Digoxin for atrial fibrillation: A drug whose time has gone? Ann Intern Med 114:573–575, 1991.
36. Goldman L, Braunwald E: General anesthesia and noncardiac surgery in patients with heart disease. In Braunwald E (ed): Heart Disease: A Textbook of Cardiovascular Medicine. Philadelphia: WB Saunders, 1992.
37. Vitelli CE, Cooper K, Rogatko A, Brennan MF: Cardiopulmonary resuscitation and the patient with cancer. J Clin Oncol 9:111–115, 1991.
38. Landry FJ, Parker JM, Phillips YY: Outcome of cardiopulmonary resuscitation in the intensive care setting. Arch Intern Med 152:2305–2308, 1992.
39. Shifren JL, Adlestein L, Finkler NJ: Asystolic cardiac arrest: A rare complication of laparoscopy. Obstet Gynecol 79:940, 1992.
40. Killip T: Anesthesia and major noncardiac surgery (editorial). JAMA 268:252–253, 1992.
41. Gardner B, Palasti S: A comparison of hospital costs and morbidity between octogenarians and other patients undergoing general surgical operations. Surg Gynecol Obstet 171:299, 1990.
42. Geokas MC (moderator): The aging process. Ann Intern Med 113:455–466, 1990.
43. Abrams WB: Cardiovascular drugs in the elderly. Chest 98:980–986, 1990.
44. Vaz FG, Seymour DG: A prospective study of elderly general surgical patients: I. Preoperative medical problems. Age Aging 18:309–315, 1989.
45. Orr JW Jr, Holloway RW, et al: Surgical staging of uterine cancer: An analysis of perioperative morbidity. Gynecol Oncol 42:209–216, 1991.
46. Kirschner CV, Deserto TM, Isaacs JH: Surgical treatment of the elderly patient with gynecologic cancer. Surgery 170:379–384, 1990.
47. Babu SC, Sharma PVP, et al: Monitor-guided responses: Operability with safety is increased in patients with peripheral vascular diseases. Arch Surg 115:1384–1386, 1980.
48. Gold S, Wong WF, Schatz IJ, Blanchette PL: Invasive treatment for coronary artery disease in the elderly. Arch Intern Med 151:1085–1088, 1991.
49. Mahar LV: Perioperative myocardial infarction in patients with coronary artery disease. J Thorac Cardiovasc Surg 76:533–537, 1978.
50. Kennedy JW, Kaiser GC, et al: Clinical and angiographic predictors of operative mortality from the collaborative study in coronary artery surgery (CASS). Circulation, 63:793–802, 1981.
51. O'Connor GT, Plume SK, Olmstead EM, et al: A regional prospective study of in-hospital mortality associated with coronary artery bypass grafting. JAMA 266:803–815, 1991.
52. Steingart RM: Managing coronary artery disease in women: What is the role of cardiac catheterization? Female Patient 17:29, 1992.
53. Huber KC, Evans MA, Bresnahan JF: Outcome of noncardiac operations in patients with severe coronary artery disease successfully treated preoperatively with coronary angioplasty. Mayo Clin Proc 67:15–21, 1992.
54. Shah KB, Kleinman BS, Rao TLK, et al: Angina and other risk factors in patients with cardiac diseases undergoing noncardiac operations. Anesth Analg 70:240–247, 1990.
55. Paraskas JA: Who needs a preoperative electrocardiogram? (editorial). Arch Intern Med 152:261–263, 1992.
56. Majid PA, Roberts R: Heart failure. In Civetta JM, Taylor RW, Kirby RR (eds): Critical Care, 2nd ed, chap 86. Philadelphia: JB Lippincott, 1992.
57. Skinner JF, Pearce ML: Surgical risk in the cardiac patient. J Chronic Dis 17:57–72, 1964.
58. Charlson ME, Mackenzie CR, Gold JP, et al: Risk for postoperative congestive heart failure. Surg Gynecol Obstet 172:95–104, 1991.
59. Deron SJ, Kotler MN: Noncardiac surgery in the cardiac patient. Am Heart J 116:831–838, 1988.
60. Lowell JA, Schifferdecker C, et al: Postoperative fluid overload: Not a benign problem. Crit Care Med 18:728–733, 1990.

61. Clavell A, Stingo A, et al: Physiological significance of endothelin: Its role in congestive heart failure. Circulation 87:V-45–V-50, 1993.

62. DiBianco R, Shabetani R, Kostuk W, et al: A comparison of oral milrinone, digoxin, and their combination in the treatment of patients with chronic heart failure. N Engl J Med 320:677, 1989.

63. Kaplan JA: Anesthesia for cardiac surgery: Clinical update. American Society of Anesthesiologists 1991 Annual Refresher Course Lectures, lecture 422. San Francisco, Oct 26–30, 1991.

64. Lawson NW: Clinical use of pressors and inotropes. American Society of Anesthesiologists 1991 Annual Refresher Course Lectures, lecture 114. San Francisco, Oct 26–30, 1991.

65. Consensus Trial Study Group: Effects of enalapril on mortality in severe congestive heart failure: Results of the Cooperative North Scandinavian Enalapril Survival Study. N Engl J Med 316:1429, 1987.

66. Berstein AD, Holt AW, Vedig AE, et al: Treatment of severe cardiogenic pulmonary edema with continuous positive airway pressure delivered by face mask. N Engl J Med 325:1825–1830, 1991.

67. Heuser D, Guggenberger H, Fretschner R: Acute blood pressure increase during the perioperative period. Am J Cardiol 63:26c–31c, 1989.

68. Longnecker D: Perioperative blood pressure control. American Society of Anesthesiologists 1990 Annual Refresher Course Lectures, lecture 211. Las Vegas, Oct 19–23, 1990.

69. Prys-Roberts C: Studies of anaesthesia in relation to hypertension: I. Cardiovascular responses of treated and untreated patients. Br J Anaesth 43(2):122–137, 1971.

70. Devault GA Jr: Therapy in hypertensive emergencies: Part 1. Vasodilators and sympatholytics. J Crit Illness 5:973–988, 1990.

71. Devault GA Jr: Hypertensive urgencies: Part 1. Sympatholytics, calcium antagonists. J Crit Illness 6:563–574, 1991.

72. Devault GA Jr: Therapy in hypertensive emergencies: Part 2. Calcium antagonists, ACE inhibitors. J Crit Illness 6:388, 1991.

73. Eisen SA, Miller DK, Woodward RS, Spitznagel E, Przybeck TR: The effect of prescribed daily dose frequency on patient medication compliance. Arch Intern Med 150:1882–1884, 1990.

74. Lesar TS, Briceland LL, Delcoure K, et al: Medication prescribing errors in a teaching hospital. JAMA 263:2329–2334, 1990.

75. Wyld R, Nimmo WS: Do patients fasting before and after operation receive their prescribed drug treatment? Br Med J 290:744, 1988.

76. Charlson ME, Mackenzie CR, Gold JP, et al: Intraoperative blood pressure: What patterns identify patients at risk for postoperative complications? Ann Surg 212:567–580, 1990.

77. Chang HJ, Bell JR, Deroo DB, et al: Physician variation in anticoagulating patients with atrial fibrillation. Arch Intern Med 150:83–86, 1990.

78. Albers G (moderator): Stroke prevention in nonvalvular atrial fibrillation. Ann Intern Med 115:727–736, 1991.

79. Artucio H, Pereira M: Cardiac arrhythmias in critically ill patients: Epidemiologic study. Crit Care Med 18:1383–1388, 1990.

80. Goldman L: Supraventricular tachyarrhythmias in hospitalized adults after surgery. Chest 73:450, 1978.

81. Stroke Prevention in Atrial Fibrillation Investigators: Predictors of thromboembolism in atrial fibrillation: II. Echocardiographic features of patients at risk. Ann Intern Med 116:6–12, 1992.

82. Guidera SA, Josephson ME: Premature ventricular contractions: Selecting the best treatments. J Crit Illness 7:1219, 1992.

83. Gettes LS: Electrolyte abnormalities underlying lethal and ventricular arrhythmias. Circulation 85(suppl I):170–176, 1992.

84. Kruse JA, Carlson RW: Rapid correction of hypokalemia using concentrated intravenous potassium chloride infusions. Arch Intern Med 150:613–617, 1990.

85. Hamill RJ, Robinson LM, Wexler HR, Moote C: Efficacy and safety of potassium infusion therapy in hypokalemic critically ill patients. Crit Care Med 19:694–699, 1991.

86. Vitez TS, Sopor LE, et al: Chronic hypokalemia and intraoperative dysrhythmias. Anesthesiology 63:130–133, 1985.

87. Zaidan JR: Pacemakers. American Society of Anesthesiologists 1991 Annual Refresher Course Lectures, lecture 173. San Francisco, Oct 26–30, 1991.

88. Kannel WB, Thom JT: Declining cardiovascular morbidity. Circulation 70:331, 1984.

89. Roizen MF: Anesthetic implications of concurrent diseases. In Miller RD (ed): Anesthesia, 3rd ed, vol 1, chap 25. New York: Churchill Livingstone, 1990.

90. Roizen MF: Preoperative evaluation. In Miller RD (ed): Anesthesia, 3rd ed, vol 1, chap 23. New York: Churchill Livingstone, 1990.

91. Thomas SJ: Anesthesia for cardiac patient undergoing non-cardiac surgery. American Society of Anesthesiologists 1991 Annual Refresher Course Lectures, lecture 175. San Francisco, Oct 26–30, 1991.

92. Tinker JH, Tarhan S: Discontinuing anticoagulant therapy in surgical patients with cardiac valve prosthesis. JAMA 239:738–741, 1978.

93. Katholi RE: Living with prosthetic heart valves: Subsequent noncardiac operations and the risk of thromboembolism of hemorrhage. Am Heart J 92:162–167, 1976.

94. Dajani AS, Bisno AL, Chung KJ, et al: Prevention of bacterial endocarditis: Recommendations by the American Heart Association. JAMA 264:2919–2922, 1990.

95. Charlson ME, Mackenzie CR, Gold JP, et al: The preoperative and intraoperative hemodynamic predictors of postoperative myocardial infarction or ischemia in patients undergoing noncardiac surgery. Ann Surg 210:637–648, 1990.

96. Gagner M: Value of preoperative physiologic assessment in outcome of patients undergoing major surgical procedures. Surg Clin North Am 71:1141–1150, 1991.

97. Detsky AS, Abrams HB, McLaughlin JR, et al: Predicting cardiac complications in patients undergoing noncardiac surgery. J Gen Crit Med 1:211, 1986.

98. Brown DL, Kirby RR: Preoperative evaluation of high risk surgical patients. In Civetta JM, Taylor RW, Kirby RR (eds): Critical Care, 2nd ed, chap 41. Philadelphia: JB Lippincott, 1992.

99. Narr BJ, Hansen RD, Warner MA: Preoperative laboratory screening in healthy Mayo patients: Cost-effective elimination of tests and unchanged outcomes. Mayo Clin Proc 66:155–159, 1991.

100. Wong T, Detsky AS: Preoperative cardiac risk assessment for patients having peripheral vascular surgery. Ann Intern Med 116:743–753, 1992.

101. Korvin CC, Pearce RH, Stanley J: Admissions screening: Clinical benefits. Ann Intern Med 83:197, 1975.

102. Olsen DM, Kane RL, Proctor PH: A controlled trial of multiphasic screening. N Engl J Med 294:925, 1976.

103. Durbridge TC, Edwards F, et al: Evaluation of benefits of screening tests done immediately on admission to hospital. Clin Chem 22:968, 1976.

104. Domoto K, Ben R, Wei JY, et al: Yield of routine annual laboratory screening in the institutionalized elderly. Am J Public Health 75:243, 1985.

105. Wood RA, Hoekelman RA: Value of the chest x-ray as a screening test for elective surgery in children. Pediatrics 67:477, 1981.

106. Paraskos JA: Who needs a preoperative electrocardiogram? (editorial) Arch Intern Med 152:261–263, 1992.

107. Gold BS, Young ML, Kinman JL, et al: The utility of preoperative electrocardiograms in the ambulatory surgical patient. Arch Intern Med 152:301–305, 1992. Cited in Paraskos JA: Who needs a preoperative electrocardiogram? Arch Intern Med 152:261–263, 1992.

108. Rabkin SW, Horne JM: Preoperative electrocardiography: Its cost-effectiveness in detecting abnormalities when a previous tracing exists. Can Med Assoc J 121:401, 1979.

109. McKee RF, Scott EM: The value of routine preoperative investigations. Ann R Coll Surg Engl 69:160, 1987.

110. Moorman JR, Hlatky MA, et al: The yield of the routine admission electrocardiogram: A study in a general medical service. Ann Intern Med 103:590, 1985.

111. Blery C, Szatan M, et al: Evaluation of a protocol for selective ordering of preoperative tests. Lancet 1:139, 1986.

112. Golub R, Cantu R, Sorrento JJ, Stein HD: Efficacy of preadmission testing in ambulatory surgical patients. Am J Surg 163:565, 1992.

113. Goldberger AL, O'Konski M: Utility of the routine electrocardiogram before surgery and on general hospital admission: Critical review and new guidelines. Ann Intern Med 105:552, 1986.

114. Carliner NH, Fisher ML, Plotnick GD, et al: Routine preoperative exercise testing in patients undergoing major noncardiac surgery. Am J Cardiol 56:51–58, 1985.

115. Tape TG, Mushlin AL: How useful are routine chest x-rays of preoperative patients at risk for postoperative chest disease? J Gen Intern Med 3:15, 1988.

116. Kopriva CJ: Perioperative ECG: Catching the danger signs. American Society of Anesthesiologists 1991 Annual Refresher Course Lectures, lecture 272. San Francisco, Oct 26–30, 1991.

117. Kazmers A, Cerqueira MD, Zierler RE: Perioperative and late outcome in patients with left ventricular ejection fraction of 35% or less who require major vascular surgery. J Vasc Surg 8:307–315, 1988.

118. Quinones MA, Verani MS, Haichin RM, et al: Exercise echocardiography vs. thallium 201 single photon emission computed tomography in evaluation of coronary artery disease: Analysis of 292 patients. Circulation 85:1026–1031, 1992.

119. Reference deleted.

120. Kahn JK, Sills MN, Corbett JR, Willerson JT: What is the current role of nuclear cardiology in clinical medicine? Chest 97:442–446, 1990.

121. Sue DY, Wasserman K: Impact of integrative cardiopulmonary exercise testing on clinical decision making. Chest 99:981–992, 1991.

122. Cutler BS, Wheeler HB, et al: Applicability and interpretation of electrocardiographic stress testing in patients with peripheral vascular disease. Am J Surg 141:501–506, 1981.

123. Pasternak PF, Imparato AM, Bear G, et al: The value of radionuclide angiography as a predictor of perioperative myocardial infarction in patients undergoing abdominal aortic aneurysm resection. J Vasc Surg 1:320–325, 1984.

124. Madlon-Kay R: Evaluation of coronary artery disease in patients having noncardiac surgery. South Med J 80:1366–1369, 1987.

125. Child JS: Use of echocardiography for patient management in chronic ischemic heart disease. Circulation 84(suppl I):I-66, 1991.

126. Cahalan MK: Non-invasive cardiovascular monitoring. American Society of Anesthesiologists 1991 Annual Refresher Course Lectures, lecture 522. San Francisco, Oct 26–30, 1991.

127. Ofili EO, Labovitz AJ: Transesophageal echocardiography: Expanding indications for ICU use. How TEE can complement—or surpass—transthoracic techniques. J Crit Illness 7:85–96, 1992.

128. Fisher EA, Stahl JA, Budd JH, Goldman ME: Transesophageal echocardiography: Procedures and clinical application. J Am Coll Cardiol 18:1333–1348, 1991.

129. Eisenberg MJ, London MJ, Leung JM, et al: Monitoring for myocardial ischemia during noncardiac surgery. JAMA 268:210–216, 1992.

130. Beller GA: Diagnostic accuracy of thallium-201 myocardial perfusion imaging. Circulation 84(suppl I):I-1–I-16, 1991.

131. Kotler TS, Diamond GA, et al: Exercise thallium-201 scintigraphy in the diagnosis and prognosis of coronary artery disease. Ann Intern Med 113:684–702, 1990.

132. Kahn JK, Sills MN, Corbett JR, Willerson JT: What is the current role of nuclear cardiology in clinical medicine? Chest 97(2):442–446, 1990.

133. Makaroun MS, Shuman-Jackson N, Rippey A, Schreiner D, Arvan S: Cardiac risk in vascular surgery: The oral dipyridamole-thallium stress test. Arch Surg 125:1610–1613, 1990.

134. Beller GA: Pharmacologic stress imaging. JAMA 265:633–638, 1991.

135. Strawn DJ, Guernsey JM: Dipyridamole thallium scanning in the evaluation of coronary artery disease in elective abdominal aortic surgery. Arch Surg 126:880–883, 1991.

136. Lette J, Waters D, Bernier H, et al: Preoperative and long-term cardiac risk assessment. Ann Surg 216:192, 1992.

137. Berman DS, Kiat H, Maddahi J: The new ^{99m}Tc myocardial perfusion imaging agents: ^{99m}Tc-sestamibi and ^{99m}Tc-teboroxime. Circulation 84(suppl I):I-17–I-121, 1991.

138. Gould KL: Clinical cardiac positron emission tomography: State of the art. Circulation 84(suppl I):I-22–I-36, 1991.

139. Nwaskowa O: Bypass surgery for chronic stable angina: Predictors of survival, benefit and strategy for patient selection. Ann Intern Med 114:1035–1049, 1991.

Complications in Gynecologic Surgery: Prevention, Recognition, and Management,
edited by James W. Orr, Jr., and Hugh M. Shingleton.
J. B. Lippincott Company, Philadelphia, © 1994.

Chapter 2

Pulmonary Complications

James W. Orr, Jr.
Robert W. Holloway
Pamela Jo Orr

In 1910, Pasteur originally described postoperative lobar collapse and pulmonary dysfunction after an abdominal operation. Since that time the majority of studies evaluating postoperative pulmonary dysfunction have focused on subclinical complications, including radiographic evidence of atelectasis, associated pleural fluid, excessive cough, or fever. With this broad definition the incidence of postoperative pulmonary complications increases dramatically to as high as 75% after abdominal surgery. Pulmonary complications necessitating intervention are less common, occurring in approximately 3% of patients following elective surgery and 10% after emergency surgical procedures.[1]

Despite the difficulty of extracting data for pulmonary risks following specific gynecologic or obstetric procedures, postoperative pulmonary complications are important causes of both acute perioperative mortality (occurring intraoperatively or within 48 hours) and late postoperative mortality (occurring within 6 weeks). Acute perioperative deaths occur in approximately 0.3% of all surgical procedures. Ten percent occur during anesthetic induction, 35% occur intraoperatively, and 55% occur postoperatively. Inadequate ventilation, aspiration, arrhythmias, drug-related myocardial suppression, and refractory hypotension are each responsible for approximately 10% to 15% of perioperative deaths. Hypoxemia contributes to more than 50% of all anesthetic deaths, and analysis of closed claims cases indicates that the most common respiratory cause is some form of inadequate ventilation, usually related to a difficult or esophageal intubation. Most of these cases occurred prior to 1980, and these risks have decreased significantly with the introduction of pulse oximetry and capnometry.[2] In fact, the American Society of Anesthesiologists has revised its standard for basic intraoperative monitoring to include the identification of carbon dioxide in expired gas to ensure correct endotracheal tube positioning. Continuous capnography is "encouraged."[3]

A significant portion of late postoperative mortality is related to pneumonia (approximately 20%) and pulmonary embolism (10%), but deaths related to nonpulmonary infection (30%), cardiac arrest (20%), renal failure (5%), hypovolemic shock (5%), sepsis (5%), and stroke (5%) also occur.[4]

Pulmonary Physiology

The human lung is composed of an intricate three-dimensional matrix of 300 million thin-walled alveoli, supported by small airways, intimately approximated to a rich network of sinusoidal capillaries that originates in pulmonary arterioles and terminates in pulmonary venules.[5] An interwoven net of collagen elastin fibers radiating from the hilum outward to the periphery suspends this matrix of alveoli, small airways, and capillaries. This radial orientation of suspensory fibers and the surface tension on alveolar air–fluid surfaces promote reduction in lung volume. Lung distention increases this "elastic" force so that the lung actually behaves as a three-dimensional spring. Pulmonary distention also creates a traction effect in the elastin collagen fibers that assists in maintaining alveoli and small airway expansion. The normal characteristics of the intrathoracic cavity resist the tendency to completely collapse. Simultaneously, intraparenchymal forces pull the diaphragm upward and the ribs inward, opposing thoracic expansion. This three-dimensional dynamic equilibrium generates a subatmospheric negative pleural pressure, maintaining uninterrupted contact between the pleural surfaces. Any break in pleural integrity permits lung collapse, diaphragmatic descent, and rib cage expansion, generating a pneumothorax.[6]

At end-expiration, lung recoil and thoracic cavity expansive forces are at resting equilibrium. Lung volume at end-expiratory equilibrium is termed functional residual capacity (FRC) (Fig. 2–1). Because elastin and collagen fiber stretch varies directly with lung volume, radial forces that maintain air spaces open are lowest at FRC, which remains relatively constant in healthy people throughout adult life. However, if lung volume is reduced below normal, radial traction becomes insufficient,

small airways open, and air spaces collapse. The lung volume at which air spaces first collapse is termed closing capacity (CC). Normally, airway closure occurs only at volumes far less than normal FRC; therefore, small airways usually remain patent throughout tidal ventilation. However, chronic degenerative diseases and normal aging reduce lung recoil radial airway traction, and at a given lung volume, small airway closure begins to occur at end-expiration. In a healthy individual in the supine position, this change occurs at approximately age 44. During pregnancy at least 50% of women experience significant small airway closure when in the supine position.[7] Increased lung volume during inspiration reopens airways and allows fresh gas flow to distal air spaces. If degenerative diseases are more severe, some small airways remain closed throughout the breathing cycle and distal air spaces will collapse.

Mechanics of Ventilation

Spontaneous ventilation involves the repetitive creation of pressure gradients between ambient mouth pressure and alveolar pressure. These gradients overcome airway flow resistance, generating gas movement into and out of the lungs. At end-expiration, pressure within the alveoli equals atmospheric pressure and gas flow ceases. During inspiration, the thoracic cavity is acutely expanded by inspiratory muscles and the volume of pulmonary parenchymal air space increases. At end-expiration, lung and chest wall forces are unbalanced because ex-

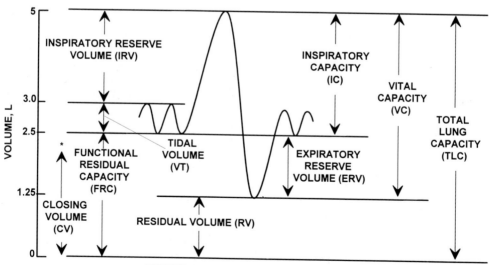

FIGURE 2–1. Important respiratory parameters.

pansion increases the tendency for the lungs to collapse and decreases the tendency for the chest cavity to spring forward. When respiratory muscles relax, this equilibrium allows lung retractile forces to reduce lung volumes and increase alveolar pressure above ambient pressure, forcing gas to flow outward until FRC is reached. This sequence is described as one spontaneous tidal volume (VT) exchange.

Pulmonary Compliance

An elastic object that has been deformed by an external force tends to restore its original resting tension. When a hollow elastic object is inflated with positive pressure, the relationship between inflation pressure is related to the change in volume, the change in pressure creating a constant, which is termed *compliance*. The anatomy of the human lung resists expansion; however, stretch and reorientation of elastic tissue only partially explain lung retraction. Surface tension in the large air–fluid interface also contributes to lung recoil. Surface tension is the force generated in a fluid surface that tends to minimize the area of an air–fluid interface. If a surface is spherical (as in a bubble), surface tension generates pressure within the sphere according to the law of Laplace. However, the unique properties of pulmonary surfactant allow lung pressure-volume relationships to deviate from those predicted by a surface tension equation. Pulmonary surfactant is a highly insoluble substance containing phospholipids, including lecithin, sphingomyelin, phosphatile choline, and phosphatile delestinol. It is secreted in part by type II alveolar cells and floats on the alveolar lining, reducing the surface tension of the air–fluid interface. As the radius of alveoli increases, the surface tension in the surfactant layer increases more than the surface tension in the underlying fluid decreases, causing a net increase in expansive alveolar surface forces.[6]

Alterations Specific to Pregnancy

The major metabolic stress imposed by pregnancy is the arithmetic sum of the mother's normal nonpregnant metabolic rate, the metabolic rate of the products of conception, and the slight increase in maternal metabolic rate associated with the physical work of carrying "extra" tissue.[7] At term, "normal" maternal metabolism increases by 20% to 30%, an amount greater than the pregnancy-associated increase in maternal surface area or weight. Maternal minute ventilation increases during preg-

nancy and the pulmonary response differs from that which occurs with the slight increase in metabolic rate during exercise or hyperthermia in the nonpregnant state. Upward displacement of the diaphragm and rib cage associated with an enlarging uterus alters the mechanics of ventilation, resulting in a decreased FRC. This change facilitates nitrogen washout, enhances inhalational anesthetic agent uptake, and limits oxygen supply. The last factor, together with the increased metabolic rate, contributes to the rapid oxygen desaturation observed in a pregnant woman during periods of apnea.

Pervasive changes also occur in the regulation of ventilation with an increased sensitivity to the respiratory nuclei in the brain stem that results in a decrease in $PaCO_2$ to 30 to 35 mm Hg as early as the sixth week of pregnancy. The kidneys respond to a low $PaCO_2$ by proportionately decreasing plasma bicarbonate. Since the carbon dioxide–bicarbonate ratio remains almost constant, pH is only slightly increased; however, the decreased buffering capacity contributes to the mild feeling of dyspnea that many women experience during pregnancy. This phenomenon can also occur in the luteal phase of a normal menstrual cycle.[7]

Pulmonary Effects of Anesthesia

Endotracheal intubation during general anesthesia results in epithelial desquamation, decreased mucous velocity, and altered bacterial clearance. Relative hypoxia, hypercarbia, increased dead space ventilation, pulmonary ventilation–perfusion mismatch, and altered chest wall mechanics are respiratory effects routinely associated with anesthesia.[4]

General anesthesia results in impaired gas exchange, in part related to effects on the chest wall and the lung itself. Associated changes in the shape and motion of the chest wall and diaphragm result in alterations in the distribution of inspired gas without a corresponding adjustment in pulmonary blood flow. A shift from abdominal to rib cage breathing occurs shortly after anesthesia induction.[8] Thus, general anesthesia creates lung units with a low ventilation–perfusion ratio and a wide alveolar–arterial oxygen difference. Altered chest wall mechanics contribute to a 20% (0.5 L) decrease in FRC. Additionally, the diaphragm, particularly the dependent part, shifts cephalad following the induction of anesthesia with inhalational agents. These functional changes in chest wall and diaphragm mechanics may be mediated by the central nervous system. Careful evaluation using computed axial tomography to determine thoracic and abdominal dimensions before and after anesthesia induction has shown a quantitative decrease in thoracic volume that is accounted for primarily by the cephalad shift of the diaphragm. Intraparenchymal pulmonary atelectatic plaques are visualized within 15 minutes after induction but rapidly resolve after the application of 10 cm H_2O positive end-expiratory pressure (PEEP). They recur within minutes of discontinuing PEEP.[1] Although gas exchange has not been evaluated in patients who develop atelectatic plaques, these findings suggest that atelectasis contributes to the decrease in FRC as well as gas exchange abnormalities found in patients undergoing anesthesia. Interestingly, anesthesia with specific agents such as intravenous (IV) ketamine has a minimal measurable effect on FRC.

Postoperative pathophysiologic pulmonary changes occur to some degree in all patients following abdominal surgery and are increased following upper abdominal incisions (Fig. 2–2). The mechanisms responsible for reduced vital capacity (VC), reduced FRC, atelectasis, and arterial hypoxemia that occur during postoperative recovery are not entirely clear. Depressed diaphragmatic and intercostal muscle function may alter pulmonary mechanics. Evidence suggests that a reflex inhibition of respiratory muscle function occurs when the operative site is close to the diaphragm and correlates with specific upper abdominal organs involved in the procedure. In fact, esophageal distention causes an immediate inhibition of diaphragm and intercostal muscle function that is abolished with bilateral cervical vagotomy. Intravenous theophylline can reverse diaphragmatic dysfunction, presumably by a direct rather than a central effect, but its possible benefit in improving postoperative lung function remains unclear.

FRC, the resting lung volume after normal expiration, is reduced by as much as 1.0 L when a subject moves from an upright to a supine position. These changes are thought to be related to the craniad displacement of the diaphragm. The postoperative effects of anesthesia further reduce FRC by approximately 0.5 L. The fact that FRC changes after upper abdominal incision do not occur until approximately 16 hours suggests that the cause of the general anesthesia–induced changes in FRC may be different from the cause of the postoperative changes. Moreover, the delay in development of reduced FRC suggests the possible therapeutic benefit of interventions that will limit changes in FRC.[9]

FRC also increases with age. Thus, subjects over

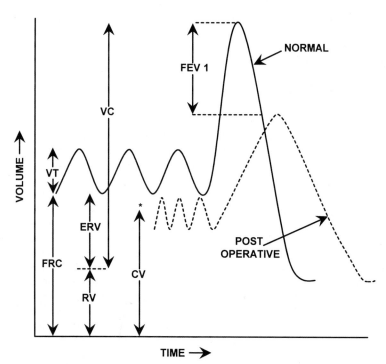

FIGURE 2–2. Effect of postoperative state on respiratory parameters.

70 years old are at significant risk for developing airway closure during ordinary breathing, as the lung volume at which airways collapse during expiration increases with age.[1] These changes place older women at increased risk for pulmonary complications.

Narcotic-associated alteration of respiratory muscle function further compounds the risk of perioperative pulmonary problems as such alterations can suppress central respiratory drive, alter diaphragmatic function, and suppress neural output, with a potential loss of airway patency or upper airway obstruction. The administration of intraoperative neuromuscular blocking agents, barbiturates, narcotics, and inhalational agents can further contribute to significant perioperative respiratory depression and even ventilatory insufficiency.

As a result of lung volume changes, relative hypoxemia, characterized by a mild decrease in carbon dioxide tension and respiratory alkalosis, is usually observed after the termination of general anesthesia. The magnitude of the decline in arterial oxygen tension varies considerably and the consequence can be insignificant in healthy individuals or profound in patients with perioperative pulmonary dysfunction. Extrinsic abnormalities of ventilation and perfusion occur with advancing age, placing the elderly at significant risk for developing perioperative hypoxemia. Significant episodic oxygen desaturation even following narcotic anesthesia and analgesia is more common in the elderly and in patients who have some airway obstruction associated with sleep. Unfortunately, respiratory rate does not correlate with the presence of hypoxemia or necessarily indicate the presence or give a clinical warning of oxygen desaturation.[10]

Arterial oxygen pressures (PaO$_2$) fall 20% to 30% after upper abdominal surgery, 10% to 18% after lower abdominal surgery, and 5% to 10% after nonabdominal surgery (Table 2–1).[11] Following upper abdominal incisions, decreases in VC of 50% to 60% are common. V$_T$ decreases by an average of 25%, accompanied by a 20% increase in respiratory rate with no net change in minute ventilation. The supine position alone accounts for a 10% to 20% reduction in postoperative lung volume. FRC and residual volume (RV) are decreased by 30% at 16 to 24 hours but usually increase to 90% of preoperative values after the fifth postoperative day. A subcostal incision for cholecystectomy results in a 40% to 50% fall in VC and FRC even in the absence of underlying lung pathology. Lower abdominal surgery is associated with a lesser (25%–30%) decrease in VC and mild, usually insignificant de-

TABLE 2–1. Postoperative Ventilatory Changes

1. ↓ Sigh or cough
   - not eliminated with narcotics
2. ↓ Vital capacity
   - lower abdominal: 30%
   - upper abdominal: 60%
3. ↓ Tidal volume: 25%
   - supine position accounts for 20%
4. ↑ Respiratory rate: 20%
   - no net change in minute ventilation
5. ↓ Functional residual capacity (FRC): 30%
   - as long as 5–7 days
   - > 40% ↓ in FRC = radiologic abnormalities
6. Diaphragmatic dysfunction
   - not contractility
   - phrenic nerve (aminophylline)
7. Closing volume
   - atelectasis, bacterial proliferation
8. Gas exchange
   - PaO$_2$ ↓ 20% lower abdomen
     ↓ 30% upper abdomen
     ↓ 10% nonabdominal
9. Mucous transport
   - impaired

creases in arterial oxygenation. Subsequently, postoperative pulmonary complications are less common following gynecologic procedures for benign indications performed with transverse incisions or vertical infraumbilical incisions.

Normal closing volumes are located between end-tidal point, FRC, and RV. When postoperative tidal breathing occurs below closing volume, alveoli become underventilated and collapse as residual gas is absorbed. Bacteria rapidly proliferate in atelectatic areas, predisposing to the development of pneumonia. Frequently, these changes are termed microatelectasis and occur in the absence of chest radiographic abnormalities. Although atelectasis commonly occurs, clinical and radiographic evidence of postoperative atelectasis is consistently present when FRC decreases to 60% or less of normal. Fortunately, this constellation of abnormalities can be reversed by repeated deep inspiration.

Additionally, many intra-abdominal surgical procedures are associated with large-volume fluid resuscitation. In specific situations (hypoalbuminemia, parenchymal lung injury), associated translocation of fluid between the intracellular and extracellular pulmonary compartments may contribute to altered pulmonary gas exchange.

Altered postanesthesia pulmonary function may persist for several hours or several days. Following extremity and perhaps vulvar surgery, lung volumes and PaO$_2$ return to normal within 24 hours. Patients undergoing upper abdominal incisions experience a more prolonged and profound period of pulmonary dysfunction that potentially increases the incidence of postoperative pulmonary complications, specifically pneumonia and respiratory failure. Postoperative pain was formerly believed to be a major contributor to abnormal pulmonary function. Postoperative pain causes patients to breathe rapidly with small tidal volumes, and without deep sighing breaths. The decrease in FRC (secondary to shallow breathing), the reduced inspiratory capacity, the reduced VC, the premature small airway collapse, and gas trapping contribute to an increased risk of pulmonary complications or infection.[11] However, pulmonary dysfunction and diaphragm dysfunction persist even with adequate analgesia. Despite this apparent link between diaphragm dysfunction and postoperative pulmonary dysfunction, diaphragmatic dysfunction has not been conclusively proved to be a basis of pulmonary dysfunction in all patients after abdominal surgery. Neither pain relief nor postoperative maneuvers to improve lung volumes have consistently prevented postoperative pulmonary dysfunction in patients following abdominal surgery. Nonetheless, the incidence and perhaps severity of postoperative pulmonary complications are decreased in patients who receive some kind of deep breathing exercise postoperatively.[11]

Reports citing preserved lung compliance and a lessened adverse effect on arterial oxygenation have suggested that a regional anesthetic should be considered the method of choice for patients with chronic lung disease. To date, despite these theoretical considerations, there is no clear clinical evidence that regional anesthesia is superior to general anesthesia in terms of maintaining normal intraoperative and postoperative pulmonary function or decreasing the risk of postoperative complications. Ravin evaluated 20 patients undergoing lower abdominal surgery who had severe preoperative ventilatory abnormalities, including a maximum voluntary ventilation less than 8 L/min and a residual volume–total lung capacity (RV/TLC) ratio greater than 45%.[12] He could not demonstrate any difference in intraoperative and postoperative PaO$_2$ between patients undergoing spinal or general anesthesia. In another report, Boutrous and Weisel[13] evaluated patients with compromised maximal expiratory flow rates (< 75 L/min) undergoing spinal or general anesthesia and could not demonstrate a difference in arterial blood gas values. Perhaps as

important, general anesthesia and intubation offers superior airway control and improves the removal of pulmonary secretions.[10]

As previously noted, normal human thermoregulation maintains a central body temperature within 0.4° C of normal. The administration of volatile inhalational agents widens thermoregulatory thresholds of effector responses that maintain body temperature, with the greatest rate of decrease in core temperature occurring immediately after the induction of anesthesia. Critical ambient temperatures greater than 21° C are necessary to maintain normothermia in patients undergoing non-body-cavity and intra-abdominal procedures. Most complications of hypothermia—i.e., dysrhythmia, increased blood viscosity, and platelet coagulation abnormalities—occur at core temperatures less than 33° C and are reversible on rewarming. However, associated postoperative shivering and elevated tissue oxygen demands of up to 300% during recovery from hypothermia necessitate adequate oxygen delivery and are of particular importance in patients with limited cardiopulmonary reserve, who may decompensate quickly when faced with the added stress of meeting this increased tissue oxygen demand. The associated increased systemic vascular resistance may contribute to hypoxemia, acidosis, and even cardiovascular collapse. These risks as well as specific preventive methods should be addressed in an attempt to decrease the incidence and severity of perioperative hypothermia. Just as with cardiac risks, patients with compromised cardiorespiratory reserve may benefit from prolonged postoperative ventilation and other interventions that inhibit shivering.

The choice of anesthetic technique as it relates to perioperative respiratory risk must remain the primary responsibility of the anesthesiologist. Obviously, surgical needs must be considered, and the information obtained from preoperative studies and medical consultation must be evaluated to determine the safest anesthetic method or technique for each individual woman.

Tests of Pulmonary Function

The spirometer was developed nearly 150 years ago, and throughout the years physicians have sought one pulmonary function test to allow assessment of operability in a patient with pulmonary compromise. Although initially intended to identify lung abnormalities, the clinical use of spirometry dates only to the mid-1950s. Spirometry has been touted as satisfying the criteria for a good screening test for lung disease,[14] and today, spirometric studies are often ordered before abdominal surgery with the goal of predicting and/or preventing postoperative pulmonary complications. The clinical yield of spirometry when compared to or in addition to a thorough history and physical examination is unknown, but it is clear that spirometry should not be considered a screening test. One critical appraisal of 130 clinical articles reportedly evaluating the use of spirometry could identify only 22% that actually investigated the use and predictive value of preoperative spirometry.[15] Unfortunately, important methodologic flaws in almost all studies preclude valid conclusions. The available evidence suggests that while preoperative studies can be used to modify perioperative care on an individual basis, spirometry's predictive power is small[15] both in patients with clinically apparent lung disease and in patients with surgically important occult pulmonary disease.

Preoperative pulmonary evaluation should focus on identifying patients with chronic air flow obstruction or restrictive lung disorders (Table 2–2). Simple spirometry is easily performed and should be considered as an initial study following the history and physical examination, as it may assist in making a specific pulmonary diagnosis and assessing the degree of impairment. The combination of all available spirometric data enhances clinical assessment, and a practical approach would combine arterial blood gas and pH measurements with information from pulmonary spirometry. Although hypoxemia suggests risk, hypercarbia indicates a higher risk of pulmonary complications and a higher likelihood of requiring postoperative mechanical ventilation. Unfortunately, a valid, reliable pulmonary risk index that incorporates clinical and spirometric variables is not available. In fact, not all studies conclude that preoperative spirometry can predict postoperative pulmonary complications.[15]

Current literature supports the conclusion that smokers and women with chronic obstructive pulmonary disease (COPD) are at increased risk for postoperative pulmonary complications; however, acute respiratory failure requiring mechanical ventilation is extremely uncommon even in high-risk groups following abdominal procedures. Although pulmonary function tests can identify a group of high-risk patients, most patients with abnormal pulmonary function tests will not develop serious postoperative pulmonary complications. Additionally, evaluating preoperative pulmonary function does not reliably identify all patients who will develop severe postoperative pulmonary complications or reliably detect which patients are more likely to need intensive care therapy postoperatively. Even with sophisticated studies available, the most important preoperative abnormality in terms of predicting postoperative pulmonary ventilation is arterial hypoxemia or hypercapnia. For this reason, we frequently use preoperative arterial blood gas studies in patients "at risk." Persistently elevated Pco_2 (>45 mm Hg) in patients who do not have neuro-

TABLE 2–2. **Comparison of Respiratory Function Test Results in COPD and Asthma**

	"Blue Bloater"	"Pink Puffer"	COPD	Asthma Acute Attack	Chronic
FEV_1	↓↓	↓↓↓	↓↓	↓↓↓	Normal or ↓
FVC	↓	↓↓	↓	↓↓	Normal or ↓
FEV_1/FVC	↓	↓↓	↓	↓↓	Normal or ↓
Reversibility	Poor	Very poor	<15%	>15% or poor	>15% or poor
TLC	Normal or ↑	↑↑	Normal or ↑	↑↑	Normal or ↑
RV	Normal or ↑	↑↑↑	Normal or ↑	↑↑↑	Normal or ↑
RV/TLC	↑	↑↑	↑	↑↑	Normal or ↑
Pao_2	↓↓	Normal	Normal or Å	↓	Normal
$Paco_2$	↑↑	↓	Normal or ↑	↓	Normal

Modified from Clark M: Obstructive airways disease in surgical practice. J R Coll Surg Edinb 34:177–184, 1989.
Abbreviations: COPD, chronic obstructive pulmonary disease; FEV_1, forced expiratory volume in 1 second; FVC, forced vital capacity; TLC, total lung capacity; RV, residual volume; Pao_2, partial pressure of oxygen in arterial blood; $Paco_2$, partial pressure of carbon dioxide in arterial blood.

muscular disease or drug-induced alveolar hypoventilation reliably predicts a high risk for pulmonary morbidity or mortality.[16]

Each patient becomes her own standard. Patients with an FEV_1, less than 800 mL have been excluded from any type of thoracic resection, while patients with an FEV_1 of 2 L or less have a moderate airway obstructive ventilatory deficit and a strong possibility of experiencing postoperative pulmonary dysfunction. FEV_1/FVC ratios (defined below) of 0.65 to 0.85 are consistent with mild obstruction. Ratios of 0.55 to 0.65 are consistent with moderate obstruction, and ratios less than 0.55 are consistent with severe airway obstruction.

Pulmonary support is frequently necessary 48 to 72 hours following surgery, when perioperative pulmonary dysfunction is pronounced. Abnormal pulmonary studies should prompt appropriate preoperative consultation, modification of the surgical approach, or both. Perioperative prophylactic measures can be designed to minimize anticipated postoperative pathophysiologic changes that would otherwise devastate a patient with compromised pulmonary function. Specific methods of intervention can decrease this risk.[4]

Forced Vital Capacity

Forced vital capacity (FVC), one of the most easily measured and highly reproducible pulmonary function values obtained during spirometric testing, represents the balance of forces generated by the respiratory muscles and mechanical properties of the lung and chest wall. A decreased FVC suggests either a restrictive ventilatory defect or a severe obstructive defect with hyperinflation. An FVC below 50% or an absolute predicted value below 1.75 to 2 L suggests an increased risk of postoperative pulmonary complications.

Ethnic differences exist, and accurate prediction formulas in whites overestimate lung volumes in Africans, Indians, and Chinese by roughly 15% to 20%.[14]

Forced Expiratory Volume in 1 Second

The forced expiratory volume in 1 second (FEV_1) is a direct measurement of air flow obstruction. FEV_1 is probably the best indicator of the patient's ability to clear postoperative secretions.[14] The ratio of FEV_1 to FVC is used as a diagnostic hallmark for obstructive lung disease. A "normal" FEV_1/FVC ratio is ≥ 0.85. The ratio of FEV_1/FVC was devel-

oped to overcome limitations caused by variations in patient morphology, and this ratio yields a percentage to interpret the degree of bronchial obstruction. However, this ratio may be "normal" in patients with severe restrictive disease and an abnormally low FVC.

Spirometric studies evaluate the ability to move air. Although other studies evaluate functional size (lung volume) or gas transfer (diffusing capacity), it is essential that the gynecologic surgeon understand the derivation of basic spirometric functions.

Mid-flow Measurements

While a reduction in FEV_1 or in the FEV_1/FVC ratio is a sensitive indicator of extensive disease, minimal degrees of lung pathology may only cause reduced flow rates in the mid and lower vital capacity range. In fact, maximum flow rates at low lung volumes are more likely to be determined by the properties of smaller, more peripheral airways in which the pathologic and presymptomatic lesions of diseases such as emphysema can first be identified before the onset of symptoms.[16]

Spirometric mid-flow measurements include maximal mid-expiratory flow rate (MMEFR) and the forced expiratory flow rate between 25% and 75% of the exhaled volume (FEF_{25-75}). Mid-flow measurements, sensitive indicators of small airway dysfunction, are always abnormal in patients with COPD. Abnormal measurements are relatively specific indicators for the risk of postoperative complications following abdominal surgery.

Routine flow rate testing includes an evaluation of air flow as well as the immediate response to nebulized bronchodilators. Bronchodilator-associated improvement in air flow suggests the need for preoperative pulmonary therapy and an improved postoperative pulmonary prognosis. Patients who demonstrate little or no response to nebulized bronchodilators may eventually improve with intensive pulmonary therapy, including the use of bronchodilators, hydration, antibiotics, and cessation of smoking. However, patients whose FEV_{25-75} does not improve after a therapeutic regimen of bronchodilators should be considered and counseled as to the associated significant risk of pulmonary complications.[17]

Maximal Voluntary Ventilation

Maximal voluntary ventilation (MVV) evaluates obstructive and restrictive physiology but is dependent on the ability of the patient to cooperate and to perform the necessary maneuvers. The nonspecificity of this test may actually make it a useful pulmonary study. The risk of pulmonary complications is significantly increased in patients with an MVV less than 50% of predicted.

Lung Volumes

Patients with abnormalities in spirometric measurements often have existing changes in lung volumes and the ratios between various lung volumes. Increases in the RV/TLC ratio or the FRC/TLC ratio indicate hyperinflation and gas trapping. An RV/TLC ratio above 0.40 retrospectively identified 8% of postoperative deaths in one study.[11] An RV/TLC ratio greater than 0.50 was associated with a 36% mortality in another study. Once hyperinflation and gas trapping are evident, the FEV_1 and possibly FVC are severely abnormal. FRC, though seldom measured, is the single most important determinant of the patient's ability to maintain oxygenation.[11] Although lung volume abnormalities suggest pulmonary risk, improvement in lung volumes following intensive bronchodilator therapy should be considered a good prognostic sign.

Diffusing Capacity

Diffusing capacity measures membrane permeability and can be decreased in restrictive or obstructive pulmonary disease. A diffusing capacity of less than 15 mL/min/mm Hg is associated with a significant risk of morbidity and mortality.

Exercise Testing

Exercise testing can be considered a diagnostic stress study designed to precipitate cardiopulmonary dysfunction. Patients who cannot complete the exercise study are at increased risk of pulmonary dysfunction.

Graded exercise testing varies in degree of sophistication. A simple test, climbing stairs at normal speed, requires an oxygen uptake of 1.5 to 2.0 L and tests the integration of cardiopulmonary and neuromuscular systems.[18]

Other sophisticated pulmonary function studies, including measurement of closing capacity and washout volume, have not been adequately studied to determine their role in stratifying pulmonary risk.

As noted, abnormal spirometric values suggest a higher risk of postoperative pulmonary complications. While this high-risk subgroup exists, to date

no studies have clearly defined the exact degree of pulmonary function abnormality at which the patient should not undergo general anesthesia and abdominal surgery. Importantly, preoperative identification of patients with abnormal pulmonary function tests allows the initiation of an intensive preoperative respiratory regimen, including bronchodilators, antibiotics, and chest physiotherapy.[19] In fact, a pulmonary "tune-up" should be considered in patients with abnormal pulmonary function tests. Preoperative admission of these patients for pulmonary treatment does not appear to be indicated, but maximal preoperative outpatient treatment seems reasonable.[11]

Given the ease and the relatively low cost of spirometry, two important clinical questions become pertinent. Which patient should undergo pulmonary testing? Which test should be performed? In the latter case, the best information can be obtained with the combination of arterial blood gas measurements and simple spirometric testing before and after bronchodilator administration. The data obtained from the spirogram assessing the risk of obstructive or restrictive physiology should be combined with the information available from the patient's history and physical examination, laboratory data, and chest radiographs. A preoperative regimen of bronchopulmonary therapy can be instituted if deemed appropriate, and in borderline cases testing can be repeated after a therapeutic interval.

The question of which patient should undergo preoperative pulmonary testing is difficult to answer. Spirometric studies are easily performed and are equally or more informative than either the electrocardiogram (ECG) or chest radiograph at approximately one half the cost. Although no firm guidelines exist, preoperative pulmonary function studies should be considered in patients with a productive cough, who are obese, who are more than 60 years old, who have a 20 pack-year smoking history, or who have historical or physical findings of cardiopulmonary disease. Testing may also be indicated for the elderly.[20] Until otherwise convincing prospective studies point to a different conclusion, there is no strong support for doing screening pulmonary function tests in asymptomatic nonsmokers before abdominal surgery.[16]

Another potentially useful approach involves devising a risk stratification accounting for all changes and other clinical modifiers that might affect abdominal surgery (Table 2–3). No outcome data have been generated, but this scale represents a reasonable approach, with attention focused on the variety of factors that must be considered in any

TABLE 2–3. **System for Classifying Risk of Pulmonary Complications**

Assessment	Points
Expiratory Spirogram	
Normal: %FVC + %FEV$_1$/FVC > 150	0
%FVC + %FEV$_1$/FVC = 100–150	1
%FVC + %FEV$_1$/FVC < 100	2
Preoperative FVC < 20 mL/kg	3
Postbronchodilator FEV$_1$/FVC < 50%	3
Cardiovascular System	
Normal	0
Controlled hypertension, myocardial infarction without sequelae for >2 yr	0
Dyspnea on exertion, orthopnea, paroxysmal nocturnal dyspnea, dependent edema, congestive heart failure, angina	1
Nervous System	
Normal	0
Confusion, obtundation, agitation, spasticity, discoordination, bulbar malfunction	1
Significant muscular weakness	1
Arterial Blood Gas Values	
Acceptable	0
Paco$_2$ > 50 mm Hg or Pao$_2$ < 60 mm Hg with room air	1
Metabolism pH > 7.5 or < 7.3	1
Recovery	
Ambulation (at minimum, sitting at bedside) expected within 36 hr	0
Complete bed confinement expected for at least 36 hr	1

*0 points = low risk; 1–2 points = moderate risk; >3 points = high risk.

Modified from Shapiro BA, Kacmarek RM, et al (eds): Clinical Application of Blood Gases, 4th ed. Chicago: Mosby–Year Book Medical Publishers, 1989.

preoperative pulmonary evaluation. Abnormalities defined with this approach are likely to prompt precautionary arrangements for an intensive care bed and an intensive postoperative plan to minimize pulmonary dysfunction or failure.[20]

Perioperative Pulmonary Morbidity

Unlike cardiovascular complications, the overall incidence and risks of clinically significant atelectasis, pneumonia, aspiration, or respiratory failure are often reported with different criteria, making it difficult to quantify risks. One of the difficulties encountered in analyzing the literature arises from the

lack of consensus as to what constitutes a pulmonary complication (Table 2–4). In retrospective studies, detection of pulmonary complications depends on the thoroughness with which clinical events are recorded. Extrapolation from existing data indicates that postoperative pulmonary infection occurs in approximately 0.4% of patients undergoing total hysterectomy for benign indications, 2% of patients following radical hysterectomy, 3% of those undergoing exenteration, and 3% of patients after ovarian debulking procedures.[4]

Specific population subsets without specific existing pulmonary problems are at increased risk. Following noncomplicated abdominal surgery, the institutionalized patient has a 13% risk of developing significant pulmonary complications (atelectasis, pneumonia) during recovery.[21] In this group and in the elderly, confusion may be the initial presentation of hypoxemia. Although confusion frequently occurs in the elderly (80%), it should not be attrib-

TABLE 2–4. **Operational Definitions of Postoperative Pulmonary Complications**

Grade	Definition
1	Dry cough Microatelectasis: abnormal lung findings and temperature >37.5° C with no identifiable extrapulmonary cause; chest roentgenogram Unexplained dyspnea
2	Productive cough New or persistent bronchospasm resulting in change in therapy Hypoxemia: alveolar – arterial gradient > 29 mm Hg and symptoms of dyspnea or wheezing Radiologically confirmed atelectasis plus temperature elevation (>37.5° C) or at abnormal lung findings Hypercarbia, transient, requiring treatment Adverse reaction to pulmonary medication
3	Pleural effusion resulting in thoracentesis Pneumonia, suspected or proved Pneumothorax Reintubation postoperatively, or intubation in someone not needing intraoperative intubation; in either case, period of ventilator dependence does not exceed 48 hr
4	Ventilatory failure: postoperative ventilator dependence exceeding 48 hr, or reintubation with subsequent period of ventilator dependence exceeding 48 hr

Modified from Kroenke K, Lawrence VA, Theroux JF, Tuley MR: Operative risk in patients with severe obstructive pulmonary disease. Arch Intern Med 152:967–971, 1992.

uted to "sundowning" but should be investigated for potentially reversible causes, including hypoxemia or hypercarbia.

Pulmonary infectious morbidity is also increased in the immunocompromised (e.g., those with malnutrition, malignancy, or other immune disorders) and in women undergoing long (>3 hours) operative procedures.[21] Prophylactic antibiotics are not effective in decreasing this pulmonary risk; however, postoperative ambulation combined with techniques to maximize deep inspiration may decrease the risk of postoperative pulmonary infection.

Atelectasis

Atelectasis, the clinical term denoting collapse of previously inflated lung tissue and alveoli, is subclassified into obstructive, compressive, contractile, and patchy. *Obstructive atelectasis,* common in the immediate postoperative period, results from complete obstruction of a pulmonary segment and results in the absorption of trapped oxygen in distal alveoli. If the affected area is sufficiently large, deflation may result in a mediastinal shift. Local pulmonary defenses are altered, and if infection intervenes, inflammatory exudate and necrotic debris may obstruct larger bronchi. Parenchymal collapse or consolidation ensues. *Compressive atelectasis* results from external lung compression by pleural effusion, pneumothorax, or an elevated diaphragm. The mediastinum shifts away from the compressed portion of the lung. *Contractile atelectasis* occurs when normal lung parenchyma is pulled toward a focus of inflammation or fibrosis that impairs normal alveolar expansion. *Patchy atelectasis* results from focal inflammation and often occurs in conjunction with surfactant denaturation and direct alveolar cell damage. Inhalation injury and adult respiratory distress syndrome (ARDS) are the most common clinical entities associated with patchy alveolar atelectasis.

Postoperative atelectasis most often occurs following a recent procedure that results in a pain-induced decrease in respiratory excursion or direct lung injury. As with any form of pulmonary dysfunction, dyspnea, tachypnea, and tachycardia are prominent clinical features of alveolar collapse, especially when it occurs acutely. The cough response, mediated in part by vagal stretch receptors in the lung, is thought to represent the mechanism responsible for the nonproductive cough. Fever is nearly always present, usually unrelated to concomitant postsurgical infection, and promptly disappears following pulmonary reinflation. If larger portions of the lung are atelectatic, dullness to percussion, decreased breath sounds, and elevation of the diaphragm may be present on physical examination.

There is no evidence that routine prophylactic postoperative mechanical ventilation prevents atelectasis. In fact, the opposite is true, as continued intubation interferes with mucociliary function and provides a route for introduction of nosocomial pathogens. Additionally, the presence of the endotracheal tube may worsen bronchospasm.[17]

Chest radiographs can but do not necessarily provide a valuable diagnostic tool. Postsurgical microatelectasis may appear as tiny bilateral, basal plate-like linear densities. However, radiographs may be "normal" or may only demonstrate a decrease in lung volume, manifested by diaphragmatic elevation. Atelectasis is most deleterious when protracted and associated with a decrease in pulmonary perfusion through the collapsed lung segment. The increased pulmonary shunt increases the risk of hypoxemia. Additionally, the collapsed lung segment is at higher risk of infection as local pulmonary clearance of bacteria is impaired. In these situations, mucous plugging of the involved lung is common; it is not only the cause but also the result of local parenchymal collapse and the adverse effects of absence of mucus clearance.

Incentive spirometry continues to be the simplest, most effective method of preventing and treating atelectasis. Intermittent positive-pressure breathing (IPPB) was replaced by blow bottles more than a decade ago, and incentive spirometers have now replaced blow bottles. Incentive spirometry remains the treatment of choice because of its simplicity and lack of treatment complications. Incentive spirometry requires sustained deep breathing, which opens lower airway passages; however, patients should be closely supervised to ensure proper use.[22] The upright position allows gravity to assist in diaphragmatic excursion. Some information suggests that periodic administration of continuous positive airway pressure (CPAP) or positive expiratory pressure by face mask is superior to incentive spirometry with respect to gas exchange, preservation of lung volumes, and the development of atelectasis after upper abdominal procedures. Unfortunately, these treatments are not as simple or well tolerated.

Holding each breath at or near full inflation allows gas to distribute into areas of low compliance. Breath holding for about 5.5 seconds is required to reduce intrasegmental pressure differences by 60%. Therefore, the most effective technique for voluntary lung inflation consists of taking at least five segmental deep breaths, each held for 5 to 6 seconds, once every waking hour.[23] Recent prospective data from Roukema et al. suggest that preoperative education in deep breathing exercises significantly decreases the risk of postoperative pulmonary complications in patients with a non-compromised pulmonary status undergoing upper abdominal surgery. In their experience, preoperative instruction combined with incentive spirometry has reduced the rate of significant postoperative pulmonary complications to 3.5%.[24]

Tracheal suction, deep breathing maneuvers, and airway humidification are also indicated for the prevention and treatment of postoperative atelectasis. Bronchoscopy is valuable for removing debris from larger airways, especially if the lobe or entire lung is collapsed.

Appropriate management of perioperative atelectasis should be aggressive and involve frequent clinical reassessment (Table 2–5). It is essential to identify and alleviate the underlying disease process even if it requires invasive techniques. A recent prospective study of ultrasound-guided thoracentesis, needle with catheter, and needle-only tap of 53 patients with free-flowing pleural effusion indicated that the ultrasound-guided method was associated with significantly fewer serious complications and fewer pneumothoraces (0/19) than the needle catheter technique (7/18) or needle-only method (3/15).[25] Thoracostomy should be considered a primary procedure to drain existing malignant pleural fluid either pre- or postoperatively. In the latter situation, pleural sclerosis with tetracycline or bleomycin should be considered when suction volumes decrease significantly. If oxygen supplementation is necessary, 1 to 6 L of nasal oxygen equals an FiO_2 of 24% to 44%.[22]

Pneumonia

More than a million cases of pneumonia occur annually in the United States. In persons older than 65, pneumonia and influenza together constitute one of the leading infectious causes of death. The traditional separation of pneumonias into hospital acquired and community acquired is not as clearcut as previously proposed. The profile of environmental pathogens causing most infectious diseases changed dramatically in the 1980s. The risks associated with developing postoperative pneumonia (Fig. 2–3) are identical to those that increase other pulmonary risks. This risk is significantly increased

TABLE 2–5. Treatment Strategies for Refractory Postoperative Atelectasis

General

Remove any obstruction to large airway (e.g., mainstem or lobar bronchus)

Control pain

Provide therapy at least every 1–2 waking hours initially

Reduce frequency of therapy as improvement occurs

Ensure adequate supervision of therapy

Deep-Breathing Techniques

Voluntary deep breathing (with incentive spirometry)
  Have patient repeat maximum lung inflations at least 5 times
  Monitor volumes achieved
  Have patient hold each breath for 5–6 sec

Intermittent positive-pressure breathing
  Use volume-oriented technique
  Provide maximum inflations in series of at least 5, repeated once or twice
  Use only to treat clinically significant atelectasis, not as prophylaxis
  Use if spontaneous inspiratory capacity is <1L (in adult)
  Document that therapy increases inspiratory capacity by at least 25%

Measures to Increase Functional Residual Capacity

Intermittent continuous positive airway pressure (CPAP) or expiratory positive airway pressure by mask
  Use adequate end-expiratory pressure (usually 10–15 cm H_2O) to increase FRC
  Administer 25–35 breaths or for 5–10 min every 1–2 waking hours initially
  Monitor constantly when occlusive mask is used

Positive end-expiratory pressure (PEEP) or CPAP by tracheal tube (continuous)
  Use adequate end-expiratory pressure (usually 10–15 cm H_2O) to increase FRC
  Continue PEEP or CPAP for at least 24 hr after resolution of atelectasis on radiographs

Modified from Postgrad Med 91:00, 1992.

in the malnourished, who often have diminished respiratory muscle strength, VC, and flow rates.[26]

A careful history of underlying illness or exposure to usual and unusual pathogens is essential and must be sought in all patients with serious pulmonary infection.[27]

The incidence of nosocomial pneumonia has been reported to be 17.5% in patients undergoing elective abdominal or thoracic procedures, 21% in patients in an ICU receiving ventilatory assistance, and 29% in patients undergoing laparotomy for intra-abdominal abscess.[28]

The prognosis for hospital-acquired pneumonia remains almost as it was 20 years ago, and mortality from nosocomial pneumonia in the SICU may

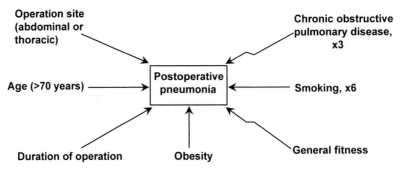

FIGURE 2-3. Important factors associated with the risk of developing postoperative pneumonia.

approach 50%.[29] Sixty percent of cases of hospital-acquired pneumonia are caused by aerobic gram-negative bacilli, specifically *Klebsiella pneumoniae, Pseudomonas aeruginosa,* and *E. coli.* Other isolates include *Staphylococcus aureus, Streptococcus pneumoniae,* and anaerobic bacteria.[29]

Once the diagnosis is suspected, culture techniques may be necessary to establish a diagnosis. Material cultured may include expectorated sputum, bronchoscopic aspirates, protected brushing specimens, transtracheal aspirates, transgastric needle aspirates, bronchoalveolar lavage products, or even lung biopsy specimens.[30] Regardless, the physician is faced with placement of antibiotics, with the choice of directed or empirical antibiotics related to the presence or absence of host defense problems. Broad-spectrum coverage in specific patient subsets (i.e., those who are ventilator dependent) may allow superinfection and may predispose to increased pulmonary morbidity.[30] The recommended empirical antimicrobial therapy should be tailored to the most likely offending organism within a given patient's scenario. Cephalosporin, aminoglycoside, antipseudomonal penicillin, and erythromycin may be given individually or in an appropriate combination to adequately treat most gram-positive and gram-negative coccal and bacillary bacteria as well as *Legionella* and *Chlamydia.* Trimethoprim–sulfamethoxazole is effective against *Pneumocystis carinii.* The fluoroquinolones cover a broad spectrum of aerobic pulmonary pathogens and have good tissue penetration. The monobactam aztreonam rather than an aminoglycoside may be used under special circumstances.[29]

Nosocomial pneumonia can be devastating. When associated with intra-abdominal sepsis, it has a mortality rate as high as 66%. One prospective evaluation of 300 patients compared the outcome of patients with nosocomial pneumonia complicating

intra-abdominal sepsis and patients with recurrent abdominal sepsis but no nosocomial pneumonia. The in-hospital mortality was 20% in the 171 patients without nosocomial pneumonia or recurrent intra-abdominal sepsis. Mortality was 17% in the 36 patients without nosocomial pneumonia in whom recurrent intra-abdominal sepsis developed, and 53% in the 47 patients with nosocomial pneumonia but no recurrent intra-abdominal sepsis. Finally, 12 patients who had both nosocomial pneumonia and recurrent intra-abdominal sepsis had a 75% mortality, suggesting that nosocomial pneumonia complicating intra-abdominal sepsis is an independent risk factor associated with significant mortality when compared to recurrent intra-abdominal sepsis.[28]

Respiratory Failure

In the absence of preexisting respiratory disease or coexisting complications, respiratory insufficiency is an unusual complication following elective gynecologic or obstetric procedures. However, this is not true of longer procedures, those requiring high-volume blood replacement, or ultraradical procedures for the treatment of gynecologic cancer. In the latter clinical situation, postoperative respiratory compromise may complicate recovery in 25% of patients.[31]

Although not common, postoperative respiratory problems may progress to inadequate ventilation as well as inadequate oxygenation. In either situation, regardless of whether it is a primary pulmonary process or one aggravated by the anesthetic or surgical procedure, the underlying process may necessitate intensive therapy, including mechanical ventilation. It therefore becomes imperative that the pelvic surgeon understand the potential indications for intubation and be comfortable with basic ventilator management.

Routine postoperative ventilatory support to minimize pulmonary complications in specific patients following selected operative procedures seems logical; however, there are no existing studies to substantiate this contention.[32] Again, published studies do not indicate that prophylactic postoperative mechanical ventilation, except when it is of duration sufficient to allow anesthetic agents to be eliminated or metabolized, is of any benefit with respect to decreased morbidity, mortality, complications, or length of stay in the ICU. When inhalational anesthesia is used rather than high-dose narcotic techniques, most patients are successfully extubated shortly after the operation, and acute perioperative reintubation is rarely necessary provided patients remain hemodynamically stable. Therefore, the decision to provide or continue postoperative mechanical ventilation should be based on the preoperative evaluation, surgical incision site, the extent of the surgical procedure, and the expected residual anesthetic effect or other factors that might impair ventilation (Table 2–6). In one recent prospective evaluation the incidence of pulmonary failure and the duration of intubation were significantly less in patients receiving perioperative epidural pain relief.[33]

There are specific indicators suggesting the presence of respiratory failure and the need for ventilation (Table 2–7). There are four indications for controlling the airway by endotracheal intubation: to maintain patency of an impaired airway, to protect an inadequate airway, to support inadequate pulmonary function, and to meet the needs of postoperative ventilation. Thus, the goals of intubation include improving gas exchange, reducing the work of breathing, and protecting airway patency.[34] There are guidelines for standards of care with acute respiratory failure and mechanical ventilatory support.[35]

Acute intervention with intubation and ventilation may become necessary any time during the postoperative period. Once ventilatory support is established, its extent and duration are guided by clinical examination and physiologic monitoring. Although pulmonary consultation is customary in those situations, it is imperative that the gynecologic surgeon understand the basics of mechanical ventilation (Table 2–8). Initial delivery of VT of 12 to 15 mL/kg of body weight is appropriate. Normal VC is 30 to 70 cc/kg of body weight, and FRC is 15 to 30 cc/kg of body weight. A compliance curve can be constructed to select the optimal VT that re-

TABLE 2–6. Preoperative Factors That Impair Ventilation

Structural defects
  Scoliosis
  Kyphosis
  Flail chest
Mechanical uncoupling
  Effusion
  Hemorrhage
  Pneumothorax
Muscular weakness
  Malnutrition
  Cachexia
  Deconditioning of muscles
  Myasthenia
  Paralysis
Obstruction to flow
  Stenosis
  Aspiration
  Trauma
  Asthma
  COPD
Increased work of breathing
  Pregnancy
  Distention
  Ascites
  Obesity
Nutritional supply–demand imbalance
  Thyroid disease
  Hypoperfusion states
Lung restriction
  Entrapped lung
  Pulmonary edema
  Pulmonary fibrosis
  Surfactant failure

Modified from Pett SB, Wernly JA: Respiratory function in surgical patients: Perioperative evaluation and management. Surg Annu 20:311–329, 1988.

sults in minimal airway closure and interference with cardiac hemodynamics. Adequate sigh volumes are approximately 40% above normal VT and are given intermittently (six per hour) to prevent atelectasis. The ventilation rate is initially set at 10 to 12 breaths per minute, with adjustments made to maintain PCO_2 between 35 and 45 mm Hg. PEEP is used to improve oxygenation in the patient with an oxygenation defect that cannot be resolved with safe (< 60% FiO_2) oxygen concentration.[34]

An initial FiO_2 of less than 60% should be considered a safe FiO_2 for long-term exposure in ventilated patients needing intensive support. Examination of the dose–time–toxicity curve in humans as it relates to hyperoxemia indicates that 100% oxygen should not be administered for more than 12 hours, 80% oxygen should not be administered for more

TABLE 2–7. **Respiratory Insufficiency**

Mechanics	Normal	Insufficiency
Respiratory rate (min)	12–20	>35
Tidal volume (cc/kg)	6	<3
Vital capacity (cc/kg)	70	<15
Inspiratory force (cm H_2O)	20–40	<20
Ventilation		
Pa_{CO_2} (mm Hg)	35–45	>55
Physiologic dead space (V_D/V_T)	0.4	>0.6
Oxygenation		
Pa_{O_2} (mm Hg)	60–95	<100 on 100% Fi_{O_2}
P_A–a_{O_2} (mm Hg)	5–15	<450 on 100% Fi_{O_2}
Pulmonary shunt (%) (Qs/Qt)	5–6	30
Perfusion		
Cardiac index	3.0 ± 0.5	<2
Mixed venous oxygen (mm Hg)	40	<30

Modified from Orr JW: Introduction to pelvic surgery: Pre- and postoperative care. In Gusberg SB: Female Genital Cancer. New York: Churchill Livingstone, 1988.

than 24 hours, and 60% oxygen should not be administered for more than 36 hours. No measurable changes in pulmonary function or blood gas exchange occur in humans during exposure to less than 50% oxygen, even for long periods.[35]

The lowest amount of PEEP that effectively oxygenates the patient is desirable. Oxygen consumption and not Pa_{O_2} should be the variable monitored when high levels of inspired oxygen or PEEP are

TABLE 2–8. **Guidelines for Setting Basic Ventilator Parameters**

Parameter	Setting
Tidal volume (V_T)	10 to 12 mL/kg
Respiratory rate	8 to 12 breaths/min
Pressure limit	5 to 10 cm H_2O above pressure required to deliver V_T
Sigh volume	$1\frac{1}{2}$ to 2 times V_T for patients with V_T <8 mL/kg
Sigh pressure limit	5 to 10 cm H_2O above pressure required to deliver sigh volume
Peak flow	Select a flow rate to provide an inspiratory to expiratory ratio of no less than 1:1
Sensitivity	–0.3 to –0.5 cm H_2O
Oxygen percentage	Fi_{O_2} necessary to achieve a Pa_{O_2} of 60 mm Hg

Modified from Gluck E, et al: Technique of instituting mechanical ventilation: Patient preparation, endotracheal intubation and monitoring. J Crit Illness 7:1325, 1992.
Abbreviations: Fi_{O_2}, fraction of inspired oxygen; Pa_{O_2}, arterial oxygen tension.

used. Normally there is minimal small airway closure during tidal breathing, as FRC is greater than the critical closing volume (CCV). However, CCV increases with age, prolonged bed rest, or intrinsic pulmonary disease, whereas FRC decreases with prolonged bed rest, anesthesia, muscle weakness, or abdominal surgery. Both of these situations increase the tendency toward small airway closure, progressive atelectasis, and resultant hypoxemia. These relationships must be considered and may be particularly important in the ventilated patient. Small airways (less than 1 mm in diameter) are most vulnerable to collapse when the lung is functioning at low volumes. As V_T falls toward CCV, dependent and compressed areas in the lung begin to collapse, and resorption of gas trapped distally can result in complete alveolar collapse (atelectasis) of a particular lung segment. At the time of alveolar collapse a mucous plug is often present as the result and not the cause of atelectasis and pooled secretions. The type of trapped gas resorbed affects the degree of atelectasis, and resorption is rapid if the gas mixture is high in oxygen and low in nitrogen content. Thus, gas mixtures administered during anesthesia predispose to atelectasis. Surfactant production begins to decrease almost immediately after the development of atelectasis, and lung reexpansion becomes more difficult as time passes, since normal surfactant function is altered, which can also predispose to atelectasis.

Once respiratory function has improved, high oxygen concentrations may be tapered quickly with Fi_{O_2} changes monitored every 5 minutes. The ability to make rapid changes may be particularly beneficial in patients who initially require high FiO_2 and may be beneficial in those patients who have severely depressed oxygenation, as PEEP therapy can also be augmented very quickly.[36]

Optimal mechanical ventilation should focus on preservation of functional lung volume and the prevention of atelectasis. This is best achieved by providing maximal ventilatory volumes. Current ventilation methods relate to the mechanism responsible for inspiration and expiration. Time-cycled ventilation terminates inspiration after a preset time interval, and volume-cycled ventilation terminates inspiration after a preset volume is delivered. Pressure-cycled ventilation terminates inspiration after a preset pressure is reached.

Pressure support ventilation assists the patient's spontaneous inspiratory effort by providing a preselected amount of positive airway pressure to each spontaneous breath and is designed to give the patient more control over her breathing pattern. Pressure support is triggered by an inspiratory effort of -0.5 to -0.1 cm H_2O, and positive airway pressure is delivered until inspiratory flow decreases to the preset value. In spontaneously breathing patients with adequate V_T, pressure support ventilation reduces the work of breathing, increases patient comfort, and increases patient control over inspiratory time, flow, and V_T. The addition of pressure support ventilation to trials of intermittent mandatory ventilation (IMV) or continuous positive airway pressure (CPAP) during weaning from the ventilator decreases respiratory work and improves the number of successful weaning trials.

Airway pressure release ventilation is a new support modality that is being evaluated in clinical trials but is not yet commercially available. The lungs are inflated with CPAP and breaths are allowed by releasing the CPAP, which allows the lung volume to fall and expiration to occur. There appears to be less derangement of cardiovascular function than is seen with conventional positive-pressure ventilation.

IMV delivers conventional positive-pressure ventilatory support with a fixed mechanical rate while allowing simultaneous unrestricted, unassisted, spontaneous breathing to occur. Any level of mechanical ventilatory support from 0 to 100% may be used in IMV. Control of ventilation is achieved by increasing the frequency of mandatory breaths until $PaCO_2$ is lowered below apneic thresholds and the patient's spontaneous respiratory efforts cease. IMV is probably the most widely used ventilatory technique in critical care at the present time. It is likely that any patient failing IMV would also fail any other form of mechanical ventilation.[37]

High-frequency ventilation is a new modality that allows adequate pulmonary gas exchange and offers the advantage of allowing effective gas transport without high airway pressure or depression of hemodynamic function. Currently, high-frequency positive-pressure ventilation with respiratory rates of 60 to 120, high-frequency jet ventilation with rates of up to 400 per minute, and high-frequency oscillation ventilation with a wide range of frequency up to 40 Hz are available. Initially, the specific advantages of high-frequency jet ventilation over conventional ventilation were thought to be a reduced incidence of barotrauma and cardiovascular depression. Unfortunately, barotrauma frequently occurs shortly after initiation despite lower peak airway pressures, indicating that this problem may actually relate to the underlying lung pathology more than to the type of ventilation.[32,38]

Ventilatory drive as well as diaphragmatic muscle strength is lost with progressive starvation, and dietary alteration may suppress ventilatory response to both hypoxic and hypercarbic challenge. These pulmonary changes in otherwise healthy individuals may approach established criteria indicating the need for mechanical ventilation that have been established for patients with neuromuscular respiratory failures. Malnutrition-associated loss of respiratory muscle strength can result in a 40% reduction in maximum voluntary ventilation and a 63% reduction in VC when compared to controls.

Although the need of supplemental nutritional therapy in many clinical situations is widely accepted and advocated, the scientific data to support nutritional supplementation during ventilatory support are lacking. In fact, the only documented effect of refeeding involves a blunting of the ventilatory drive associated with starvation. Metabolic demands and nutritional needs are altered following most surgical procedures. One report evaluating surgical patients who required more than 3 days of postoperative mechanical ventilation indicated that 10 of 11 patients were successfully weaned and extubated when nutritional support was included in their therapeutic regimen. In contrast, only 8 of 22 patients were successfully weaned and extubated when nutritional support was not included in their therapeutic regimen. Interestingly, no difference in successful weaning was evident in medical patients, regardless of the institution of nutritional support.[39]

Although hyperalimentation has not been shown to benefit patients with respiratory failure, clinical consensus suggesting its potential benefit in respiratory failure, along with other indications including improved response to infection and improved healing, warrants its use. However, there are documented disadvantages to overfeeding, as very high caloric intake and carbohydrate loading can be detrimental and increase $PaCO_2$.

Nutritional support during ventilatory support can be expensive, is not without risk, and necessitates careful monitoring by experienced personnel. Enteral nutritional support can be justified in the patient with an intact functional intestinal tract, as it is less expensive and less invasive. An important point to remember is the frequently encountered impact of ventilation that occurs with increased nutrition, particularly high carbohydrate loads, which can elevate carbon dioxide production and may interfere with successful weaning from the ventilator.

Arterial blood gas measurements are the standard of monitoring during ventilator care. These invasive procedures require an indwelling arterial catheter or arterial puncture, placing the patient at risk for significant blood loss as well as predisposing the patient to the potential risks of an arterial catheter. In most clinical situations, the direct measurement of PaO_2 has been replaced by pulse oximetry. Pulse oximetry was accidentally discovered in 1972 in Japan by investigators seeking a method for measuring cardiac output. Pulse oximetry computes a ratio of the pulsatile variations and optical densities of tissues at two wavelengths of red light at 660 nm and infrared light at 10 to 940 nm. Pulse oximeters have been extensively evaluated and determined to be accurate in both laboratory and clinical settings. As of January 1990, pulse oximetry became an ASA standard for basic intraoperative monitoring, and it is now mandated in several states. Oximeters have been judged unacceptable if alarms can be turned off.[40] Specific situations (Table 2–9) including extreme hypoxemia (SO_2 <70%) can affect oximeter accuracy. Although accurate, studies evaluating acute changes in SO_2 indicate that response time can vary from 0.1 second to as long as 50 seconds when monitoring acute changes in SaO_2 and that ear probes have a faster and more accurate response than finger probes.

Fully saturated hemoglobin (at a value of 13 g/dL) carries 18.07 mL of oxygen. If PaO_2 is 100 mm Hg, hemoglobin is essentially fully saturated, and an additional 0.31 mL can be dissolved in the plasma, resulting in a total oxygen content of 18.38 mL. Therefore, 98.3% of arterial blood oxygen is carried by hemoglobin and only 1.7% is dissolved in plasma. A drop in PaO_2 to 75 mm Hg is associ-

TABLE 2–9. **Pulse Oximetry Limitations**

Dyshemoglobinemias
  CO_2
  Methemoglobin
  Fetal hemoglobin
  Carboxyhemoglobin
Dyes, pigments
  Methylene blue
  Bilirubin
Low perfusion
Anemia
Increased venous pulsation
External light source

ated with a total oxygen content of 17.4 mL and a concomitant fall of SaO_2 to 95%. In this situation the quotient of total oxygen content (17.4/18.38) is 0.95, and total oxygen content changes in the same amount as arterial saturation. If PaO_2 and SaO_2 are maintained in the range of the normal oxyhemoglobin dissociation curve, concomitant changes allow changes in SaO_2 to be used clinically in many situations without the necessity to determine PaO_2 or to calculate total oxygen content. Oximetry saturation less than 70% suggests that the PaO_2 is less than 40 mm Hg. On the other hand, high levels of saturation give no information about PaO_2, as hemoglobin is fully saturated at a PaO_2 of 150 mm Hg. Therefore, in the stable patient given supplemental oxygen, regardless of method, large changes in PaO_2 (up to 600 mm Hg) can occur without a noted change in saturation.[41]

Continuous mixed venous oximetry or pulse oximetry are tools of potentially great utility and are considered the standard of care for intraoperative and recovery room management. Additional uses during transport (particularly in those at high risk) diagnostic procedures, ventilator dependence, or just high-risk postoperative patients have become common and yield useful information. Perioperative use suggests a 53% incidence of hypoxia during cardiac catherization.[41] Evidence suggests that pulse oximetry potentially increases safety. During routine gynecologic surgery in which oximetry readings were not made available to the anesthesiologist, 10% of patients experienced desaturation to less than 90% and 5% desaturated to less than 85%. Pulse oximetry monitoring has been successfully used as an important monitor during anesthesia; however, its role in postoperative care remains to be determined.

Continuous oximetry monitoring in general care

units suggests that 75% of patients experience at least one episode of desaturation to less than 90% and 58% experience episodes of desaturation to less than 85%. These episodes are not well documented in nursing notes (30%) or physician notes (7%), and management by respiratory therapy occurred in only 20% of patients who desaturated to less than 90% and 26% of those who desaturated to less than 85%. This tool, if used successfully, should assist and result in changes in physician-directed respiratory care.[42]

Successful ventilation includes the ability to wean patients when mechanical support is no longer necessary. A number of direct and indirect measurements of pulmonary function have been proposed for guidelines to predict successful weaning from mechanical ventilatory support (Table 2–10). The value of an index for weaning from mechanical ventilation lies in its ability to predict respiratory endurance, which reflects the ability of the respiratory capacity to meet respiratory demands, the resistive load from airways or endotracheal tube resistance, and the elastic load from con-

TABLE 2–10. Weaning from Mechanical Ventilation

Pathophysiologic Determinants of Outcome
Failure of respiratory muscle pump
  Decreased neuromuscular capacity
  Increased respiratory load or demands
Physiologic factors
Impaired oxygenation
  Hypoventilation
  Impaired pulmonary gas exchange
  Decreased oxygen content of venous blood

Indices Used to Predict Weaning Outcome
Oxygenation (gas exchange) indices:
  Alveolar–arterial oxygen tension difference
  Arterial/alveolar oxygen tension ratio
  Arterial/fractional inspired oxygen ratio
Vital capacity
Maximum inspiratory pressure
Minute ventilation
Maximum voluntary ventilation
Respiratory system compliance
Airway occlusion pressure
Breathing pattern:
  Respiratory frequency
  Tidal volume
  Rib cage–abdominal motion
Work of breathing

Modified from J Crit Illness 5(8), 1990.

ditions of decreased compliance. A VC of 10 mL/kg and a negative inspiratory force of at least – 20 mm H_2O are useful predictors of successful weaning. A maximum voluntary ventilation greater than twice the resting level and a minute ventilation of less than 10 L/min are also predictive. Maximal static inspiratory pressure (P_i max) is measured when inspiratory muscles are at optimal length and near residual volume. A P_i max of 25 mm H_2O or less indicates severe impairment of deep breathing. Similarly, maximal static expiratory pressure (P_e max) is measured when expiratory muscles are optimally stretched after a full inspiration to near total lung capacity. A P_e max of less than +40 mm Hg suggests a severely impaired coughing reflex.[43] One recently evaluated parameter is the rapid shallow breathing (RSP) index, which evaluates the ratio of respiratory rate divided by tidal volume in liters. Patients with an RSP index of 105 are almost always successfully weaned (sensitivity = 0.97%).[44] Tidal volumes greater than 325 mL have a sensitivity of 0.97%, and a maximum expiratory index of ≥15 mL has a sensitivity of 100% (Yang).[45]

Regardless of methods of ventilation and parameters for weaning, all medical personnel must remember that patients receiving mechanical ventilation, even on a short-term basis, need enormous emotional support. Constant conversation and reassurance are important to ensure that patient needs will be met. This care includes constant evaluation for signs of pain or discomfort, and patients should be given adequate amounts of analgesia and sedatives. Methods of communication should be provided for patients who are unable to speak or to move extremities.[46]

Adult Respiratory Distress Syndrome

In the past 10 years the reported death rate for patients with ARDS has decreased from approximately 80% to 50%. The term ARDS does not define a specific disease process. Instead, the lung exhibits a generalized response and clinical appearance resulting from a spectrum of causes. True sepsisassociated ARDS is characterized by an increase in extravascular lung water and a decrease in oxygenation with normal pulmonary capillary wedge pressures.[47]

ARDS can occur within a few minutes to a few days following any insult, including shock, gram-negative sepsis, or aspiration. Many factors, including alterations in complement activity, prostaglandin function, neutrophil hyperstimulation, and platelet activity, have been proposed to contribute to the development of ARDS. In ARDS, alveolar capillary membrane injury produces a "leak" and a clinical hypoxemia that remains uncorrected even though FiO_2 is increased when mechanical ventilation is used. Pulmonary capillary wedge pressure is usually normal. Intubation, oxygenation, and mechanical ventilation are crucial in the management of ARDS. Identification of an underlying abnormality in the postoperative patient requires a careful search for pulmonary or intra-abdominal infection. It has become clear that available antimicrobial agents directed against gram-negative organisms are less than completely successful. Efforts have now focused on the bacterial products, namely cell wall endotoxin, as data suggest that when endotoxemia is present, irrespective of the blood level, the incidence of ARDS appeared to be significantly higher than when endotoxin is not isolated.

The release of endotoxin ultimately stimulates the release of other cytokines such as tumor necrosis factor (TNF), IL-5, and IL-1. TNF can directly alter capillary permeability. Another mediator, platelet-activating factor (PAF), is derived from neutrophils, eosinophils, monocytes, macrophages, platelets, and endothelial cells. Stimulation of the arachidonic acid cascade by complement or other factors can affect pulmonary function.[47]

When present, large tidal volumes (12–15 mL/kg) are used to assist in inflating stiff or partially collapsed alveoli. Severe right-to-left shunting is corrected by adding PEEP, not allowing end-expiratory pressure to fall to normal atmospheric pressure. PEEP levels are raised in increments of 3 to 5 cm H_2O in an attempt to open atelectatic alveoli. Proper use entails the least amount of PEEP needed to obtain a PaO_2 of 60 mm Hg or more and an FiO_2 of 50% or less without interfering with venous return.[48] Excessive PEEP overdistends alveoli, causing compression of alveolar capillary vessels or resulting in barotrauma such as pneumothorax, pneumomediastinum, or interstitial emphysema. In the presence of severe anemia, transfusion of packed red cells is useful; however, colloid or crystalloid is an acceptable replacement. The latter is less expensive. Regardless, the patient should be well hydrated in order to maintain cardiac filling pressures, blood pressure, urine output, and tissue perfusion.[47]

Despite considerable clinical experience with different therapeutic approaches, definitive answers to improve outcome have not been forthcoming. Newer therapeutic agents attempt to decrease neutrophil chemo-attraction via polyclonal antibody to C_{5a} or to increase immunity by infusing human antiserum directed against endotoxin. Neutrophil function inhibitors, such as prostaglandin E and monoclonal antibody to TNF, have also been tried.[49] Two different types of monoclonal antibodies have been developed against the lipid moiety found in endotoxin. A multi-institutional double-blind placebo-controlled trial demonstrated no difference in the incidence of ARDS, disseminated intravascular coagulopathy, or hepatic or renal failure in patients treated with placebo and those given human monoclonal antibody. However, in the subset of patients who were in shock prior to reception of the drug, the death rate was considerably lower (33%) than in those who received placebo (57%). During sepsis, endothelial cells contract, widening intracellular clefts. A significant change in the diameter of these gaps can result in large unmanageable influxes of fluid into the interstitial space.

Pulmonary Risk Assessment

Depending on selection criteria, pulmonary complications may occur in 85% of surgical procedures. This nearly universal occurrence of perioperative pulmonary dysfunction following abdominal surgery suggests an important role for pulmonary risk assessment and the recognition of specific patients at risk (Table 2–11).

A careful history and physical examination are paramount in determining pulmonary risk (Table 2–12). Important information obtained during the history and physical examination include exercise tolerance; the presence of dyspnea, cough, or

TABLE 2–11. **Pulmonary Complications: Risk Factors**

Obesity: risk increased 5–10×
  Pronounced decrease in VC; diaphragmatic dysfunction and
    myocardial dysfunction
Smoking
  20 pack-years, productive cough
  Fewer than 20% quit
Anesthesia
  3.0 hr
  Spinal = general
Surgical
  Incision placement
  Nasogastric tube
Age
  > 60 yr
Pulmonary disease risk increased 6–10×
Asthma

Modified from Jackson C: Arch Intern Med 148:2120, 1988.

TABLE 2–12. **Surgical Risk Factors for Patients with Chronic Lung Disease**

General
    Smoking
    Age
    Obesity
    Inanition
    Altered mental status
    Neuromuscular
Pulmonary
    Wheezing
    Sputum production
    Dyspnea
    Tachypnea
    Edema
Cardiac
    Left ventricular failure
    Right ventricular failure
Operative procedure
    Upper abdominal incision
    Extensive surgery
    Prolonged anesthesia

productive sputum; any recent respiratory tract infection; hemoptysis or wheezing; prior use of bronchodilators or corticosteroids; pulmonary complications with previous surgery; smoking history; age; breathing frequency and form; and body habitus (Fig. 2–4).[16] Other important historical factors such as specific drug exposures cannot be overlooked. The reported incidence of bleomycin-induced fibrosis is as high as 33%, and pulmonary toxicity is increased with chest irradiation, smoking, and hypoxia. Although no distinct pathognomonic signs or symptoms exist, patients with bleomycin toxicity usually present with dyspnea, tachypnea, and nonproductive cough with rales initially at the base and then throughout the lungs. In 1978, the first report of postanesthetic pulmonary complications related to bleomycin administration was published. The report indicated that patients needed a lowered FiO_2 intraoperatively.[50]

The social history should concentrate on special environmental problems or exposures (i.e., cobalt or asbestos) that might be important.[51] The importance of a careful history and physical examination has been described in 128 asbestos workers. Although clinical factors suggested a pulmonary cause, the authors found "unexpectedly" that 37% of those with reduced exercise capacity had a cardiac rather than a ventilatory limitation identified during testing.[52]

Easily elicited physical findings can be helpful. The time it takes to forcibly exhale VC is normally less than 4 seconds. Therefore, longer times are associated with air flow obstruction. Hyperinflation may also be detected at the bedside. At residual volume (the volume of air remaining in the lungs after maximal expiration), the diaphragm is generally percussible posteriorly at the level of the bottom of the scapula and descends 4 to 6 inches on maximal inspiration. However, in obstructive lung disease with hyperinflation, the diaphragm is below the scapula at residual volume and fails to descend normally on inspiration to total lung capacity. An increase in circumference of the thoracic cage also suggests hyperinflation. The bedside estimate of the ratio of the time for inspiration/expiration is normally 1:2.[53]

Simple exercise maneuvers can assist in determining which patient might benefit from additional pulmonary testing. In one study, patients who were unable to climb three flights (76 steps) of stairs had an FEV_1 below 1.7 L, while 97% of patients who completed more than three flights of stairs had an FEV_1 above 1.7 L. Climbing five or more flights corresponded to an FEV_1 above 2.3 L. The ability to blow out a match at 6 inches was associated with an FEV_1 above 1.5 L and an MVV above 60 L/min.[54]

Chest radiography is the most frequent radiographic study performed in the United States. The primary rationale for obtaining preoperative chest radiographs is to detect serious cardiac or respiratory abnormalities that might place patients at risk for perioperative death or other serious complications. Obtaining preoperative chest radiographs to establish a preoperative baseline for comparison has no scientific merit and a negligible effect on patient management. In fact, when compared to history and physical examination, there exists no documented benefit of routine preoperative chest radiographs in the detection of clinical abnormalities. Routine preoperative chest radiographs offer little patient benefit in terms of increasing life expectancy or preventing morbidity.[48] In an attempt to determine whether clinical criteria alone are sufficient to identify patients who would not benefit from preoperative chest radiographs, a retrospective analysis of 136 preoperative patients over the age of 59 was performed. Thirty-four percent of the patients *without* risk factors and 62% of those in the high-risk group were found to have significant abnormalities on the chest radiograph. The difference was not statistically significant between patients over the age of 70 (49% abnormal) and those in the age group of 60 to 70 years (59%).[55]

One study evaluated follow-up chest radiographs

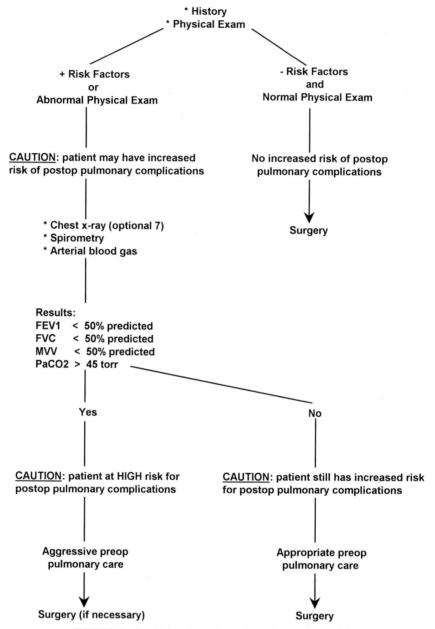

FIGURE 2–4. Algorithm to determine perioperative pulmonary risks.

in 117 hospitalized (non-ICU) patients. Unexpected findings (25.4%) were frequent and highly valued, with 21% classified as having a definite influence on therapy and 36% having a possible influence on therapy. New diagnoses were found in 14.5%, progression of a known abnormality in 13.7%, diagnoses were ruled out in 44.5%, 17% provided reassurance, and 6.8% provided no new information.[56]

Seventy-four patients who required intubation and mechanical ventilation were evaluated to determine the efficacy of daily routine chest radiographs. A total of 538 chest radiographs were examined, of which 354 (65.8%) failed to disclose either new or major findings. New, minor findings were disclosed in 163 radiographs, 40% of which were anticipated by bedside assessment. However, in 13 (17.6%) of 74 patients, new major findings were discovered only by daily chest radiography. It would appear that while a large percentage of routine radiographs will not disclose new findings, routine daily studies have a substantial impact on the management of intubated, mechanically ventilated patients in the ICU.[57]

Historical Factors

Smoking

Approximately 20% of U.S. women abuse tobacco. Although this percentage has continued to decline, the absolute numbers constitute a significant population of high-risk patients. Postoperative pulmonary complications occur in 33% of smokers, who are at greater risk for pneumonia, fever, productive cough, and abnormal chest findings when undergoing elective surgical procedures. Cigarette smoking increases the risk of developing pneumonia by a factor of two and quadruples the pulmonary risk if the patient is a smoker with evidence of COPD.[8]

Cigarette smoking adversely affects both the cardiovascular and respiratory systems, decreases PaO_2, increases tissue oxygen extraction, and lowers mixed venous oxygen tension. Smokers have significantly elevated levels of carboxyhemoglobin related to the brand of cigarette used, the depth of inhalation, the number of "puffs" taken, and their level of ventilation while they are smoking. The level of carboxyhemoglobin elevation in smokers ranges from 3% to 15% and reduces the amount of hemoglobin available to bond oxygen, producing a decrease in arterial oxygen content and a shift to the left in the oxyhemoglobin saturation curve. Patients at greatest risk for significantly elevated carboxyhemoglobin levels include those who smoke avidly, late at night, and then undergo an early morning operation. Therefore, at a minimum it is recommended that smokers stop smoking for at least 12 to 14 hours preoperatively in order to ensure three half-lives of carboxyhemoglobin clearance and a lower carboxyhemoglobin level during and immediately following anesthesia.[58]

Although all smokers are at increased risk, a 20 pack-year history is a significant threshold for increased risk of postoperative pulmonary complications. A history of 20 pack-years, or consumption of more than 20 cigarettes per day, appears to be the threshold for increased risk, but the presence of a productive cough is probably more important.[11] A history of more than 40 pack-years of smoking suggests the need for spirometry and a strong suspicion of obstructive lung disease.

Previous recommendations to discontinue smoking 2 to 4 weeks preoperatively were based only on observations that a 5-day abstinence did not protect against postoperative pulmonary complications. To be of benefit, the preoperative duration of smoking cessation should be prolonged. A significant decrease in postoperative pulmonary complications occurs only in patients who have stopped smoking for at least 8 weeks preoperatively. This 8-week smoke-free interval is consistent with data indicating that this same interval of abstinence is required to effect improvement in small airway function, closing volumes, sputum production, and tracheobronchial clearance of radiolabeled particles.

Encouraging smoking cessation is worthwhile, even though only 20% of smokers will quit when advised to do so by the physician before an elective operation. In an evaluation of 200 patients undergoing CABG, patients who had stopped smoking for 2 months or less had a pulmonary complication rate almost four times that of patients who had stopped for more than 2 months (57% vs. 14%). Patients who had stopped smoking for more than 6 months had rates similar to those who had never smoked (11%). Preoperative pulmonary dysfunction increased with independent risk factors, increased pack-years of smoking, prolonged surgical time, and the use of enflurane.[59]

Some studies have suggested that smokers have a decreased incidence of postoperative deep venous thrombosis, suggesting that patients who stop smoking preoperatively may be at a higher risk for developing thrombophlebitis. Although this information may be valid, we believe that the trade-off risk for pulmonary complications, both in incidence and in severity, is high enough that cessation should be encouraged. Obviously, mechanical or chemical antithrombotic prophylaxis should be considered in both smokers and nonsmokers.[11]

Chronic Obstructive Pulmonary Disease

The energy cost of breathing is 1% to 5% in healthy persons. COPD results in increased airway resistance and hyperinflation, which increase the energy cost of breathing to 15% of total oxygen consumption.[60]

A survey by the College of General Practitioners indicated that 80% of women aged 40 to 64 years have chronic bronchitis.[61] Complications occur three times more frequently in patients with cough or chronic lung disease.[8] Most investigators have concluded that postoperative pulmonary complications including fever, atelectasis, pneumonia, and exacerbation of bronchitis and respiratory failure occur more commonly two to six times in patients with COPD.[11] Patients with COPD are at increased risk for developing postoperative pulmonary complications than those with restrictive lung disease where cough and respiratory flow rates are preserved.

Although the clinical history remains important, a number of reports suggest that patients with COPD and abnormal pulmonary function tests are at higher risk for developing postoperative pulmonary complications than is the normal population. However, pulmonary function test abnormality has reliably demonstrated the ability to quantitate that risk. Specific values are associated with an increased risk. In fact, no degree of spirometric abnormality can be considered absolutely prohibitive for a nonthoracic procedure until FEV_1 reaches values below 450 mL. As previously stated, a PCO_2 above 45 mm Hg seems to be predictive of high risk of morbidity and mortality.[11]

Anesthesia and surgery-induced alterations in pulmonary physiology predispose the pulmonary parenchyma to a number of complications. In patients with significant predisposing factors (Table 2–12) or abnormal pulmonary function tests (Table 2–13), diligent preoperative preparation and postoperative care (Table 2–14) may decrease the rate of pulmonary complications. Perioperative respiratory care must emphasize sustained maximum inspiration to increase alveolar inflation and maintain a near normal FRC. Positive-pressure breathing using blow bottles and endotracheal stimulation is only variably effective and may in fact be harmful. Incentive spirometry appears to be the most effective and potentially most cost-effective postoperative maneuver to decrease the risk of perioperative atelectasis and should be a routine part of perioperative care in those at risk. Unfortunately, alveoli remain inflated for only an hour, and any effective pulmonary maneuver or treatment must be scheduled on a frequent (hourly) basis during the patient's waking hours.[4] Antibiotics have been advocated for those patients with chronic purulent sputum, and elective surgery should be postponed until a full course of antibiotics is completed.[8]

Preoperative education as to the importance of deep breathing, coughing, and the appropriate use of the incentive spirometer is more effective than attempting to teach or implement these principles during postoperative convalescence in the presence of pain.[11] In specific situations, continuation of

TABLE 2–13. **Pulmonary Function Criteria Suggesting Increased Risk of Postoperative Complications**

Spirometric Function	Abdominal Surgery
FVC	<70% predicted or <2 L
	<75% predicted or <1.7 L
	< 70% predicted
FEV_1	<70% predicted or <1.2 L
FEV_1/FVC	<65%
FVC	
FEF_{25-75}	<50% predicted or <1.6 L
MEFR	<200 L/min
MVV	<50% predicted or <28 L/min
RV	Increased >47%
Dco	<50% predicted
$PaCO_2$	>45 mm Hg
PAP	
PVR	190 dyne • sec • cm^5
	1 L/min
Vo_2	<1 L/min
	<15 ml/kg/min

Modified from Gass GD, Olsen GN: Preoperative pulmonary function testing to predict postoperative morbidity and mortality. Chest 89:127–135, 1986.

aminophylline into the postoperative period may be particularly beneficial in upper abdominal surgical procedures, as aminophylline may improve diaphragmatic function in the immediate postoperative period.[11]

Postoperative prophylactic lung expansion ma-

TABLE 2–14. **Perioperative Prophylactic Pulmonary Maneuvers**

Cessation of smoking

Bronchodilators (preoperative and postoperative)

Chest physiotherapy and postural drainage (preoperative and postoperative)

Preoperative education in use of incentive spirometer and deep breathing exercises

Preoperative incentive spirometry and deep breathing exercises

Preoperative antibiotics if sputum is purulent

Preoperative corticosteroids in cases of refractory bronchospasm

Early postoperative ambulation

Antiembolic prophylaxis

Adequate analgesia

Reproduced from Houston MC, et al: Preoperative medical consultation and evaluation of surgical risk. South Med J 80:1385–1397, 1987.

neuvers should include early ambulation, as the upright position alone increases FRC by 10% to 20%. Routine chest physiotherapy is of little benefit; however, there is a role for chest physiotherapy in the treatment of severe lobar atelectasis or in clinical situations characterized by sputum production in excess of 30 mL/day.[11]

Stein and Cassar[62] evaluated patients with an FEV_1/FVC ratio below 0.70, an end-tidal PCO_2 above 45 mm Hg, or a maximal expiratory flow rate below 200 L/min and found that failure to receive a perioperative preventive regimen of bronchodilators, chest physiotherapy, and postural drainage resulted in a 60% risk of developing postoperative pulmonary complications. In contrast, the risk of postoperative pulmonary complications in patients with normal values and those with abnormal values but who were placed on a postoperative preventive regimen was markedly decreased (21% and 10%, respectively).[11]

Another recent study of 170 consecutive operations performed in 89 patients with severe obstructive pulmonary disease (defined as an FEV_1 less than 50% of predicted) reported postoperative pulmonary complications in 31 operations (29%), primarily related to the type and duration of surgery, with the risk increasing to 56% after major abdominal procedures. The incidence was 4% for procedures lasting less than 1 hour, 23% for operations between 1 to 2 hours, 38% for procedures lasting 2 to 4 hours, and 73% for procedures of more than 4 hours. The mortality in this study was 5.6% and the incidence of ventilatory failure, both fatal and nonfatal, was 5.6%.[63]

A prospective evaluation of 153 patients without pulmonary compromise randomized patients into a control group of 84 patients who were not instructed in breathing exercises and a therapy group of 69 patients who had preoperative and postoperative breathing exercises supervised by a physical therapist. The incidence of postoperative complications as evaluated with chest radiographs, arterial blood gas values, and temperature elevation was less (19%) in the treatment group than in the control group (60%). Only 4% of patients in the treatment group had clinical evidence of pulmonary dysfunction, compared to 35% in the control group. Preoperative pulmonary function test values were not predictive.[24]

Another study indicated that only 4% of patients who underwent physical therapy had postoperative clinical evidence of pulmonary dysfunction, compared to 35% of patients in the group that did not receive physical therapy.[24]

Perioperative IPPB, chest physiotherapy, and updraft nebulizer treatments are time-consuming to administer and are no more beneficial than postoperative incentive spirometry, irrespective of the presence of lung disease and the use of CPAP delivered by mask, in preventing complications. Moreover, self-administered incentive spirometry is so simple and inexpensive that it has become a routine treatment for many patients undergoing abdominal procedures.[16] Because alveoli, once inflated, tend to remain inflated for only an hour, these maneuvers should be repeated on an hourly basis. Pulmonary complications have been reduced from 30% in controls to 10% in treated patients using postlaparotomy incentive spirometry. However, complication rates did not change in one study that included only patients with a "low risk" of pulmonary complications.[8]

Although not routinely prescribed, IPPB may be beneficial for those women who cannot or will not take deep inspirations.[23]

Bronchospastic Disorders

Asthma affects 4% to 5% of the population.[61] Perioperative bronchospasm may occur unpredictably. However, women with bronchospastic disorders, asthma, or COPD have increased airway reactivity to a number of chemical, pharmacologic, and physical stimuli. In fact, the frequency of perioperative bronchospasm related to airway manipulation and tracheal intubation of asthmatic patients is six times that of normal controls.

Wheezing, the principal clinical finding present during perioperative bronchospasm, may result from many pathologic conditions (Table 2–14). As airway resistance increases, air trapping (autopositive end-expiratory pressure) may occur, with resultant decreases in venous return and even hypotension secondary to increased intrathoracic pressure.[2]

Perioperative concerns for patients with asthma should focus on the factors likely to result in exacerbation of bronchospasm and the problems of poor wound healing or adrenal insufficiency in those patients who are steroid dependent. To date, patient classification by asthma severity is not predictive of the risk of postoperative bronchospasm or other pulmonary complications. However, the risk of postoperative pulmonary complications is related to the site of operation and duration of anesthesia.[11]

Although no studies clearly demonstrate the asthmatic to be at higher risk for postoperative pulmonary complications, endotracheal intubation and handling of the viscera are probably the two most important factors that potentially precipitate bronchospasm during general anesthesia. Tracheal intubation initiates bronchospasm in 7% of asthmatics. Regional anesthesia should be considered if possible, as asthmatics receiving general anesthesia without intubation have an incidence of bronchospasm similar to that of patients receiving regional anesthesia. While all of the inhalational agents are equally effective in preventing or reversing bronchospasm, halothane is considered the anesthetic of choice for asthmatics because of its rapid induction, lack of salivation, increased lung compliance, and fewer postoperative complications.[11] Unfortunately, this agent is more likely to induce ventricular arrhythmias than enflurane or isoflurane. Thiopental has no effect on bronchomotor tone, and ketamine prevents antigen-induced increases in pulmonary resistance in experimental models of asthma and should be considered for induction. Ketamine affects bronchodilation both directly and by release of endogenous catecholamines and is the IV induction agent of choice in the patient who is actively wheezing.[2] The use of *d*-tubocurare is discouraged because it is associated with histamine release.

Although narcotic effects have not been well studied in asthmatics, morphine has been associated with histamine release, and some recommend avoiding its use in asthmatics.[10]

TREATMENT. The goal of preoperative preparation of asthmatic patients includes optimizing pulmonary function and eliminating clinical wheezing. The latter is important, as the risk of pulmonary complications is reduced in patients who are free of preoperative wheezing.[11] In specific situations, the addition of or an increase in steroid dose may be required 7 to 10 days preoperatively. If surgery is emergent, the surgeon should proceed in the presence of mild wheezing, realizing the relatively low postoperative risk of a severe exacerbation of asthma.[11]

Sympathetic agents continue as the mainstay of the treatment of patients with bronchospasm. β-agonists lead to an increase in the intracellular concentration of cyclic adenosine monophosphate, relaxing bronchial smooth muscle and decreasing airway resistance. A secondary action involves inhibiting other mediators from mast cells. Bronchial dilation results from the stimulation of β_2 receptors in the lung. Agents such as epinephrine and isuprel stimulate both β_2 and β_1 receptors; the latter is associated with significant tachycardia. When given by metered-dose inhaler, most β-agonists have peak effects in the first 10 to 30 minutes, with efficacy waning in about 3 hours.[17] Delivery by nebulizer or aerosol metered-dose inhaler produces less systemic absorption while minimizing side effects (tremor, palpitation, tachycardia, hypokalemia, hypoglycemia, tachyphylaxis, uterine relaxation, pulmonary edema). Agents that are predominantly β_2-agonists (albuterol, metaproterenol, terbutaline), are preferable; however, they may produce β_1 side effects when administered in high doses or by IV or subcutaneous route.[2] Clinically useful β_2-selective drugs include metaproterenol and albuterol, both of which are well tolerated and have long half-lives of approximately 5 to 6 hours. Another medication (an atropine-like compound), ipratropium bromide, blocks the parasympathetic system, allowing sympathetic system predominance. Anticholinergic agents block muscarinic receptors, interfering with vagal cholinergic tone and blocking cholinergic reflex bronchoconstriction, and are more effective in patients with COPD than in the asthmatic. The advent of ipratropium bromide, a poorly absorbed inhaled anticholinergic, has made this class of drug an important adjunctive therapy.[17] Respiratory therapists administer these drugs usually in an aerosol solution and can advise the obstetrician-gynecologist of the recommended dilutions and methods of delivery. Despite the long half-life (5–6 hours) these medications can be repeated at 4-hour intervals in the compromised patient.

Corticosteroids are efficacious in the treatment of acute asthma, as steroids potentiate the effects of epinephrine by inhibiting its breakdown by catechol methyl transferase and preventing and reversing pulmonary receptor down-regulation. Inhaled steroids require weeks to become fully effective. The onset of action for systemic steroids is achieved in less than 12 hours.[17] The potent anti-inflammatory action of corticosteroids has led some experts to advocate their earlier use in the treatment of patients with chronic asthma.[2] Steroids can be used perioperatively in the absence of active infection. Their potential adverse effects on wound healing should be considered and may alter intraoperative decisions, including type of suture material or closure. Any patient recently treated (within 1 year) with steroids should receive supplementation with perioperative stress dosages administered parenterally.

Obesity

Obese patients are eight times more likely to develop pulmonary complications, with the reported incidence of pulmonary complications in the obese varying from 3.9% to 95%.[11] Unfortunately, assessment for surgical risk of postoperative pulmonary complications related to obesity is limited by the paucity of prospective data, the failure of many studies to define obesity, and the lack of a uniform definition of complications. Previous reports suggest an extremely high (20%) mortality in very obese women (>300 lb) undergoing hysterectomy for endometrial cancer.[64] Although this study has often been cited in evidence of an increased operative mortality, the figure represents only one death among five such women. The average mortality in morbidly obese women undergoing abdominal hysterectomy approaches 1%.[65]

Obese patients have a more marked decrease in postoperative VC and a lower baseline for postoperative oxygenation. The associated postoperative hypoxemia, which may last 4 to 6 days after intraabdominal procedures, presents a universal hazard in the morbidly obese patient. In one prospective study obesity, defined as a weight 10% above the Metropolitan Life Insurance table of weights, was the most important risk factor associated with clinically significant atelectasis following upper abdominal surgery. Pulmonary complications occurred in 53% of obese patients and 9% of normal-weight patients.[11]

The increased energy expenditure in the morbidly obese patient coupled with the metabolic activity of fat increases the basal body rate, oxygen consumption, and CO_2 production. Fat loads the body wall, reducing respiratory compliance and static lung volumes, particularly expiratory reserve volume (ERV) and FRC. FRC may fall within closing capacity during respiration, producing profound ventilation–perfusion mismatches and anatomic shunts that are further accentuated by the supine position.[66]

Circulating blood volume, plasma volume, and cardiac output rise proportionately with weight,[66] and the hemodynamic status of uncomplicated obesity is one of both increased afterload and preload.

Obese women also have significantly higher gastric volumes (42.3 mL compared to 14.7 mL) and lower pH (1.7 compared to 3.7) than nonobese women. In fact, 75% of morbidly obese patients have a gastric volume greater than 25 mL and a gastric pH below 2.5, placing them at higher risk for aspiration. Appropriate preoperative medication and perioperative attention to intubation and extubation are mandatory.[66]

Before elective surgery, the most important step the physician can take on behalf of the obese patient is to encourage and even insist on preoperative weight loss. A weight loss as small as 10% to 15%

may have a dramatic benefit on cardiopulmonary and metabolic functions. Changes in VC, ERV, MRV, and right-to-left shunting as well as other pulmonary functions are dramatically improved with weight loss. Although evidence of left ventricular dysfunction persists after weight loss, hypertension, total blood volume, pulmonary blood volume, stroke volume, and left ventricular stroke work are all reduced.[66]

Patients with obesity hypoventilation syndrome are an extremely high-risk subset of patients more likely to exhibit severe cardiopulmonary derangements than obese patients without the obesity hypoventilation syndrome. Although fewer than 10% of the morbidly obese have the obesity hypoventilation syndrome, it may be prudent to postpone a nonemergency operation in this group of patients. Weight loss of as little as 10 to 20 kg may bring about a significant improvement in PaO_2 and $PaCO_2$.

Preoperative arterial blood gas measurements and pulmonary function tests should be considered in all obese patients. Any extent of hypoxemia in a morbidly obese patient should prompt consideration of continuous postoperative SO_2 monitoring. Assessment of thyroid function should be part of the routine evaluation of morbidly obese patients, and a preoperative sleep study may disclose a common pattern of obstructive sleep apnea. Postoperative head-of-bed elevation and prophylactic measures such as incentive spirometry should be used. Early ambulation is essential, and affixing a trapeze bar over the bed may be beneficial in improving postoperative mobility.[11] Antiembolic prophylaxis and an intensive postoperative pulmonary regimen are appropriate.

Age

Elderly patients are more likely to undergo major urgent or emergency procedures, with mortality rates four to five times those of elective procedures (Table 2–15). This may reflect either poor physiologic reserves, inaccessibility of medical care, or the reluctance of surgeons and anesthesiologists to subject elderly patients to elective surgery (Table 2–15).[53]

Elderly patients have a diminished cough reflex and a lessened ability to clear secretions, as well as diminished airway protective reflexes.[67] Associated degenerative changes in connective tissue collagen and elastin fibers, decreases in chest wall compliance, and decrease in lung tissue elastic recoil result in reduced VC and air flow rates. There is an increase in small airway closing volume, causing

TABLE 2–15. **Preoperative Risk Factors and Postoperative Respiratory Complications in the Elderly**

Preoperative Risk Factor	Relative Risk of Postoperative Respiratory Complication
Age > 75 yr	↑ approximately 1.5×
Male sex	↑ 1.3–4×
Smoking	↑ 1.5–7×
>120% ideal weight	↑ 2×
Emergency surgery	↑ 1.5–2.5×
Dyspnea on minimal exercise (NYHA class III or IV)	↑ 2×
ASA class 3 or 4	↑ 2–5×
Incision near diaphragm	↑ 2×
Past respiratory history or recent symptoms	↑ 2×
Acute respiratory disease	↑ 2–3×
Peak flow 250 L/min	↑ 1.5–2×
FEV_1/FVC 70%	↑ approximately 2–3×

Modified from Seymour DG: Aspects of surgery in the elderly: Preoperative medical assessment. Br J Hosp Med, February 1987, pp 102–112.

physiologic shunting and arterial hypoxemia, and an increased reliance on diaphragmatic breathing.[68]

Age-related pulmonary alterations include thoracic cage changes, reflected by an increased rigidity and decreased volume, as well as changes in the lung parenchyma. Expiratory muscle strength and endurance decrease. Measures of pulmonary function show an increase in FRC, RV, and dead space, as well as a decrease in FEV and PEFR.[69]

These changes culminate in an incidence of postoperative respiratory complications in the elderly general surgical population varying between 20% and 40%. Additionally, between one sixth and one third of all postoperative deaths in patients over 65 are in part related to a respiratory etiology.[70]

Among patients more than 80 years old who underwent upper abdominal or thoracic operations, 24% and 57% affected required controlled ventilation within 24 hours postoperatively. When underlying physical status and pulmonary function are considered, however, age alone does not seem to confer an independent risk of mortality or pulmonary complications, and surgical decisions should not be made on the basis of age alone.[8,70]

Viral Infections

Upper respiratory tract infection (URI) impairs pulmonary function.[8] Following a recent URI children are two to seven times more likely to have a respiratory-related adverse perioperative pulmonary event following intubation.[71] Normal adult subjects with viral respiratory tract infections may demon-

strate persistent increased airway reactivity for as long as 7 weeks after complete symptomatic recovery. Management of patients with a recent or current URI prior to elective surgery is controversial. There is no conclusive evidence that anesthesia after a recent URI in an otherwise healthy adult patient results in a higher rate of respiratory complications[2]; however, patient management, including timing of anesthesia and technique, should be related to extent of infection, the radicality of the procedure, the emergency or nonemergency nature, as well as the duration of the planned surgical procedure. It would seem prudent to postpone nonemergency procedures to allow parenchymal recovery.

Surgical Factors

Incision

Although postoperative pulmonary complications can occur in any patient, including those with a normal pulmonary history and examination, the risk is greatly influenced by incision site. Decreases in VC, altered diaphragmatic excursion, changes in regional ventilation with a shift of ventilation from the bases of the lungs to the apices, and restriction of lung expansion after abdominal surgery results in a postoperative shift from predominantly abdominal to rib cage breathing. Following nonabdominal surgery, the risk of subsequent pulmonary complications is less than 1%. As the incision site approaches the diaphragm, the incidence of complications increases, approaching 30% with an upper abdominal incision. In general, vertical incisions are associated with an increased risk for, and greater severity of, atelectasis and hypoxemia than are horizontal incisions.[11] Vertical laparotomies that cross several dermatomes seem to be associated with more pain and a higher incidence of pneumonia than are horizontal incisions.[8] Although choice of incision site should be related to a number of factors, we believe that the role of the transverse incision should be further explored in many noncustomary situations, particularly in high-risk patients.

Although most women tolerate any type of incision, planning may allow "alteration" or consideration of a different type of incision or a different placement of the incision.

Duration of Surgery

In-hospital mortality increases from 1.6% for operative procedures lasting less than 2 hours to 7% for procedures lasting 2 to 6 hours, to 14% for procedures lasting 6 to 20 hours.[11] Although the etiology of morbidity and mortality differ, surgical procedures lasting more than 3 hours are associated with a twofold increased risk of pulmonary complications. It is imperative that the surgical team work diligently to complete the operative procedure as efficiently as possible.

Gastric Intubation

Prolonged (>24 hours) nasogastric suction alters gastroesophageal competency and is one factor strongly associated with the development of postoperative pulmonary complications.[11] When coupled with the fact that prophylactic gastric suction does not decrease operative morbidity, prevent ileus, or hasten the return of bowel function,[4] there appears to be little benefit from the routine prophylactic use of nasogastric tubes following an abdominal procedure.

Aspiration

Aspiration of acidic material damages type I membranous pneumocytes responsible for surfactant production and produces an intense bronchorrhea. Consequently, type II pneumocytes, or granulopneumocytes, proliferate in an exudative response, to the exclusion of type I pneumocytes. Surfactant levels decrease. The subsequent alveolar capillary block results in decreased lung compliance, an increased risk of superimposed infection, and additional parenchymal damage.

Silent or active aspiration can occur in any patient during any phase of the surgical patient's hospital stay; however, patients receiving postoperative sedation, general anesthesia, long-term sedation, or major regional blocks are all at high risk. Reports indicate that as many as 16% to 27% of all anesthetized patients have evidence of silent aspiration, which can be facilitated by a number of mechanisms, including gastric insufflation during anesthetic induction, altered lower esophageal sphincter relaxation, or intraoperative manipulation. Parameters suggesting a significantly increased risk of perioperative aspiration include a gastric pH at or below 2.5 and a gastric volume greater than 25 mL.[72] Metoclopramide, a dopamine$_2$ inhibitor, augments lower esophageal sphincter tone and stimulates gastric motility, and cimetidine, a well-known H$_2$ antihistamine, reduces gastric acidity.[73] In women undergoing gynecologic surgery, the combination of metoclopramide and cimetidine results in a mean gastric pH of 6.9 and a mean gastric volume of 2 mL. These aspiration risks are less than in controls, as metoclopramide alone reduces the risk of aspiration related to volume and cimetidine alone reduces the risk related to pH.

Unrecognized bronchopulmonary aspiration in patients who clinically present with dyspnea, tachycardia, cyanosis, rales, and rhonchi and with laboratory findings of hypoxemia and interstitial fluid has a mortality rate of 40% to 80%. Active aspiration is the most common cause of aspiration in ICU.[72] If aspiration is suspected or diagnosed, treatment is directed toward maintenance of arterial oxygenation, broad-spectrum antibiotic coverage, and support.

Postoperative Analgesia

The most important consideration during the postoperative period of patients at risk for postoperative pulmonary complications is pain management. Pain is associated with decreased VT, tachypnea, and decreased FRC. Efforts should be made to decrease narcotic requirements, which might include the use of parenteral Toradol. Central apnea, obstructive apnea, and paradoxical breathing are common to patients receiving postoperative narcotic analgesia, as narcotics and inhalational anesthetics both suppress central drive. The upper airway is especially prone to functional alteration and is particularly affected by narcotics; airway patency can be compromised.

Pain associated with chest wall injury or a recent surgical procedure in the torso predisposes to the shallow breathing that is a major cause of postoperative atelectasis. Infiltration of the surgical incision with a local anesthetic or epidural anesthesia of the involved area in the postoperative period relieves the pain and permits increased ventilatory effort without discomfort.

Patient-controlled analgesia (PCA), an effective means of postoperative pain control, is not well accepted by all patients, requires additional expensive equipment, and has not been demonstrated to improve pulmonary mechanics. In a randomized prospective trial of 230 women undergoing abdominal hysterectomy with intermittant morphine infusion (control) or continuous (0.5, 1.0, or 2.0 mg/hr) morphine infusion, those receiving continuous morphine infusion received significantly more opioid medication 9 to 72 hours after the operation than those who received no infusion. The continuous morphine infusion did not significantly decrease the number of patient demands of supplemental bolus doses administered compared with the control group. Overall, 84% of patients who completed the 72-hour study were able to achieve adequate analgesia without requiring changes in the PCA regimen or experiencing major side effects.[74]

Regional anesthesia when used effectively and without supplemental IV drugs may reduce the incidence of postoperative pulmonary complications. Numerous authors have demonstrated that postoperative epidural administration of opiates for local anesthesia results in significant improvement in lung function as compared with systemic analgesia after upper abdominal surgery. Studies using VC as an indication of lung function demonstrated that VC was 15% to 20% greater with epidural analgesia than with systemic administration of analgesic agents. The mean improvement in lung function was 15%. All authors reported a parallel improvement in FEV_1 associated with epidural analgesia. Freedom from pain leads to a 15% to 20% improvement in VC.[75] Epidural and intrathecal techniques are of special interest to both the anesthesiologist and surgeon for delivering both intraoperative and postoperative analgesics. Small doses of narcotic can effect profound and prolonged analgesia; however, respiratory depression can occur, especially if parenteral narcotics are administered concurrently. In addition to improved respiratory function, epidural anesthesia results in a lower incidence of thromboembolic phenomena, a decrease in intraoperative blood loss, a decrease in perioperative catabolism, earlier ambulation, and a decrease in the need for postoperative sedatives.

Respiratory depression occurs in 4% to 7% of patients receiving intrathecal morphine and in 0.9% to 4% of patients receiving epidural morphine. Spinal opioids produce a progressive 20% to 30% decrease in the slope of the CO_2 response curves.[2] Associated respiratory depression occurs in a bimodal fashion. The initial effect occurs within hours of dosing and is secondary to vascular absorption and the rapid delivery of opioids to the brain by way of the basivertebral plexus. The delayed effect (6–8 hours) is thought to be related to drug migration rostrally, and occasionally, respiratory depression may occur up to 24 hours after drug administration. Continued monitoring at additional expense may be necessary.[20]

Advances in anesthesia, surgical technique, and perioperative care have made operative intervention possible in the majority of patients with serious underlying cardiopulmonary disease who previously might have been denied the benefits of a surgical procedure.

References

1. Hedenstierna G: Mechanisms of postoperative pulmonary dysfunction. Acta Chir Scand Suppl 550:152–158, 1988.
2. Entrup MH, Davis FG: Perioperative complications of anesthesia. Surg Clin North Am 71:1151–1173, 1991.
3. Good ML: Capnography: A comprehensive review. American Society of Anesthesiologists 1991 Annual Refresher Course Lectures, lecture 431. San Francisco, Oct 26–30, 1991.
4. Orr JW Jr: Introduction to pelvic surgery: Pre and post operative care. In Gusberg S (ed): Female Genital Cancer. London: Churchill Livingstone, 1988.
5. Huddleston VB: Postoperative problems: Current nursing management. Pulmonary problems. Crit Care Nurs Clin North Am 2:527–536, 1990.
6. Mecca RD: Essentials of pulmonary physiology. In Civetta JM, Taylor RW, Kirby RR (eds): Critical Care, 2nd ed, chap 92. Philadelphia: JB Lippincott, 1992.
7. Caton D: Pregnancy: Essential physiologic concerns. In Civetta JM, Taylor RW, Kirby RR (eds): Critical Care, 2nd ed, chap 64. Philadelphia: JB Lippincott, 1992.
8. Mohr DN, Jett JR: Preoperative evaluation of pulmonary risk factors. J Gen Intern Med 3:277–287, 1988.
9. Craig DB: Postoperative recovery of pulmonary function. Anesth Analg 60:46, 1981.
10. Wiener-Kronish JP: Preoperative evaluation. In Murray JF, Nadel JA (eds): Textbook of Respiratory Medicine, chap 32. Philadelphia: WB Saunders, 1988.
11. Jackson CV: Preoperative pulmonary evaluation. Arch Intern Med 148:21–27, 1988.
12. Ravin MB: Comparison of spinal and general anesthesia for lower abdominal surgery in patients with chronic obstructive pulmonary disease. Anesthesiology 35:319–322, 1971.
13. Boutrous AR, Weisel M: Comparison of effects of three anaesthetic techniques on patients with severe pulmonary obstructive disease. Can Anaesth Soc J 18:286–292, 1971.
14. Iber C: Pulmonary function testing in clinical practice. Contemp Intern Med, May 1990, p 31.

15. Lawrence VA, Page CP, Harris GD: Preoperative spirometry before abdominal operations: A critical appraisal of its predictive value. Arch Intern Med 149:280–285, 1989.
16. Zibrak JD, O'Donnell CR, Marton K: Indications for pulmonary function testing. Ann Intern Med 112:763–771, 1990.
17. Bishop MJ: Respiratory disease: When to delay surgery and how to proceed. American Society of Anesthesiologists 1991 Annual Refresher Course Lectures, lecture 224. San Francisco, Oct 26–30, 1991.
18. Pett SB Jr, Wernly JA: Respiratory function in surgical patients: Perioperative evaluation and management. Surg Annu 20:311–329, 1988.
19. Gass GD, Olsen GN: Preoperative pulmonary function testing to predict postoperative morbidity and mortality. Chest 89:127, 1989.
20. Boysen PG: Preoperative pulmonary function testing. In Civetta JM, Taylor RW, Kirby RR (eds): Critical Care, 2nd ed, chap 40. Philadelphia: JB Lippincott, 1992.
21. Orr JW Jr: Intraoperative and postoperative care. In Copeland LC (ed): Textbook of Gynecology. Philadelphia: WB Saunders, 1992.
22. Nolan TE, Gallup DG: The gynecologist and surgical respiratory care. Female Patient 17:15, 1992.
23. O'Donohue WJ Jr: Postoperative pulmonary complications: When are preventive and therapeutic measures necessary? Postgrad Med 91:167–175, 1992.
24. Roukema JA, Carol EJ, Prins JG: The prevention of pulmonary complications after upper abdominal surgery in patients with noncompromised pulmonary status. Arch Surg 123:30–34, 1988.
25. Grogan DE, Irwin RS, Channick R, et al: Complications associated with thoracentesis: A prospective, randomized study comparing three different approaches. Arch Intern Med 150:873–877, 1990.
26. Windsor JA, Hill GL: Risk factors for postoperative pneumonia. Ann Surg 208:209, 1988.
27. Spence TH: Pneumonia. In Civetta JM, Taylor RW, Kirby RR (eds): Critical Care, 2nd ed, chap 40. Philadelphia: JB Lippincott, 1992.
28. Mustard RA, Bohnen JMA, Rosati C, Schouten D: Pneumonia complicating abdominal sepsis. Arch Surg 126:170–175, 1991.
29. Burchard K: Diagnosis and treatment of pneumonia in the surgical intensive care unit. Surgery Gynecol Obstet 171s:35–40, 1990.
30. Meduri GU: Ventilator-associated pneumonia in patients with respiratory failure: A diagnostic approach. Chest 97:1208–1219, 1990.
31. Gertanner RE, Decampo T, Alleyn JN, Averette HE: Routine intensive care for pelvic exenterative operations. Surg Gynecol Obstet 153:657–661, 1981.
32. Rochon RB, Mozingo DW, Weigelt JA: New modes of mechanical ventilation. Surg Clin North Am 71:843–858, 1991.
33. Schwieger I, Gamulin Z, Suter PM: Lung function during anesthesia and respiratory insufficiency in the postoperative period: Physiological and clinical implications. Acta Anaesthesiol Scand 33:527–534, 1989.
34. Schuster DP: A physiologic approach to initiating, maintaining, and withdrawing mechanical ventilatory support during acute respiratory failure. Am J Med 88:268–278, 1990.
35. Task Force on Guidelines, Society of Critical Care Medicine: Guidelines for standards of care for patients with acute respiratory failure on mechanical ventilatory support. Crit Care Med 19:275–278, 1991.
35a. Bostek CC: Oxygen toxicity: An introduction. J Am Assoc Nurse Anesthetists 57:231–237, 1989.
36. Civetta JM: Bedside use of arterial and venous oximetry. In Civetta JM, Taylor RW, Kirby RR (eds): Critical Care, 2nd ed, chap 25. Philadelphia: JB Lippincott, 1992.
37. Downs JB: What's new in mechanical ventilation. American Society of Anesthesiologists 1991 Annual Refresher Course Lectures, lecture 411. San Francisco, Oct 26–30, 1991.
38. Clevenger FW, Acosta JA, Osler TM, et al: Barotrauma associated with high-frequency jet ventilation for hypoxic salvage. Arch Surg 125:1542–1545, 1990.
39. Bassili HR, Deitel M: Effect of nutritional support on weaning patients off mechanical ventilators. JPEN J Parenter Enter Nutr 5(2):161–163, 1981.
40. Severinghaus JW: Oximetry: What does it tell you? American Society of Anesthesiologists 1991 Annual Refresher Course Lectures, lecture 266. San Francisco, Oct 26–30, 1991.
41. Schnapp LM, Cohen NH: Pulse oximetry, uses and abuses. Chest 98:1244–1250, 1990.
42. Bowton DL, Scuderi PE, Harris L, Haponik EF: Pulse oximetry monitoring outside the intensive care unit: Progress or problem:? Ann Intern Med 115:450–454, 1991.
43. Benumof JL: Respiratory physiology and respiratory function during anesthesia. In Miller RD (ed): Anesthesia, 3rd ed. New York: Churchill Livingstone, 1990.
44. Cohen NH: Respiratory monitoring in the intensive care unit. American Society of Anesthesiologists 1991 Annual Refresher Course Lectures, lecture 142. San Francisco, Oct 26–30, 1991.
45. Yang KL, Tobin MJ: Prediction of success in weaning from mechanical ventilation. ACP J Club 115(2):52, 1991.
46. Kelly BJ, Luce JM: The diagnosis and management of neuromuscular diseases causing respiratory failure. Chest 99:1485–1496, 1991.
47. Gallagher TJ: Adult respiratory distress syndrome. American Society of Anesthesiologists 1991 Annual Refresher Course Lectures, lecture 115. San Francisco, Oct 26–30, 1991.
48. Fowkes FGR: The value of routine preoperative chest x-rays. Br J Hosp Med, February 1986, p 120.
49. Crocco JA. Adult respiratory distress syndrome. New York State J Med 86:508–510, 1986.
50. Waid-Jones MI, Coursin DB: Perioperative considerations for patients treated with bleomycin. Chest 99:993–999, 1991.
51. Cugell DW, Morgan WKC, Perkins DG, Rubin A: The respiratory effects of cobalt. Arch Intern Med 150:177–183, 1990.
52. Sue DY, Wasserman K: Impact of integrative cardiopulmonary exercise testing on clinical decision making. Chest 99:981–992, 1991.
53. Klein JT, Rosen MJ: Preoperative evaluation of pulmonary status. Mt Sinai J Med 58:37–40, 1991.
54. Bonekat HW, Chu CS, Shigeoka JW: Preoperative pulmonary assessment of the surgical patient. Mo Med 85(11):729–736, 1988.
55. Boghosian SG, Mooradian AD: Usefulness of routine preoperative chest roentgenograms in elderly patients. J Am Geriatr Soc 35:142–146, 1987.
56. Berlowitz DR, Ghalill K, Moskowitz MA: The use of follow-up chest roentgenograms among hospitalized patients. Arch Intern Med 149:821–825, 1989.
57. Hall JB, Shite SR, Karrison T: Efficacy of daily routine chest 19:689–693, 1991.

58. Anderson ME, Belani KG: Short-term preoperative smoking abstinence. Am Fam Physician 41:1191–1194, 1990.

59. Warner MA, Offord KP, Warner ME, et al: Role of preoperative cessation of smoking and other factors in postoperative pulmonary complications: A blinded prospective study of coronary artery bypass patients. Mayo Clin Proc 64:609–616, 1989.

60. Tobin MJ: Respiratory muscle dysfunction: When to anticipate, how to minimize. How overload and weakness contribute to respiratory fatigue. J Crit Illness 6(7):711–722, 1991.

61. Clark RA: Obstructive airways disease in surgical practice. J R Coll Surg Edinb 34:177–184, 1989.

62. Stein M, Cassara EL: Preoperative pulmonary evaluation and therapy on surgery patients. JAMA 258:927–930, 1970.

63. Kroenke K, Lawrence VA, Theroux JF, Tuley MR: Operative risk in patients with severe obstructive pulmonary disease. Arch Intern Med 152:967–971, 1992.

64. Prem KA, Mensheha NM, McKelvey JL: Operative treatment of adenocarcinoma of the endometrium in obese women. Am J Obstet Gynecol 92:16–22, 1965.

65. Pitkin RM: Abdominal hysterectomy in obese women. Surg Gynecol Obstet 142:532–536, 1976.

66. Pasulka PS, Bistrian BR, Benotti PN, Blackburn GL: The risks of surgery in obese patients. Ann Intern Med 104:540–546, 1986.

67. Hotchkiss RS: Perioperative management of patient with chronic obstructive pulmonary disease. Int Anesthesiol Clin 26:134–142, 1988.

68. Manning FC: Preoperative evaluation of the elderly patient. Am Fam Physician 39:123–126, 1989.

69. Galazka SS: Preoperative evaluation of the elderly surgical patient. J Fam Pract 27:622–632, 1988.

70. Seymour DG: Aspects of surgery in the elderly: Preoperative medical assessment. Br J Hosp Med, February 1987, pp 102–112.

71. Hirshman CA: Anesthesia for patients with reactive airway disease. American Society of Anesthesiologists 1991 Annual Refresher Course Lectures, lecture 144. San Francisco, Oct 26–30, 1991.

72. Locicero J III: Bronchopulmonary aspiration. Surg Clin Nocta Am 69:71, 1989.

73. Gipson SL, Stovall TG, Elkins TE, Crumrine RS: Pharmacologic reduction of the risk of aspiration. South Med J 79(11):1356, 1986.

74. Parker RK, Holtmann B, White PF: Patient-controlled analgesia. Does a concurrent opioid infusion improve pain management after surgery? JAMA 266:1947–1952, 1991.

75. Sydow FW: The influence of anesthesia and postoperative analgesic management of lung function. Acta Chir Scand Suppl 550:159–168, 1988.

Complications in Gynecologic Surgery: Prevention, Recognition, and Management,
edited by James W. Orr, Jr., and Hugh M. Shingleton.
J. B. Lippincott Company, Philadelphia, © 1994.

Chapter 3

Hematologic Complications

Daniel L. Clarke-Pearson
Gustavo Rodriguez

Preoperative Preparation

Evaluation and Screening for Coexisting Hematologic Disorders

The majority of bleeding complications associated with gynecologic procedures are surgically related rather than secondary to congenital or acquired hematologic disorders. Nonetheless, even with appropriate medical management and meticulous surgical technique, unexpected hemorrhagic complications will occasionally be encountered. A thorough history, physical examination, and a directed preoperative hematologic evaluation can identify patients with a coagulation defect and reduce these hemorrhagic risks to a minimum.

The physiology of hemostasis includes a normally functioning vascular system, an adequate number of properly functioning platelets, as well as an intact coagulation cascade.[1] The immediate primary response to vessel injury is vasoconstriction. Platelets then adhere to the subendothelial structures of injured vessels. Their activation releases vasoactive substances, including 5-hydroxytryptophan, catecholamines, and platelet factor 3, which induce platelet aggregation and fusion, promoting the formation of a platelet plug. Concomitantly the coagulation cascade is triggered, resulting in formation of fibrin to stabilize and reinforce the platelet plug. Ineffective hemostasis can result from defects in any one of the three constituents of the coagulation mechanism. Defects in the vascular system and in platelets characteristically result in ineffective hemostasis immediately following vessel injury (Table 3–1).[2] Defects in the coagulation cascade result in bleeding that starts several hours to days after the initial vessel injury.

Defective hemostasis is most commonly related to deficiencies in the function or number of circulating platelets. Many drugs adversely affect platelet function, the most common groups being the nonsteroidal anti-inflammatory preparations and the β-lactam antibiotics (Table 3–2).[3] Platelet dysfunction can also occur in systemic conditions, including chronic renal failure, liver disease, disseminated intravascular coagulation, chronic myeloproliferative disorders, leukemia, dysproteinemias, systemic lupus erythematosus, and idiopathic thrombocytopenia purpura. Excessive bleeding also occurs in the presence of thrombocytopenia. Thrombocytopenia can be induced by many drugs and clinical conditions and is often acquired rather than hereditary (Table 3–3).[4,5] Spontaneous bleeding can occur with platelet counts below $20,000/mm^3$.

Defects in the coagulation cascade are unusual and are more often acquired than hereditary. Hemophilia A and B are X-linked recessive disorders predominantly affecting males and are associated with deficiencies in factors VIII and IX, respectively. Von Willebrand's disease, which can affect both

TABLE 3–1. **Comparison of the Clinical Characteristics of Platelet and Clotting Factor Disorders**

	Platelet Disorder	**Clotting Factor Disorder**
Site of bleeding	Skin, mucous membranes (nose, gums, vaginal, gastrointestinal, etc.)	Deep/soft tissue (e.g., muscles, joints)
Bleeding after cuts and scratches	Yes	No
Petechiae	Yes	No
Ecchymoses	Small, superficial	Large, deep (often palpable)
Hemarthroses	Rare	Common
Bleeding after surgery	Immediate, usually mild	Delayed (several hours or 1–2 d), then severe

Adapted from Koutts J: Clinching the diagnosis: Assessment of hemostatic function. J Pathol 17:643–647, 1985.

males and females, is a rare autosomal dominant disorder in which a deficiency in von Willebrand's factor antigen results in inadequate functioning of the factor VIII complex as well as improper adherence of platelets to the endothelium of vessels. The most common acquired coagulation factor deficiencies are those of the vitamin K–dependent coagulation factors (II, VII, IX, X). Deficiencies in these factors can result from impaired hepatic synthesis, which may occur in patients taking Coumadin or with liver disease, and from impaired absorption of vitamin K, which can occur in patients who have undergone surgical resection of the distal ileum. In addition, impaired synthesis of vitamin K–dependent factors can occur in patients taking broad-spectrum antibiotics, which have an adverse effect on gut flora, an important source of vitamin K. Deficiencies in the vitamin K–dependent factors will result in a prolonged prothrombin time (PT).

Routine coagulation screening preoperatively in patients with no history or physical findings indicative of a bleeding disorder is unwarranted both because of the low prevalence of true coagulopathies in asymptomatic patients and because of the low specificity of coagulation tests. The arbitrary normal upper limit for the prothrombin and partial thromboplastin (PTT) times is set at two standard deviations above the population mean. Therefore, the prevalence of an abnormally elevated PT or PTT should be expected to be slightly greater than 2% in any screened population. The incidence of a congenital coagulation factor deficiency in the general population has been estimated at 5 in 100,000 women, comprising mainly patients with von Willebrand's disease.[6] At a cost of $10 per PT and PTT test, the cost of diagnosis of a congenital coagulation factor deficiency in women would be in excess of $200,000 per case found. Acquired coagulation factor deficiencies are also uncommon, especially in the absence of historical or physical findings suggestive of a bleeding disorder. There-

fore, routine screening in normal patients is not warranted. In patients with historical or physical findings suggestive of a bleeding disorder, however, the specificity of the PT and PTT for diagnosing a true coagulation disorder is increased. In these patients the prevalence of an identifiable defect may be as high as 7% to 40%,[6-8] and a preoperative coagulation laboratory evaluation is warranted.

The efficacy of routine preoperative screening for coagulation abnormalities has been evaluated in several large prospective studies. All suggest that routine screening in asymptomatic patients with no historical factors suggesting a bleeding tendency is not useful. Watel et al. evaluated PT and PTT in 10,229 patients preoperatively and found 134 patients with abnormalities (1.35%).[8] When the test was repeated, only 37 patients (0.36%) had a persistently prolonged PTT.[9] Thus, 72% (97/134) of the abnormal values on initial screening were falsely elevated. When historical variables were considered in preoperative screening, Eisenberg et al. found that only 1.8% (9/480) patients) with a normal history had an abnormal PT or PTT.[7] In contrast, 18% of patients with historical risk factors had documented coagulation abnormalities. Other investigators have indicated that the preoperative bleeding time was prolonged in 110 of 1,941 screened patients.[10] However, on repeated testing, 50% of the initially abnormal bleeding times were normal. Furthermore, 75% of patients with an abnormal study had identifiable risk factors. Importantly, an abnormal coagulation study result does not necessarily imply an increased risk of perioperative bleeding. In fact, at least two groups have been unable to correlate bleeding time with operative blood loss.[11,12] Nearly all patients who have abnormalities of coagulation can be identified from a history of Coumadin use, liver disease, or other conditions (Table 3–4). The efficient use of laboratory resources mandates that preoperative screening be confined to individuals at risk.

TABLE 3–2. **Drugs That Inhibit Platelet Function**

Nonsteroidal Anti-Inflammatory Drugs
Aspirin
Indomethacin (Indocin)
Ibuprofen (Advil, Motrin, Nuprin, Rufen)
Naproxen (Naprosyn)

β-Lactam Antibiotics
Penicillins
Cephalosporins

Other Drugs
Antibiotics
Nitrofurantoin (Furadantin, Macrodantin)
Drugs that increase platelet cAMP concentration
Dipyridamole (Persantine)
Anticoagulant
Heparin
Plasma expanders
Dextrans
Hydroxyethyl starch (Hetastarch)
Cardiovascular drugs
Nitroglycerin
Isosorbide dinitrate (Isordil, Dilatrate)
Propranolol (Inderal)
Nitroprusside (Nitropress)
Nifedipine (Procardia)
Verapamil (Calan, Isoptin)
Diltiazem (Cardizem)
Quinidine
Psychotropic drugs
Tricyclic antidepressants
Phenothiazines
Anesthetics
Local
Dibucaine (Lidocaine)
Tetracaine (Carbocaine)
General
Halothane (Fluothane)
Oncologic Drugs
Mithramycin
Daunorubicin
BCNU
Miscellaneous drugs
Clofibrate (Atromid-S)
Antihistamines
Diphenhydramine
Chlorpheniramine
Radiographic contrast
Foods and food additives
Ethanol
Ajoene (garlic component)
Cumin
Onion Extract

Adapted from George JN, Shattil SJ: Acquired disorders of platelet function. In Hoffman R, et al (eds): Hematology: Basic Principles and Practice. New York: Churchill Livingstone, 1991.

TABLE 3–3. **Classification of Thrombocytopenia**

I. Primary idiopathic thrombocytopenia
  A. Acute
  B. Chronic
II. Secondary thrombocytopenia
  A. Ionizing radiation
  B. Malignant marrow infiltration
  C. Leukemia
  D. Disseminated intravascular coagulation
  E. Viral infection
III. Drug-induced thrombocytopenia
  A. Suppression of platelet production
    1. Myelosuppressive drugs
      a. Severe: cytosine arabinoside, daunorubicin, carboplatin
      b. Moderate: cyclophosphamide, busulfan, methotrexate, 6-mercaptopurine
      c. Mild: vinca alkaloids
    2. Thiazide diuretic
    3. Ethanol
    4. Estrogens
  B. Immunologic platelet destruction
    1. Clinical suspicion plus convincing experimental evidence
      a. Antibiotics: sulfathiazole, novobinocin, *p*-aminosalicylate
      b. Cinchona alkaloids: quinidine, quinine
      c. Food: beans
      d. Sedatives, hypnotics, anticonvulsants: apronalide, carbamazepine
      e. Digitoxin
      f. Methyldopa
      g. Stibophen
    2. Clinical suspicion (major drugs implicated)
      a. Aspirin
      b. Chlorpropamide
      c. Chloroquine
      d. Chlorothiazide and hydrochlorothiazide
      e. Gold salts
      f. Insecticides
      g. Sulfadiazine, sulfisoxazole, sulfamerazine, sulfamethazine, sulfamethoxypyridazine, sulfamethoxazole, sulfatholamide

Adapted from Rizza CR: Haemostasis and blood coagulation. In Kyle J, et al (eds): Scientific Foundations of Surgery, 4th ed. Chicago: Year Book Medical Publishers, 1989; and Handin RI: Disorders of the platelet and vessel wall. In Wilson E, et al (eds): Harrison's Principles of Internal Medicine, 12th ed.

TABLE 3–4. Historical Factors Associated with Coagulation Defects

Alcohol abuse

Liver disease

Personal or family history of bleeding tendency, especially with surgery or childbirth

Prior need for transfusions

Severe menorrhagia

Frequent nosebleeds

Easy bruising

Spontaneous hemarthrosis

Von Willebrand's disease

Chronic renal disease

Systemic lupus erythematosus

Idiopathic thrombocytopenia

History of ileal resection or small bowel bypass

Anticoagulant use (Coumadin, heparin)

Use of antiplatelet drugs (see Tables 3–2 and 3–3)

Therefore, the most important aspect for preoperative identification of patients with coagulation disorders is the history and physical examination. A thorough history will identify most patients with a bleeding tendency and should include documentation of all current or recently ingested medications, with particular emphasis on the nonsteroidal anti-inflammatory drugs, β-lactam antibiotics, and oral anticoagulants. Any drug that causes platelet dysfunction or thrombocytopenia should be noted (see Table 3–2). The history should elicit any prior patient visits to other physicians for bleeding problems, any prior need for transfusions, or any history of anemia. Decreased availability of vitamin K, either through inadequate synthesis of the vitamin K–dependent coagulation factors or inadequate absorption of vitamin K, can be suggested by a past history of liver disease, malnutrition, bowel disorders, or the recent use of broad-spectrum antibiotics. A family history of hemorrhagic complications should be noted. Inquiry should be made regarding any bleeding complications associated with prior surgical procedures or childbirth, as the best clinical test of the coagulation system may be the patient's ability to tolerate a surgical procedure or obstetric delivery without hemorrhage. In addition, severe menorrhagia, which may come to light during a detailed menstrual history, may suggest the presence of von Willebrand's disease and platelet or other coagulation disorders.

In patients who describe a history of bleeding disorders, the extent and type of bleeding should be ascertained. For example, in patients who describe epistaxis, the frequency and spontaneity of nosebleeds should be determined. Although many patients will describe gingival bleeding during dental hygiene, a history of spontaneous or nocturnal gingival bleeding may suggest a coagulopathy. Large bruises that develop spontaneously are more likely to be associated with a bleeding disorder than small bruises resulting from trauma. A history of spontaneous hemarthroses or muscle hemorrhage may suggest severe hemophilia or other factor deficiency, whereas a history of epistaxis, gingival bleeding, and menorrhagia will often be elicited from patients with a platelet dysfunction or von Willebrand's disease.

The physical examination should be directed toward a search for any cutaneous abnormalities, particularly petechia or ecchymoses in the lower extremities. In addition, the mucous membranes should be inspected for evidence of telangiectases. If the history and physical examination suggest a possible bleeding disorder or if the history is unreliable, preoperative screening should be done with a platelet count, bleeding time, PT, and PTT. The platelet count and bleeding time should reveal any evidence of thrombocytopenia or platelet dysfunction. A prolonged bleeding time may also be present in patients with von Willebrand's disease, although the bleeding time in these patients may be normal unless von Willebrand's factor antigen is present in a very low amount. The PT is sensitive for a deficiency in factor VII, any other vitamin K–dependent factors, and factors in the common pathway (Fig. 3–1). The PTT should reveal any deficiency in factors of the intrinsic system or the common pathway. If the PT, PTT, platelet count, and bleeding time are all within normal limits, no further testing is warranted. In some patients with a prolonged PT, parenteral replacement of vitamin K will correct the abnormality. If severe coagulation abnormalities are present, a hematology consult should be obtained. Appropriate evaluation and correction of the coagulation defect with appropriate blood products should be undertaken preoperatively.

In summary, both prospective and retrospective studies have shown that the prevalence of abnormal screening coagulation tests (PT, PTT, platelet count, bleeding time) is low, the number of false positive tests is high, and physician knowledge of abnormal results rarely leads to a change in patient management. The majority of true coagulation abnormalities can be predicted from the history and physical examination. Most surgical bleeding complications are due to mechanical defects rather than

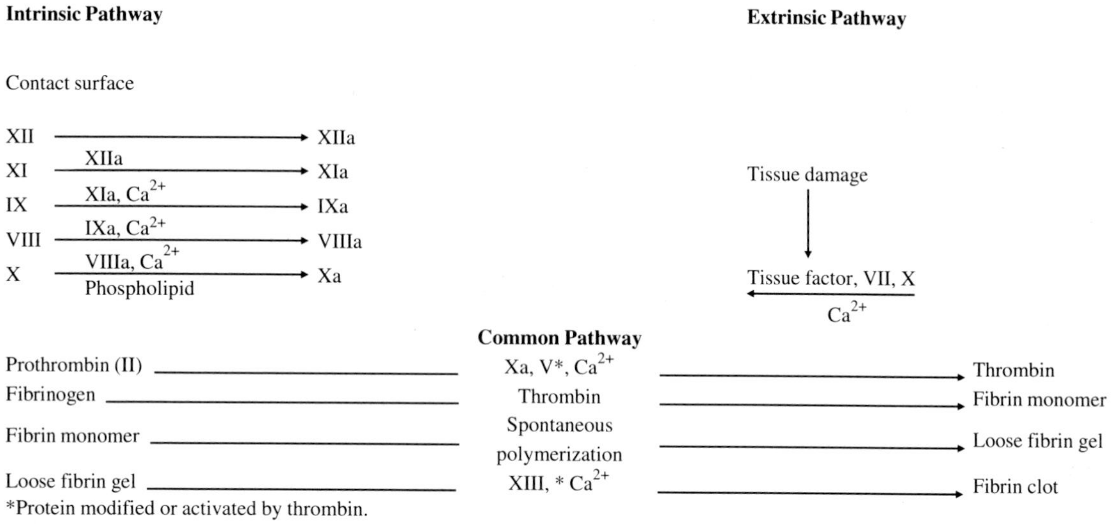

Intrinsic Pathway   **Extrinsic Pathway**

Contact surface

XII $\longrightarrow$ XIIa

XI $\xrightarrow{\text{XIIa}}$ XIa   Tissue damage

IX $\xrightarrow{\text{XIa, Ca}^{2+}}$ IXa

VIII $\xrightarrow{\text{IXa, Ca}^{2+}}$ VIIIa

X $\xrightarrow[\text{Phospholipid}]{\text{VIIIa, Ca}^{2+}}$ Xa   Tissue factor, VII, X

$\overleftarrow{\hspace{3cm}}$
Ca^{2+}

Common Pathway

Prothrombin (II) _____ $Xa, V*, Ca^{2+}$ _____ Thrombin

Fibrinogen _____ Thrombin _____ Fibrin monomer

Fibrin monomer _____ Spontaneous
polymerization _____ Loose fibrin gel

Loose fibrin gel _____ $XIII, * Ca^{2+}$ _____ Fibrin clot

*Protein modified or activated by thrombin.

FIGURE 3–1. Coagulation cascade. (Modified from Keller JW: Disorders of coagulation. In Lubin MF (ed): Medical Management of the Surgical Patient, 2nd ed, chap 27. Stoneham, Mass: Butterworth, 1988.)

to severe coagulopathies and can be corrected surgically.

Preoperative Blood Product Preparation

Careful preparation and efficient use of blood products is imperative in order to decrease the risk of iatrogenic spread of blood-borne viral diseases, avoid transfusion reactions, and limit costs. Blood transfusion not only carries a risk of spread of disease but also carries a slight risk of causing isoimmunization, which can complicate future blood component crossmatching. In general, with the exception of extremely young or old patients, those in poor health, or those with compromised cardiopulmonary status, most surgical patients undergoing elective surgery can tolerate moderate blood loss on the order of one unit. With modest blood loss, hemodynamic stability can often be maintained with the use of crystalloid and colloid fluids. Except for unique circumstances, red blood cell transfusion is rarely required unless the transfusion requirement is at least two units of blood.

Over 600 red cell blood group antigens have been identified. Of these, 250 represent important antigenic targets for a humoral immune response that can result in significant hemolysis. Fortunately, the overwhelming majority of patients (97%–98%) have negative antibody screening tests and can be safely transfused with blood compatible for ABO and Rh type. For the remaining 2%–3% of patients,

a positive antibody screen dictates additional evaluation to identify alloantibodies capable of significant red blood cell lysis in vivo.

A type and screen test determines the patient's ABO and Rh blood type and screens the plasma for the presence of circulating atypical red cell antibodies. The test can usually be performed in less than 1 hour if no atypical antibodies are discovered. If atypical antibodies are present, however, results may not be available for 24 hours or more. Although the type and screen does not test for every possible anti-red cell antibody, the overwhelming majority of clinically significant anti-red cell antibodies will be detected by this test. Oberman et al.[13] found only eight significant antibodies in over 80,000 crossmatches performed on blood from 14,000 patients who had negative antibody screens. Heisto[14] similarly detected only 15 antibodies in over 70,000 crossmatches performed on 24,000 patients with negative antibody screens. It has thus been predicted that the type and screen system prevents incompatible transfusions in over 99.9% of cases.

A type and crossmatch screen includes, in addition to ABO and Rh typing and antibody screen, a crossmatch test, which is essentially a type-specific blood compatibility test. Because the actual type-specific unit of blood to be infused is tested against the blood recipient's serum, rare antibodies not detected by the antibody screening will be noted. Blood can be typed and crossmatched within 15 to 20 minutes in patients who have a negative antibody screen, negating the need for routine type and crossmatching of blood preoperatively in patients in whom the likelihood of transfusion is low. Clearly, if there is a reasonable likelihood that a blood transfusion will be necessary, blood should be typed and crossmatched. Furthermore, if atypical antibodies are discovered in the type and screen, delays in crossmatching are common, and it may be prudent to have blood available and crossmatched preoperatively.

As a result of several retrospective studies performed in the 1970s, it became clear that numerous elective surgical procedures rarely resulted in the requirement for perioperative transfusion.[15,16] Attempts to minimize wasteful crossmatching of blood for elective surgical procedures resulted in implementation of maximal surgical blood order schedules (MSBOS). The goal of an MSBOS is to increase blood bank efficiency by decreasing the number of units crossmatched but not used. The crossmatch to transfusion ratio (C/T) has been suggested as a means by which to judge the efficiency of routine crossmatching orders. A C/T ratio of 2–3:1 is an optimal goal. The ratio indicates that 30% to 50% of blood that is crossmatched is actually used. Retrospective analysis of any institution's crossmatching and transfusing practices can be performed to estimate the C/T ratio for any elective surgical procedure. It is recommended that blood be typed and screened for procedures with a C/T ratio routinely above 3:1 while routine preoperative crossmatching be performed for procedures associated with a greater likelihood of transfusion. Ultimately, the optimal blood order schedule needs to be tailored to an individual surgeon's or institution's experience. The use of a suggested MSBOS for gynecology (Table 3–5) can result in significant cost savings. At our institution, the type and screen study routinely costs $51.00, and a type and crossmatch costs an additional $436.00 per unit of blood.

Intraoperative Bleeding

Surgical Management

Bleeding in the course of pelvic surgery can be vexing for the gynecologic surgeon and can lead to increased morbidity and mortality for the patient. Even the most meticulous and careful surgeon operating on ideal patients will occasionally encounter intraoperative bleeding. The pelvic surgeon is well advised to have a plan of action for managing particular bleeding problems in an expeditious manner.

TABLE 3–5. Suggested Maximal Surgical Blood Order Schedule for Elective Gynecologic Procedures

	No. of Units
Type and Screen	
Simple vaginal or abdominal hysterectomy	
Oophorectomy	
Ovarian wedge resection	
Tuboplasty, tubal ligation	
Laparoscopy	
Dilation and curettage	
Elective abortion	
Type and Cross	*No. of Units*
Complicated hysterectomy	2
Pelvic mass	2–4
Ovarian cancer	2–4
Myomectomy	2
Radical hysterectomy	4
Pelvic exenteration	6
Radical vulvectomy	2
Type and screen positive for atypical antibodies	2
Coagulopathy or bleeding disorder	2+

Several clinical factors are associated with intraoperative bleeding and can be identified preoperatively. These factors include

- Obesity
- Large pelvic mass
- Adhesions
- Cancer
- Prior radiation therapy

Recognition of these high-risk factors allows the surgeon to prepare for the possibility of intraoperative bleeding. In some instances the presence of specific risk factors may lead to alternative surgical or even nonsurgical modes of managing a particular clinical problem.

A clinical characteristic commonly associated with intraoperative bleeding is obesity. Because of the more difficult visual exposure the obese patient is at increased risk for intraoperative bleeding. For example, when we analyzed and compared the morbidity of radical hysterectomy with pelvic lymphadenectomy in patients weighing in excess of 80 kg and those weighing less than 80 kg, we found a significantly increased operating time and greater intraoperative blood loss in the obese.[17] Although increased operating time and increased blood loss are thought to be interrelated, our multivariate logistic regression analysis found these two clinical variables to be independent. Other potential factors that render pelvic surgery more difficult and increase the risk of bleeding include extensive pelvic adhesions, severe endometriosis, or pelvic inflammatory disease. A large leiomyomatous or adnexal mass may obstruct visualization of the deep pelvis and contribute to increased operative bleeding. Patients with cancer, especially those with advanced ovarian cancer, and patients undergoing radical surgery for gynecologic malignancy are at particularly increased risk for intraoperative bleeding. Previous pelvic radiation therapy causes significant retroperitoneal fibrosis, making dissection of the pelvic floor more difficult and increasing the risk of injury to the pelvic blood supply.

Understanding the effects of these preoperative variables should assist the surgeon in preparing surgery. In a particular case, he or she may desire to have blood available that has been typed and crossmatched for the patient preoperatively. The usual recommendations for type and screen versus type and crossmatch, outlined in the previous section, serve only as guidelines for routine cases and require modification based on clinical parameters suggesting a bleeding risk.

Intraoperative Factors

Several intraoperative factors are associated with an increase in intraoperative bleeding. Surgical exposure is critical to provide adequate visualization for the surgeon to work safely as well as to provide exposure for quick control of bleeding. Therefore, an improper surgical incision may increase the risk as well as the difficulty in controlling intraoperative bleeding, should it occur. The low midline vertical incision offers the most flexibility for the pelvic surgeon in that the incision can be extended cephalad as necessary to gain adequate exposure to both the pelvis and upper abdomen. The popular Pfannenstiel low transverse abdominal incision usually provides adequate exposure for routine gynecologic surgery. However, in specific situations the lateral pelvic wall or the deep pelvis must be exposed, and the Pfannenstiel incision is inadequate. In this circumstance, the astute surgeon might convert the Pfannenstiel incision to a Cherney incision by dividing the tendinous insertion of the rectus muscle along the pubic symphysis to allow adequate exposure for more extensive or difficult pelvic surgery through a transverse incision. Surgical exposure can also be enhanced by proper selection of self-retaining or table-stabilized retractors with blades of adequate depth to provide pelvic exposure. We have found the Bookwalter retractor to

allow superb retraction and visualization when performing difficult abdominal and pelvic surgery. This table-stabilized retractor provides flexibility in the number, depth, size, and position of retraction blades, thereby making exposure of the surgical field excellent in the most difficult situations. Most important, the surgeon must not hesitate to seek assistance from colleagues or surgical technicians if additional assistance with retraction is required.

Surgical technique is critical in preventing or reducing intraoperative blood loss. The surgeon must be thoroughly familiar with the pelvic anatomy and the vascular anatomy of the surgical field. The most hazardous vascular anatomy of the pelvis is hidden in the retroperitoneal space. Gynecologists performing procedures for benign disease are advised to increase their knowledge and skill by exploring the retroperitoneal spaces (especially the paravesical and pararectal spaces) to identify the major vasculature and ureter that traverse the lateral pelvic side wall. Familiarity with this anatomy will better prepare them to manage the more difficult surgical situation when significant bleeding is encountered.

Other aspects of surgical technique critical to reducing intraoperative blood loss include the following. (1) Sharp dissection of the pelvic tissues and skeletonization of the vascular supply to the uterus and ovary results in smaller vascular pedicles with minimal tissue volume, reducing the risk of ligature slippage. (2) Sharp dissection, especially in the retroperitoneal spaces or in advancing the bladder flap, is encouraged. Blunt dissection increases the risk of a venous plexus injury, and increases surface bleeding and even frank hemorrhage from the pelvic vessels. Sharp dissection facilitates the surgeon's ability to isolate, clamp, and ligate individual pelvic vessels. Careful blunt surgical dissection is advised only in the avascular retroperitoneal spaces; however, care must be taken to detect and avoid injury to aberrant vascular anatomy. (3) Vascular pedicles should incorporate only enough tissue to load the distal half of the clamp. "Overloaded" pedicles are more likely to bleed from slipping out of the proximal half of the clamp. Additionally, large tissue pedicles incorporated into a single tie are more likely to slip from the tie and result in delayed postoperative bleeding. (4) Needle placement in vascular pedicles is critical. Needles should be placed at the tip of the clamp in order to incorporate all tissue. (5) Ligatures placed on vascular pedicles should not be held and used for traction, as the pull-tug reaction is likely to loosen the ligature or pull it partially or completely off the vascular pedicle.

Hypotensive anesthetic techniques have been used to decrease intraoperative blood loss. Powell and associates found that hypotensive anesthesia during radical hysterectomy with pelvic lymphadenectomy was associated with a significant reduction in intraoperative blood loss.[18] In their report, the need for perioperative blood transfusion was reduced from 81% to 11.5% in patients receiving hypotensive anesthesia. However, many anesthesiologists are not skilled in or enthusiastic about hypotensive anesthesia. Additionally, the presence of heart disease or other coexisting problems may contraindicate its use. These two problems make hypotensive anesthesia unavailable in many clinical situations.

The management of intraoperative hemorrhage can prove a harrowing experience even for the most experienced surgeon. A systematic approach to the management of intraoperative bleeding is crucial to a successful outcome, and a "game plan" should be established prior to entering the operating room. The surgeon must remain calm when massive intraoperative bleeding is encountered and provide the leadership and skills necessary to establish hemostasis. If a bleeding area cannot be immediately controlled with a suture or clip, then direct pressure on the bleeding site should be used until other definitive measures are available. Direct pressure on most bleeding sites from the surgeon's finger, a small laparotomy pack, or a sponge stick is usually sufficient to stop bleeding temporarily. After the bleeding is controlled with direct pressure, the surgeon should ascertain the adequacy of surgical exposure. If necessary, the surgical incision should be extended or modified. Adequate retraction and additional staff assistance to expose the bleeding area should be obtained. Communication with the anesthesiologist to ensure adequate muscle relaxation and volume resuscitation is necessary before hemostasis is attempted. If initial blood loss results in an unstable patient, the surgeon should use pressure techniques to allow the anesthesiologist time to resuscitate the patient with appropriate intravenous (IV) fluid, blood products, additional IV catheters for transfusion, and the use of vasoactive agents if necessary.

If initial attempts at hemostasis are not successful, the surgeon and anesthesiologist should continue to communicate in order to anticipate additional volume requirements. Requesting additional units of packed red cells or other blood products such as platelets or fresh frozen plasma is appropriate. It should be remembered that approximately 40 to 45 minutes is needed to thaw fresh frozen plasma. Anticipating the patient's future blood product requirements may avoid the development of severe anemia, coagulopathy, or other complications.

In most cases of arterial bleeding, the pulsation of blood can be recognized. Rapid accumulation of blood in the surgical field occurs with a transected artery, and adequate suction apparatus should be available to maintain visualization of the surgical field. Small vessel arterial bleeding is usually easily identified, isolated, and controlled with a clamp. A hemostatic clip or suture is then used to ensure hemostasis. In most instances we prefer to apply hemoclips if the bleeding vessel can be controlled with a clamp or Debakey pickups. Placing a suture deep in the pelvis increases the risk of adjacent vessel injury. Contrarily, the indiscriminate application of clips to a general area of bleeding without identification and control of the specific bleeding site may result in incomplete hemostasis and a cluttered surgical field. It can be extremely difficult to use a clamp or secure a suture in an area where many clips have been placed. Injury to larger arteries such as the aorta or the common or external iliac artery may require vascular surgical techniques, as these arteries cannot be safely ligated without a significant risk of loss of a lower extremity. The skills of a vascular surgeon may be required. The gynecologic surgeon should maintain hemostasis by direct arterial compression or use of noncrushing vascular clamps until a decision is made to suture, patch, or graft the arterial laceration.

Venous bleeding from the pelvic floor is the most common cause of hemorrhage from gynecologic surgery and can prove a formidable challenge for even the most experienced pelvic surgeon. Pelvic venous drainage is comprised of a myriad of venous plexuses, and deep pelvic bleeding is rarely from the end of a single vessel. Clamping or ligating a bleeding venous plexus can be difficult. Exposure of the bleeding field requires adequate suction devices and assistance. If possible, the specific bleeding site should be identified, clamped or clipped with hemoclips, or sutured. However, if initial attempts at control are unsuccessful, the surgeon must use other available resources. During all of these efforts, the adjacent pelvic anatomy, including the ureter, rectum, bladder, and other pelvic nerves or blood vessels, must be identified and protected. In many instances of deep pelvic venous bleeding, direct fingertip pressure followed by the placement of a large figure-of-eight suture using a large tapered needle (such as a CT-1) will incorporate the injured venous plexus and adjacent tissues, achieving hemostasis.

Ligature of more proximal large veins (such as the hypogastric vein) is of little value in reducing distal bleeding and in fact may aggravate bleeding by increasing venous pressure in the distal pelvis. Alternatively, the arterial pulse pressure to the pelvis can be significantly reduced by bilateral ligation of the hypogastric arteries. This technique should be mastered by all pelvic surgeons. In many instances hypogastric artery ligation can sufficiently reduce local blood pressure to allow control of venous bleeding by pressure and normal clotting mechanisms. Burchell[19] reported that hypogastric artery ligation led to a 24% reduction in pelvic blood pressure and an approximately 50% reduction in pelvic blood flow. Further, the pulse pressure (the difference between the systolic and diastolic pressure) fell by 85% following bilateral internal iliac artery ligation. Ligation of the anterior division of the hypogastric artery will provide sufficient control of the arterial supply to the pelvic viscera where most bleeding arises and avoid the risks associated with ligating the posterior division of the hypogastric artery. Unfortunately, in many clinical situations, the pelvic anatomy may be significantly distorted by hematoma, edema, and surgical trauma, making isolation of the anterior trunk of the hypogastric artery difficult. In these dire cases where hemostasis must be achieved, ligation of the main trunk of the hypogastric artery is acceptable despite the risk of other complications associated with ligating the entire hypogastric arterial supply. Several authors have reported an increased frequency of fistula formation as a result of impaired tissue perfusion, or pain in the buttocks due to decreased circulation to the gluteal arteries. Hypogastric artery ligation is associated with an increased risk of ureteral injury or iliac venous injury. These risks can be decreased by anatomic dissection and stricture identification. Despite these risks, hypogastric artery ligation may be a lifesaving technique and should be considered when other methods to control pelvic bleeding have failed.

Other adjuncts to assist in the control of surgical site bleeding include electrocautery or thrombostatic agents such as Gelfoam, Avitene, and topical thrombin. The surgical pharmaceuticals may be particularly helpful in controlling a raw surface venous ooze that may be encountered during the debulking of advanced ovarian carcinoma or in extended retroperitoneal dissection performed in some radical cancer operations or with the dissection of endometriosis. These agents are ineffective in the presence of brisk bleeding, which does not allow the agent to remain in proximity to the bleeding vessels for an adequate period to promote thrombogenesis. Some authors have noted an apparently increased incidence of retroperitoneal fibrosis and ureteral stricturing following the use of thrombostatic agents. It has also been suggested that retroperitoneal infection may be increased after use of these agents.

Finally, pelvic packs may be necessary to control profound venous bleeding and complete the surgical procedure. In these situations, pelvic packing allows for correction of the intraoperative coagulopathy and allows hemostasis to occur by a normal clotting mechanism of the involved venous plexus. A 2-inch gauze firmly packed directly into the bleeding site, filling the pelvis and exiting through a low lateral abdominal incision, may successfully control bleeding. We partially advance the pack 24 hours postoperatively and remove the entire pack by the third postoperative day. Alternatively, the Logotheopulos umbrella pack may be placed in the pelvis, exiting via an open vaginal cuff.[20] Additional traction on the "parachute" pack provides additional pressure to tamponade pelvic floor bleeding sites. Our experience with this pack is limited.

The need for additional surgical assistance cannot be overemphasized when massive blood loss is encountered. The surgeon must remain calm and direct a purposeful surgical effort to achieve hemostasis. Finally, when massive blood loss (>5,000 mL) has been encountered, replacement of coagulation factors and platelets is paramount and should be instituted early. The laboratory coagulation profile should be followed serially during the immediate postoperative period to ascertain hemostatic competence or the need for additional replacement.

In our experience, the most common site of severe intraoperative bleeding involves venous bleeding from the deep pelvis and lateral pelvic side wall. However, the increasing trend toward utilization of laparoscopic surgery for more difficult pelvic operations may result in other sources of perioperative bleeding. To date, hemorrhagic complications associated with laparoscopy are related to venous or arterial puncture injury at the time of trocar insertion. Puncture injuries to the great vessels may be retroperitoneal and go unrecognized. An enlarging hematoma may be the first clue to the presence of vascular injury. Further, unrecognized vascular retroperitoneal injury may be recognized by the anesthesiologist when the patient becomes hypotensive. Successful management requires recognition, immediate open exploration, and control of the bleeding site. Large arterial injuries may require consultation with a vascular surgeon to determine the most appropriate repair. Less frequently, excessive bleeding may result from traction-related venous plexus injury incurred during pelvic dissection.

Presacral venous plexus bleeding is often encountered during sacrocolpopexy to correct vaginal prolapse.[21] The nature of these sacral veins, which traverse the sacrum and enter the sacral foramina, often precludes the successful use of traditional techniques, including cautery, clamping, ligation, and hemostatic clips. Bone wax, Gelfoam, and Avitene combined with direct pressure may not be successful. In this situation, sterile thumbtacks placed directly in the sacrum over the bleeding site will tamponade the venous bleeding and may be lifesaving. Timmons et al.[22] have described a device used to obtain better leverage and push the thumbtack into place with direct pressure.

Finally, bleeding is commonly encountered during pelvic and aortic lymph node dissection. A thorough understanding of the retroperitoneal vascular anatomy is critical to minimize injury to adjacent vessels while attempting to control bleeding.

Blood Product Replacement

The infectious and other transfusion risks as well as the limited supply of blood products make it imperative that blood products be processed efficiently and used pragmatically. Only in rare cases of massive blood loss is whole blood transfusion necessary or indicated. Administration of whole blood exposes patients to large volumes of plasma and can increase the risk of citrate reactions, allergic responses, or intravascular volume overload. Individual cellular blood components can be prescribed commensurate with patient need. In most instances donor blood is separated into individual cellular blood components and plasma fractions. This process better supplies specialized blood products necessary for the management of hematologic disorders and support of immunocompromised patients.

Blood components and plasma fractions are prepared from donor blood through processes involving centrifugation, washing, and freezing. Centrifugal separation of freshly collected whole blood produces platelet and red cell concentrates. This process also yields plasma, which can either be frozen fresh or used for production of cryoprecipitate. The latter process involves thawing of fresh frozen plasma, extraction of supernatant, and refreezing of the insoluble residual precipitate. Factor VIII concentrate, albumin, immunoglobulin preparations, and prothrombin complex concentrates can be prepared by fractionation of pooled fresh frozen plasma. Occasionally, when transfusions are necessary for patients with rare alloantibodies, blood products can be prepared through apheresis of blood from individual HLA-matched donors.

Red Cell Transfusion

Red cells can be administered in a variety of preparations, including whole blood, red blood cells, leukocyte-poor red cells, washed red cells, and frozen and deglycerolized red cells (Table 3–6). Centrifugation of whole blood yields a red cell concentrate with a hematocrit of 70% to 80%, but fails to remove the majority of leukocytes and platelet debris. Leukocyte-poor red cells can be prepared from red cell concentrate through a number of techniques, including red cell washing, further centrifugation, and filtration. The most popular method used in the preparation and reconstitution of red cells involves the freezing of red cells in 40% glycerol, followed by thawing and washing to remove the glycerol.

TABLE 3–6. **Red Blood Cell Products**

Components	Volume	Red Cell Content	Plasma Content	Hct.
Whole blood	450 mL blood + 63 mL CPDA-1	200 mL	250 mL	0.40
Red blood cells	>200 mL	200 mL	60–90 mL	0.70–0.80
Leukocyte-poor red cells	Approx. 200 mL	>160 mL	40–60 mL	0.70–0.80
Washed red cells	Approx. 200 mL	180 mL	—	As desired
Frozen and deglycerolized red cells	Approx. 200 mL	180 mL	—	As desired

Adapted from Schroeder ML, Rayner H: Transfusion of blood components. In Lee GR, et al (eds): Winthrobe's Clinical Hematology, 9th ed, vol 1, chap 21. Malvern, PA: Lea & Fabiger, 1983.

This process removes approximately 90% of the leukocytes present in red blood cell concentrate.

Hypovolemia related to blood loss is the most common indication for red blood cell transfusion. Healthy adults tolerate a 20% loss of the circulating blood volume (1,000 mL) without the need for blood transfusion if adequate fluid resuscitation is performed. Larger volumes of blood loss are associated with hemodynamic effects that include tachycardia and postural hypotension, or shock when losses exceed 30% to 40% of blood volume. Whenever possible, type-specific blood should be administered aseptically, using a large-bore IV line containing a filter. If very rapid transfusion is required, normal saline with 5% albumin can be added to decrease the viscosity of the red cell concentrate.

Platelet Transfusion

Platelets, like red cells, are extracted from whole blood by centrifugation. Centrifugation of whole blood at 1,000 G for 10 minutes yields platelet-rich plasma, which can be further centrifuged to produce both platelet-poor plasma and a sediment that contains approximately 5×10^{10} platelets. Three types of platelet products are available: platelet concentrates pooled from several donors, platelet pheresis units drawn from random unmatched donors, and platelet pheresis units drawn from donors preselected by HLA typing. Random pheresis and pooled platelet concentrates are issued interchangeably, depending on availability, whereas single-donor HLA type platelets are usually administered to recipients who are alloimmunized.

In general, the platelet count should rise by 5,000 to 8,000/mL for each unit of platelets administered. Transfused platelets should survive for 9 to 10 days in the circulation. However, in clinical situations in which platelets are actively catabolized (including cases of disseminated intravascular coagulation or autoimmune destruction of platelets), platelet survival will be decreased, resulting in a nominal effect of transfused platelets on the posttransfusion platelet count.

Prophylactic platelet transfusion is indicated to prevent spontaneous bleeding in individuals with severe thrombocytopenia. Spontaneous hemorrhage can occur when the platelet count falls below 20,000/mL. It can also occur at higher platelet counts in individuals with connective tissue disease, coagulopathy, or in individuals who have ingested drugs that can adversely affect platelet function (see Table 3–2). In these individuals, pro-phylactic platelet transfusion should be considered even when platelet counts are greater than 20,000/mL.

Platelet transfusion is indicated for individuals with active bleeding secondary to or worsened by a quantitative or qualitative platelet defect. This can include surgical patients who have suffered significant intraoperative blood loss and who have a dilutional or consumptive thrombocytopenia. Patients undergoing open heart surgery who are placed on a pump for more than 2 hours often experience both platelet dysfunction and thrombocytopenia, requiring platelet transfusion if the platelet count is less than 60,000/mL.[23] Patients with circulating antiplatelet antibodies occasionally require platelet transfusion. However, the transfused platelets are usually of transient benefit and are rapidly destroyed. In these patients, steroids and immunoglobulin administration may occasionally effect a rapid increase in the platelet count. Conversely, thrombocytopenia resulting from decreased platelet production related to previous radiotherapy or chemotherapy usually responds to platelet transfusions.

In all situations, the actual decision to transfuse platelets may involve a number of factors. Acutely, methods to effect cessation of bleeding in a patient with severe thrombocytopenia must also be implemented. Associated abnormalities in other coagulation factors should also be corrected.

Granulocyte Transfusion

Granulocyte products are difficult to produce, are associated with a number of adverse effects, including febrile reactions and severe respiratory distress, and can induce development of HLA-specific alloantibodies. In the past, granulocyte transfusion was used in selected patients with severe neutropenia, such as those treated with chemotherapy or radiotherapy. However, the therapeutic role of granulocyte transfusion is questionable, and, given the recent advances in chemotherapy administration and the development of colony-stimulating factors such as granulocyte colony-stimulating factor and granulocyte-macrophage colony-stimulating factor for bone marrow support, granulocyte transfusion will rarely be necessary in the future.

Plasma and Plasma Derivatives

Plasma transfusion used to expand volume, particularly for the treatment of hemorrhagic shock, became popular during World War II. Plasma contains all coagulation factors as well as immunoglobulin and albumin. Plasma destined for use as replacement of labile coagulation factors V and VIII requires freezing. Factor IX is also labile, but stored unfrozen plasma maintains at least 50% activity. The remaining coagulation factors are stable and do not require frozen storage. Albumin can be prepared from plasma with cold ethanol fractionation. It is usually available as a 5% solution or a 25% solution. Heat treatment of albumin eliminates the risk of transmission of blood-borne viruses, such as hepatitis B and C, and human immunodeficiency virus (HIV). Cryoprecipitate is derived from plasma and is rich in factor VIII and fibrinogen (Table 3–7).

Plasma transfusion is indicated for the treatment of coagulopathies associated with quantitative deficiencies in individual coagulation factors, or in conditions such as sepsis in which there is a deficiency in multiple coagulation factors. A deficiency in intrinsic pathway coagulation factors can occur with vitamin K deficiency or warfarin overdosage and is usually best treated with vitamin K. The therapeutic effect of vitamin K is not immediate, and benefits may require 8 to 12 hours. If necessary, stored plasma can be used to rapidly correct deficiencies of the nonlabile vitamin K–dependent coagulation factors. Indications for the use of fresh frozen plasma instead of stored or single-donor plasma include the treatment of thrombotic thrombocytopenic purpura and replacement of the labile coagulation factors V and VIII. Hemophilic patients lacking factor VIII or patients with von Willebrand's disease are most appropriately treated with cryoprecipitate, which is rich in factor VII.

Plasma and albumin are rarely required for volume replacement. Most patients who are hypovolemic as a result of bleeding can be adequately resuscitated with appropriate crystalloid infusion. Finally, neither plasma nor albumin is of benefit for nutritional support in severely malnourished patients.

Management of Postoperative Hemorrhage

Bleeding requiring reoperation is an infrequent complication associated with pelvic surgery. Fehrman reported that 0.8% of all patients at his institution required reoperation for posthysterectomy hemorrhage.[24] In a similar report from the Mayo Clinic, Smith and Pratt noted that reoperation for postoperative bleeding was necessary in seven (0.6%) of 1,219 patients after vaginal hysterectomy.[25] Even though postoperative hemorrhage occurs in less than 1% of patients, this life-threatening problem must be addressed in any postoperative patient with signs and symptoms suggesting significant bleeding. Recognition and management of postoperative bleeding should not be delayed because of the surgeon's confidence that this complication cannot be encountered in his or her patient. Postoperative bleeding may be immediate, may be recognized in the recovery room or within the first 24 postoperative hours, or may be delayed a week to 10 days following the surgical procedure. The initial management of all postoperative patients should include routine monitoring of vital signs and other clinical parameters that may indicate intravascular volume changes or depletion. Hypotension, tachycardia, diminishing urine output, or falling hematocrit are classic signs of postoperative bleeding. The symptoms of postoperative bleeding may be subtle and only reflected in the vital signs or laboratory parameters. On the other hand, excessive abdominal or pelvic pain, abdominal distention, or shoulder or scapular pain should suggest the possibility of postoperative intraperitoneal bleeding and should be evaluated appropriately. In addition to monitoring of vital signs and hematocrit, a search of the abdomen or pelvis for hematoma or free fluid, coupled with paracentesis or culdocentesis, may assist in the identification of postoperative bleeding. Once evidence of postoperative bleeding

TABLE 3–7. **Plasma and Derivatives**

Components	Usual Volume	Contents
Fresh frozen plasma	>200 mL	All factors
Single-donor (stored) plasma	>200 mL	Factor VIII deficient; factor V decreased
Cryoprecipitate	10–15 mL	Factor VIII (>80 units), fibrinogen (100–350 mg)
Albumin	Varies	5% and 25%
Immunoglobulin	Varies	Varies
Coagulation factor concentrates	Lyophilized	Varies

Adapted from Schroeder ML, Rayner H: Transfusion of blood components. In Lee GR, et al (eds): Winthrobe's Clinical Hematology, 9th ed, vol 1, chap 21. Malvern, PA: Lea & Febiger, 1983.

is identified and the diagnosis established, additional evaluation is mandatory.

The patient who underwent a difficult initial surgical procedure associated with intraoperative hemorrhage is at high risk for developing postoperative bleeding. In our experience, approximately one half of all patients reoperated on for bleeding also experienced intraoperative hemorrhage. Although incomplete control of intraoperative bleeding is a possibility, it is important to exclude postoperative disseminated intravascular coagulation (depletion of coagulation factors and platelets) in the patient who experienced intraoperative hemorrhage. The other half of patients who develop significant postoperative bleeding are usually a "surprise" following an uncomplicated surgical procedure. In most instances, we find a uterine, vaginal, or ovarian vessel vascular pedicle responsible for intraperitoneal, retroperitoneal, and/or vaginal bleeding. The evaluation of any patient suspected of having postoperative bleeding involves assessment of platelet count, PT, PTT, and fibrinogen levels. If a coagulopathy is present, appropriate correction with blood products should be undertaken as soon as possible.

The most easily recognized and managed postoperative bleeding complication is associated with vaginal cuff bleeding, which usually arises from the vaginal artery located near the lateral vaginal angle. Unfortunately, on some occasions vaginal angle bleeding results in intraperitoneal or retroperitoneal blood loss with little external vaginal bleeding. In patients suspected of having vaginal cuff bleeding, immediate vaginal examination is advised, along with bimanual and rectovaginal examinations searching for evidence of a hematoma. A bleeding vessel at the vaginal cuff may be easily controlled with transvaginal suture ligation. These pedicles should incorporate the vaginal mucosa and the vaginal artery but avoid the bladder, ureter, or rectum. Occasionally a transvaginal approach to this problem is unsuccessful and exploratory laparotomy or laparoscopy may be necessary to assess the extent of the bleeding or to achieve hemostasis. Significant arterial vaginal cuff bleeding is not likely to be successfully controlled with vaginal packing alone. We consider vaginal packing as a temporizing measure to control bleeding until the patient can be returned to the operating room.

Delayed vaginal cuff bleeding secondary to suture absorption or cuff trauma due to coitus or other factors may also occur unexpectedly. It usually manifests with bright red bleeding. Postoperative vaginal bleeding may also be associated with spontaneous drainage of a cuff hematoma that becomes apparent only after the vaginal cuff sutures are absorbed. Hematoma drainage is characterized by old blood that drains continuously over several days. In either situation, the patient should be carefully examined. Any active bleeding should be controlled with suture ligatures or cautery.

Intraperitoneal and retroperitoneal postoperative bleeding may be difficult to recognize. In our experience many patients with this problem remain stable for 12 to 24 hours postoperatively and then develop hypotension and other clinical evidence of bleeding. Initial management includes replacement of red blood cells and necessary coagulation products and increased IV fluid volumes. In extreme situations, military anti-shock trousers may be necessary to support the patient until she can be returned to the operating room.[26–28] In patients with hemodynamically significant postoperative bleeding, exploratory laparotomy should be pursued expeditiously rather than attempting the time-consuming procedure of arteriography with embolization. It is our feeling that in emergency situations, the patient is better managed by a team of surgeons, anesthesiologists, and operating room nurses, and not in the radiology suite (the role of and indications for arterial embolization are discussed later in this chapter).

Exploratory laparotomy should usually be performed through an ample midline incision to allow complete exploration of the pelvis and abdomen. Any intra-abdominal or pelvic blood clots should be evacuated and all peritoneal and retroperitoneal surfaces should be inspected to identify a bleeding source. All previous vascular pedicles must be reinspected. Immediate control of obvious bleeding sites should be performed appropriately. Reoperation and ligation of bleeding sites is difficult secondary to the edematous and friable tissues. The entire abdominal cavity should be explored to exclude any possibility that additional bleeding will occur from a traumatized liver or spleen or a retracted ovarian pedicle.

In many instances of posthysterectomy bleeding, bleeding from pelvic side wall vessels, which may be retracted into the retroperitoneum, is obscured by hematoma and edema. Thus, identification of the specific bleeding site is difficult and sometimes impossible. In these situations, continued dissection through hematoma and blood-stained tissues may result in additional bleeding. The best alternative may be bilateral hypogastric artery ligation.[29] In addition, externalized pelvic packs which are removed over the first 72 postoperative hours may be necessary. Other approaches to the management of large, raw, oozing surfaces involve the use of Avitene or Gelfoam soaked in thrombin. A new agent, fibrin glue, has been reported to be of value.

In patients who experience postoperative bleeding with the uterus in place (following cesarean section or myomectomy), several authors have advised ligating the uterine vessels and/or ovarian vessels. If the bleeding seems to originate from the uterus or uterine vessels, the uterine-ovarian anastomosis at the uterine cornua should be ligated, sparing the infundibulopelvic ligament and preserving ovarian blood supply.[24]

Patients explored for postoperative bleeding are at increased risk for infectious complications, disseminated intravascular coagulation, shock lung, injury to adjacent organs, prolonged ileus, and retroperitoneal fibrosis. They need careful observation following reoperation.

Some patients initially thought to have postoperative bleeding may stabilize with medical management alone. The success of medical management is a judgment call. In many instances a venous bleeding site may be tamponaded secondary to a retroperitoneal hematoma. Fortunately, hematomas can often be confirmed with ultrasound or CT scanning. In the hemodynamically stable patient, the next clinical management question involves the need for or benefit from hematoma evacuation. Pelvic or retroperitoneal hematomas are an ideal site for infection or abscess formation. On the other hand, if there is no evidence of infection and the patient remains asymptomatic, observation is appropriate and hematoma resolution is expected. However, drainage should be considered if the hematoma is symptomatic, causes ureteral obstruction, or becomes infected. CT-directed catheter placement, vaginal cuff opening, or exploratory laparotomy by a transperitoneal or retroperitoneal approach, depending on the location and size of the hematoma, may be necessary in patients who do not respond to conservative management.

In some instances, nonsurgical management of postoperative bleeding may be appropriate. For example, patients who are extremely poor surgical risks or who are known to have anatomy making surgical control of bleeding difficult (or in whom a variety of bleeding sites are possible, such as patients with gastrointestinal bleeding), arteriography with intra-arterial embolization of the bleeding vessel should be considered.[30–32] We have encountered particular difficulties in patients who develop lower gastrointestinal tract bleeding after extensive prior surgery and pelvic radiation therapy. In these situations the site of bleeding is uncertain as bleeding may originate from the hypogastric artery, the external iliac artery, the inferior hemorrhoidal artery, or the branches of the superior mesenteric artery.

Arteriography may disclose the responsible bleeding source and allow immediate embolization of the vessel with Gelfoam plugs, metal coils, or preformed clot. Intra-arterial embolization has also been particularly helpful in patients who continue to bleed following reexploration.[30] However, arterial embolization does carry risks, which include infarction of tissue distal to the artery embolized, infection, vesicovaginal fistula, thrombosis of the femoral artery, and toxicity associated with the use of large volumes of IV or intra-arterial contrast medium. O'Hanlan et al. described six patients who underwent arteriographically directed arterial embolization to control postoperative bleeding. Bleeding in three of the six patients was successfully managed by this method; however, three patients needed operation to control the bleeding despite arteriographic embolization.[32] Obviously, the success of arterial embolization relates not only to the specific bleeding site but also to the experience of the interventional radiologist.

Another medical approach to the management of postoperative bleeding involves the use of military anti-shock trousers.[26–28] We have successfully used MAST trousers to temporarily support an unstable patient before performing definitive surgery or arterial embolization. However, there are reported cases in which use of the MAST trousers and medical management resulted in a successful outcome without surgical intervention.[32a] It is likely that the tamponade provided by the abdominal portion of the MAST trousers resulted in bleeding control and medical correction of the coagulopathy resulted in clotting of the bleeding site.

Postoperative Venous Thromboembolism

Risk Factors

Deep venous thrombosis (DVT) and pulmonary embolism (PE) represent significant complications in postoperative gynecologic patients. The magnitude of these problems is relevant to the gynecologist because 40% of all deaths following gynecologic surgery can be directly attributed to PE.[33] PE is also the second leading cause of death in women who undergo induced abortion[34] and the most frequent cause of postoperative death in patients with uterine[35] or cervical carcinoma.[36]

The causal factors of venous thrombosis were first proposed by Virchow in 1858 and include a hypercoagulable state, venous stasis, and injury to the vessel intima. Two prospective studies have evaluated risk factors associated with the postoperative occurrence of DVT after gynecologic surgery. Clayton et al.[37] studied risk factors in 124 patients undergoing vaginal and abdominal surgery for benign gynecologic disease. On logistic regression analysis, the five factors found to be associated with the development of postoperative DVT were age, varicose veins, percent overweight, euglobulin lysis time, and serum fibrin–related antigen. Clarke-Pearson et al. prospectively assessed the risk factors associated with venous thromboembolic complications in 411 patients undergoing major abdominal and pelvic surgery.[38] Of these patients, 84% had gynecologic malignancies. Preoperative risk factors identified included age, nonwhite race, increasing stage of malignancy, a history of DVT, lower extremity edema or venous stasis changes, varicose veins, weight, and a history of radiation therapy. Intraoperative factors associated with postoperative DVT included increased anesthesia time, increased blood loss, and intraoperative transfusion requirements. The recognition of risk factors associated with postoperative venous thromboembolism should allow the clinician to stratify patients into low-risk, medium-risk, and high-risk groups.

Prophylactic Methods

Over the past two decades a number of prophylactic methods have been demonstrated in clinical trials to result in a significant reduction in the incidence of DVT.[38a] A few studies have demonstrated a reduction in fatal PE. The ideal prophylactic method should be effective, free of significant side effects, well accepted by the patient and nursing staff, widely applicable to most patient groups, and inexpensive.

The use of small doses of subcutaneously administered heparin to prevent DVT and PE is the most widely studied of all prophylactic methods. Over 25 controlled trials have demonstrated that heparin given subcutaneously 2 hours preoperatively and every 8 to 12 hours postoperatively is effective in reducing the incidence of DVT. The value of low-dose heparin in preventing fatal PE was established by a randomized, controlled, multicenter international trial that demonstrated a reduction in fatal PE in general surgery patients receiving postoperative low-dose heparin every 8 hours.[39]

Trials of low-dose heparin following gynecologic surgery are limited, and differences in patient selection and length of follow-up have not allowed a clear consensus to be established regarding the value of low-dose heparin in all groups of patients. Three randomized controlled studies in gynecologic patients used an identical regimen of low-dose heparin administration: 5,000 units given subcutaneously 2 hours preoperatively and every 12 hours for 7 days postoperatively. The trials reported by Ballard et al.[40] and Taberner et al.[41] were conducted in patients with benign gynecologic conditions (98%). All patients were over 40 years of age, and follow-up was discontinued at the time of hospital discharge. The American study[42] evaluated a larger group of patients on a gynecologic oncology unit. Only 16% had benign gynecologic conditions, and follow-up encompassed the first 6 postoperative weeks.

The study by Taberner et al.[41] recorded a 23% incidence of DVT in the control group, compared with a 6% incidence in patients treated with low-dose heparin. This difference was statistically significant ($p < 0.05$). Unfortunately, although the trial was randomized, the control group included a large number of patients with malignancy. When the cancer patients were excluded from trial analysis, there was no statistically significant value to the use of low-dose heparin in patients with benign conditions. Ballard's study also evaluated a group of patients with benign gynecologic diseases.[40] The nontreated control group had a 29% incidence of DVT, compared with a 3.6% incidence in patients treated with low-dose heparin ($p < 0.001$). A randomized trial of patients undergoing major abdominal and pelvic surgery on a gynecologic oncology service[42] failed to demonstrate a difference in the incidence of thromboembolic complications between the control group (12.4%) and the group treated with low-dose heparin (14.8%). In summary, only Ballard et al. reported a beneficial effect of low-dose postoperative heparin administered at 12-hour intervals following gynecologic surgery. Taberner et al.[41] in patients with benign gynecologic conditions and Clarke-Pearson et al.[42] in gynecologic oncology patients did not find this low-dose heparin regimen to be of benefit.

In a subsequent trial,[43] two more intense heparin regimens were evaluated in high-risk gynecologic oncology patients. In this study, heparin was administered in a regimen of either 5,000 units subcutaneously 2 hours preoperatively and every 8 hours postoperatively or 5,000 units subcutaneously every 8 hours preoperatively (a minimum of three preoperative doses) and every 8 hours postoperatively. Both of these prophylaxis regimens significantly reduced the incidence of postoperative DVT.

Although low-dose heparin is considered to have no effect on measurable coagulation parameters, most large series have noted an increase in the bleeding complication rate, particularly in the incidence of wound hematoma. As many as 10% to 15% of otherwise healthy patients develop a prolonged activated partial thromboplastin time (aPTT) after 5,000 units of heparin have been given subcutaneously.[44] These transiently anticoagulated patients have also been noted in one carefully monitored trial of low-dose heparin in gynecology. It was these patients in whom the major postoperative bleeding complications were encountered. Dockerty et al. also found that estimated blood loss increased from 246 mL to 401 mL in patients undergoing total abdominal hysterectomy who were treated with low-dose heparin.[45] Retrospective studies have suggested that low-dose heparin contributed to an increased occurrence of lymphocysts,[46,47] and a prospective study demonstrated a twofold increase in retroperitoneal lymph drainage volume in patients treated with low-dose heparin.[44] Finally, thrombocytopenia, although relatively rare, can be associated with low-dose heparin use and has been reported to occur in 6% of gynecologic patients treated prophylactically. Although many authors feel that monitoring coagulation parameters is not necessary for effective and safe low-dose heparin use, periodic postoperative assessment of aPTT and platelet count seems prudent to maximize the identification of the 22% of patients who will have either a prolonged aPTT or thrombocytopenia and who are most likely to develop major clinical hemorrhagic complications.

Venous stasis of the lower extremity has been seen on the operating table and continues postoperatively for a varying duration. Many authors feel that the combination of stasis occurring in the capacitance veins of the calf during surgery and the hypercoagulable state induced by surgery is the primary factor contributing to the development of acute postoperative DVT. Prospective studies of the natural history of postoperative venous thrombosis indicate that the calf veins are the predominant site of thrombi and that most thrombi develop with 24 hours of surgery.[48] Reduction of venous stasis in the perioperative period by various methods has been less extensively investigated than pharmacologic methods such as low-dose heparin. However, a growing body of literature supports the important role that mechanical prophylactic methods may play in the prevention of postoperative DVT.

Although probably of only modest benefit, reducing stasis by short preoperative hospital stays and early postoperative ambulation should be attempted in all patients. Elevating the foot of the bed by 20 degrees raises the calf above the heart level, thereby allowing gravity to drain the calf veins, and should further reduce stasis. More active forms of mechanical prophylaxis include elastic gradient compression stockings and external pneumatic leg compression.

In a survey of U.S. general surgeons, gradient elastic stockings were second only to low-dose heparin as the prophylactic method of choice in high-risk and moderate- to high-risk surgical patients.[49] The simplicity and the absence of significant side effects of elastic stockings are probably the two most important reasons that they are included in the routine postoperative orders of many surgeons. Controlled studies of gradient elastic stockings are limited but do suggest modest benefit when the stockings are properly fitted.[50] Poorly fitted stockings may be hazardous to some patients, as a tourniquet effect may develop at the knee or midthigh.[35] Unfortunately, variations in human anatomy do not allow perfect fit for all patients to stocking sizes manufactured.

Most reported studies on reducing postoperative venous stasis examined intermittent external compression of the leg by pneumatically inflated sleeves placed around the calf and/or leg during intraoperative and postoperative periods. Various pneumatic compression devices and leg sleeve designs are available, and the current literature has not demonstrated the superiority of any single system. The single-chambered calf compression device has been the most extensively studied and appears to significantly reduce the incidence of DVT, on par with the effect of low-dose heparin. In addition to increasing venous flow and pulsatile emptying of the calf veins, external pneumatic compression apparently augments endogenous fibrinolysis, which may result in lysis of very early thrombi before they become clinically significant.[51]

The duration of postoperative external pneumatic compression has differed in various trials. Several investigators have found external pneumatic compression to be effective when used only in the operating room, or in the operating room and for the first 24 hours postoperatively.[52,53]

External pneumatic compression in patients undergoing major surgery for gynecologic malignancy has been found to reduce the incidence of postoperative venous thromboembolic complications by nearly threefold.[54] Calf compression was applied intraoperatively and for the first 5 days postoperatively. In a subsequent trial of similar patients that was designed to evaluate whether external pneumatic compression might produce similar benefits when used only intraoperatively and for the first 24 hours postoperatively, there was no reduction in the incidence of DVT in the treatment group versus controls.[55] It appears that patients with a gynecologic malignancy remain at risk for stasis and a hypercoagulable state for a longer period of time than general surgical patients. If compression is to be effective, it must be used for at least 5 days postoperatively.

While patient tolerance has been cited as a drawback to the use of this equipment, external pneumatic leg compression has no significant side effects or risks. Only four patients of the nearly 600 we have treated with external pneumatic compression requested removal because of discomfort. The equipment is easily managed by the nursing staff, and although the initial capital outlay for external pneumatic compressors may seem large, Salzman and Davies calculated that the cost per patient of this prophylactic method is slightly less than that of low-dose heparin given for 7 days postoperatively.[56]

Diagnosis and Treatment of Postoperative Deep Venous Thrombosis and Pulmonary Embolism

Despite the identification of high-risk patients and the use of prophylactic venous thromboembolism regimens, venous thromboembolic complications will occasionally occur. Therefore, early recognition and immediate treatment of DVT and PE is critical. Most pulmonary emboli arise from the deep venous system of the leg, although the pelvic veins are a known source of fatal PE after gynecologic surgery. The diagnosis of lower extremity DVT requires a high level of suspicion and appropriate diagnostic studies. The signs and symptoms of lower extremity DVT include pain, edema, erythema, and prominent vascular pattern of the superficial veins. These signs and symptoms are relatively nonspecific. In fact, 50% to 80% of patients with these symptoms will not have DVT.[57] Conversely, approximately 80% of patients with symptomatic PE have no signs or symptoms of lower extremity thrombosis.[58] The lack of specificity when signs and symptoms are recognized indicates the need for additional diagnostic tests to establish the diagnosis of DVT. The reference standard for the diagnosis of DVT has been contrast venography. Unfortunately, this study is moderately uncomfortable, requires the injection of a contrast agent,

which may cause an allergic reaction or renal injury, and is associated with a 5% risk of phlebitis.[59] Newer diagnostic tests are less invasive while maintaining a high accuracy rate in most patients. Impedance plethysmography is a noninvasive study that measures the change in electrical impedance of the lower extremity when venous blood flow and volume are altered by an occlusive cuff on the thigh. This study may be performed at the bedside and repeated as often as necessary without any patient risk. Correlation with venographic findings in symptomatic patients approaches 95%,[60,61] and this test is sensitive for the identification of deep venous thrombi in the popliteal, femoral, and external iliac segments. It is less accurate (30%) in identifying calf vein thrombosis and does not identify thrombi occurring in the internal iliac venous system. False positive results are primarily related to extrinsic venous compression, which may occur when a large pelvic mass compresses the external iliac or common iliac vein.

Although it is slightly less accurate than impedance plethysmography, Doppler ultrasonography has also been used for the noninvasive diagnosis of DVT. The variable interpretation of audible venous flow patterns, which may be somewhat subjective, accounts for this decreased accuracy.[62] B-mode duplex Doppler imaging is more effective in the diagnosis of symptomatic venous thrombosis, especially when it originates in the proximal lower extremity. With duplex Doppler imaging, the femoral vein can be visualized and clots may be seen directly.[63] Compression of the vein with the ultrasound probe tip allows assessment of venous collapsibility. The presence of a thrombus diminishes vein wall collapsibility. Color–flow studies have also been added to this imaging technique. Doppler imaging is less accurate in the evaluation of the calf venous system and the pelvic veins.

Magnetic resonance imaging can accurately show thrombi in the deep venous system.[64] The primary drawback to MRI is the time involved in examining the lower extremity and pelvis as well as the expense of this technology.

All of these diagnostic studies are accurate when performed by a skilled technologist and in most patients probably could replace routine contrast venography.

The treatment of postoperative DVT requires the immediate institution of anticoagulant therapy. Heparin should be initiated with a bolus of 5,000 units IV, followed by continuous IV infusion of 1,000 units/hr. Approximately 4 hours after initiation of heparin therapy, the aPTT should be measured to assess the adequacy of the anticoagulant effect. In general, prolongation of the aPTT 1.5 to 2.0 times the control value is an indication of appropriate anticoagulant therapy. The goals of anticoagulant therapy include preventing clot propagation or embolization and preventing rethrombosis in a high-risk patient; the risks are primarily bleeding complications.[65] Oral maintenance therapy with sodium warfarin (Coumadin) is advised for at least 3 months. Standard treatment regimens call for the use of IV heparin for 10 days, followed by Coumadin for 3 months.[66] However, a randomized trial evaluated a 10-day regimen of heparin versus a 5-day regimen of heparin and found the 5-day regimen to be equally effective in treating acute thrombosis and preventing rethrombosis.[67] Therefore, it is recommended that IV heparin be maintained for 5 days and that oral Coumadin be initiated during that time. The goals of Coumadin therapy are to achieve an oral dose of medication that will prolong the PT to approximately 1½ times control value. Initially, PT levels should be measured on a daily basis until an appropriate dose of Coumadin is established. Thereafter the PT is checked every 1 to 2 weeks during the 3 months of therapy. Anticoagulant therapy may be discontinued in 3 months if the cause of the DVT episode (such as an acute surgical event or trauma) has been eliminated.

The major hazard of anticoagulant therapy in the postoperative patient is an increased risk of bleeding complications. It is therefore important that PTT, PT, platelet count, and hematocrit be followed carefully and that the anticoagulant does not drastically place the patient in a hypocoagulable state. Heparin-induced thrombocytopenia is a rare complication associated with heparin use and has been reported in association with both low-dose heparin given prophylactically as well as with standard anticoagulant doses.[68] Therefore, periodic evaluation of the platelet count during heparin therapy is advised. Thrombolytic therapy (streptokinase or urokinase) has been advocated by some investigators for the treatment of acute DVT. However, the risk of bleeding complications in a surgical site contraindicates thrombolytic therapy in the postoperative patient.

The diagnosis of PE also requires a high index of suspicion, as many of the signs and symptoms are associated with other, more common pulmonary complications following surgery.[69] The classic findings of pleuritic chest pain, hemoptysis, shortness of breath, tachycardia, and tachypnea should alert the physician to the possibility of PE. Many times, however, the signs are much more subtle and may only be suggested by a persistent tachycardia or a slight elevation in the respiratory rate. Patients suspected of pulmonary embolism should be evaluated initially by chest x-ray, electrocardiogram, and arterial blood gas measurements. Any evidence of an abnormality should be further evaluated by a ventilation–perfusion lung scan, searching for evidence of decreased perfusion in areas of adequate ventilation. Unfortunately, a high percentage of lung scans may be interpreted as "indeterminate." In this setting, careful clinical evaluation and judgment are required to determine the necessity of pulmonary arteriography to document or exclude a PE.

Immediate anticoagulant therapy identical to that outlined for the treatment of DVT should be initiated. Respiratory support including oxygen and bronchodilators and an intensive care setting may be necessary. Massive PEs are usually quickly fatal, although on rare occasions pulmonary embolectomy has been successfully performed. The use of pulmonary artery catheterization with the administration of thrombolytic agents bears further evaluation and may be important in the patient with a massive PE. If anticoagulant therapy is ineffective in preventing rethrombosis and repeated embolization from the lower extremities or pelvis, vena cava interruption may be necessary.[70] This may be accomplished through the percutaneous placement of a vena cava umbrella, filter, or the use of a large clip to obstruct the vena cava above the level of the thrombosis. In most cases, however, anticoagulant therapy is sufficient to prevent repeat thrombosis and embolism and to allow the patient's own endogenous thrombolytic mechanisms to lyse the pulmonary embolus.

References

1. Keller JW: Disorders of coagulation. In Lubin MF (ed): Medical Management of the Surgical Patient, 2nd ed, chap 27. Stoneham, Mass: Butterworth, 1988.
2. Koutts J: Clinching the diagnosis: Assessment of hemostatic function. J Pathol 17:643–647, 1985.
3. George JN, Shattil SJ: Acquired disorders of platelet function. In Hoffman R, Benz EJ, Shattil SJ, Furie B, Cohen HJ (eds): Hematology: Basic Principles and Practice, pp 1528–1546. New York: Churchill Livingstone, 1991.
4. Rizza CR: Haemostasis and blood coagulation. In Kyle J, Carey L (eds): Scientific Foundations of Surgery, 4th ed, pp 280–290. Chicago: Year Book Medical Publishers, 1989.
5. Handin RI: Disorders of the platelet and vessel wall. In Wilson E, Braunwald E, Ibselbacher KJ, et al (eds): Harrison's Principles of Internal Medicine, 12th ed, vol 2, pp 1500–1505. New York: McGraw-Hill, 1991.
6. Suchman AL, Griner PF: Diagnostic uses of the activated

partial thromboplastin time and prothrombin time. Ann Intern Med 104:810–816, 1986.

7. Eisenberg JM, Clarke JR, Sussman SA: Prothrombin and partial thromboplastin times as preoperative screening tests. Arch Surg 117:48–51, 1982.

8. Watel A, Jude B, Caron C, Vandeputte H, Gaeremynck E, et al: Successes and failures of the activated partial thromboplastin time in the preoperative evaluation. Ann Fr Anesth Reanim 5:35–39, 1986.

9. Barber A, Green D, Galluzzo T, Ts'ao CH: The bleeding time as a preoperative screening test. Am J Med 78:761–764, 1985.

10. Eika C, Havig O, Godal HC: The value of preoperative haemostatic screening. Scand J Haematol 21:349–354, 1978.

11. Burns ER, Billett HH, Frater RW, Sisto DA: The preoperative bleeding time as a predictor of postoperative hemorrhage after cardiopulmonary bypass. J Thorac Cardiovasc Surg 92:310–312, 1986.

12. Finley BE: Acute coagulopathy in pregnancy. Med Clin North Am 73:723–743, 1989.

13. Oberman HA, Barnes BA, Friedman BA: The risk of abbreviating the major crossmatch in urgent or massive transfusion. Transfusion 18:137–141, 1978.

14. Heisto H: Pretransfusion blood group serology: Limited value of the antiglobulin phase of the crossmatch when a careful screening test for unexpected antibodies is performed. Transfusion 19:761–763, 1979.

15. Mintz PD, Nordine RB, Henry JB, Webb WR: Expected hemotherapy in elective surgery. NY State J Med 76:532–537, 1976.

16. Friedman BA, Oberman HA, Chadwick AR, Kingdon KI: The maximum surgical blood order schedule and surgical blood use in the United States. Transfusion 16:380–387, 1976.

17. Soisson AP, Soper JT, Berchuck A, Dodge R, Clarke-Pearson DL: Radical hysterectomy in obese women, Obstet Gynecol 80:940–943, 1992.

18. Powell JL, Mogelnicki SR, Franklain EW III, Chambers DA, Burrell MO: A deliberate hypotensive technique for decreasing blood loss during radical hysterectomy and pelvic lymphadenectomy. Am J Obstet Gynecol 147:196–202, 1983.

19. Burchell RC: Physiology of internal iliac artery ligation. J Obstet Gynaecol Br Commonw 75:642–651, 1968.

20. Cassels JW, Greenberg H, Otterson WN: Pelvic tamponade in peripheral hemorrhage. J Reprod Med 30:689–692, 1985.

21. Sutton GP, Addison WA, Livengood CH, Hammond CB: Life-threatening hemorrhage complicating sacral colpopexy. Am J Obstet Gynecol 140:836–837, 1981.

22. Timmons MC, Kohler MF, Addison WA: Thumbtack use for control of presacral bleeding, with description of an instrument for thumbtack application. Obstet Gynecol 78:313, 1991.

23. Schroeder ML, Rayner H: Transfusion of blood components. In Lee GR, Bithell TC, Foerster John, Athens JW, Leukins JN (eds): Winthrobe's Clinical Hematology, 9th ed, vol 1, pp 651–700. Malvern, PA: Lea & Febiger, 1983.

24. Fehrman H: Surgical management of life-threatening obstetric and gynecologic hemorrhage. Acta Obstet Gynaecol Scand 67:125–128, 1988.

25. Smith RD, Pratt JH: Serious bleeding following vaginal or abdominal hysterectomy. Obstet Gynecol 26:593–595, 1965.

26. Hall M, Marshall JR: The gravity suit: A major advance in management of gynecologic blood loss. Obstet Gynecol 53:247–250, 1979.

27. Kaback KK, Sanders AB, Meislin HW: MAST suit update. JAMA 252:2598–2603, 1984.

28. Guerre EF, O'Keeffe DF, Elliott JP, Gilsdorf R, Newman R: Uncontrollable intra-abdominal hemorrhage treated with packing and use of a MAST suit. J Reprod Med 32:230–232, 1987.

29. Clark SL, Phelan JP, Yeh S, Bruce SR, Paul RH: Hypogastric artery ligation for obstetrical hemorrhage. Obstet Gynecol 66:353–356, 1985.

30. Heaston DK, Mineau DE, Brown BJ, Miller FJ: Transcatheter arterial embolization for control of persistent massive puerperal hemorrhage after bilateral surgical hypogastric artery ligation. AJR 133:152–154, 1979.

31. Rosenthal DM, Colapinto R: Angiographic arterial embolization in the management of post-operative vaginal hemorrhage. Am J Obstet Gynecol 151:227–231, 1983.

32. O'Hanlan KA, Trambert J, Rodriguez-Rodriguez L, Goldberg GL, Runowicz CD: Arterial embolization in the management of abdominal and retroperitoneal hemorrhage. Gynecol Oncol 34:131–135, 1989.

32a. Guerre EF, O'Keefe DF, Elliott JP, Gilsdorf R, Newman R: Uncontrollable intraabdominal hemorrhage treated with packing and use of a MAST suit. J Reprod Med 32:230–232, 1987.

33. Jeffcoate TNA, Tindall VR: Venous thrombosis and embolism in obstetrics and gynecology. Aust NZ J Obstet Gynaecol 5:119–130, 1965.

34. Kimball AM, Hallum AV, Cates W: Deaths caused by pulmonary thromboembolism after legally induced abortion. Am J Obstet Gynecol 132:169–174, 1978.

35. Clarke-Pearson DL, Jelovsek FR, Creasman WT: Thromboembolism complicating surgery for cervical and uterine malignancy: Incidence, risk factors, and prophylaxis. Obstet Gynecol 61:87–94, 1983.

36. Creasman WT, Weed JC Jr: Radical hysterectomy. In Schaefer G, Graber EA (eds): Complications in Obstetrics and Gynecologic Surgery, pp 389–398. Hagerstown, Md: Harper and Row, 1981.

37. Clayton JK, Anderson JA, McNicol GP: Preoperative prediction of postoperative deep vein thrombosis. Br Med J 2:910–916, 1976.

38. Clarke-Pearson DL, DeLong E, Synan IS, Coleman RE, Creasman WT: A prospective study of risk factors associated with postoperative venous thromboembolism in gynecology. Obstet Gynecol 69:146–150, 1987.

38a. Goldhaber SZ (ed): Prevention of Venous Thromboembolism. New York: Marcel Dekker, 1993.

39. Kakkar VV: Prevention of fatal postoperative pulmonary embolism by low dose heparin: An international multicenter trial. Lancet 2:145–151, 1975.

40. Ballard M, Bradley-Watson PJ, Johnstone ED: Low doses of subcutaneous heparin in the prevention of deep venous thrombosis after gynaecologic surgery. J Obstet Gynaecol Br Commonw 80:469–472, 1973.

41. Taberner DA, Poller L, Burslem RW: Oral anticoagulants controlled by the British comparative thromboplastin versus low dose heparin in prophylaxis of deep vein thrombosis. Br Med J 1:272–274, 1978.

42. Clarke-Pearson DL, Coleman RE, Synan IS: Venous thromboembolism prophylaxis in gynecologic oncology: A prospective controlled trial of low-dose heparin. Am J Obstet Gynecol 145:606–613, 1983.

43. Clarke-Pearson DL, DeLong E, Synan IS, Coleman RE: A controlled trial of two low-dose heparin regimens for the

prevention of postoperative deep vein thrombosis. Obstet Gynecol 75:684–689, 1990.

44. Clarke-Pearson DL, DeLong E, Synan IS, Coleman RE, Creasman WT: Complications of low-dose heparin prophylaxis in gynecologic oncology surgery. Obstet Gynecol 64:689–694, 1984.

45. Dockerty PW, Goodman JDS, Hill JG: The effect of low-dose heparin on blood loss at abdominal hysterectomy. Br J Obstet Gynaecol 90:759–762, 1983.

46. Catalona WJ, Kadmon D, Crane DB: Effect of mini-dose heparin on lymphocele formation following extraperitoneal pelvic lymphadenectomy. J Urol 123:890–895, 1979.

47. Piver MS, Malfetano JH, Lele SB: Prophylactic anticoagulation as a possible cause of inguinal lymphocyst after radical vulvectomy and inguinal lymphadenectomy. Obstet Gynecol 62:17–21, 1983.

48. Clarke-Pearson DL, Synan IS, Coleman RE, Hinshaw W, Creasman WT: The natural history of postoperative venous thromboembolism in gynecologic oncology: A prospective study of 382 patients. Am J Obstet Gynecol 148:1051–1054, 1984.

49. Conti, S, Daschbach M: Venous thromboembolism prophylaxis: A survey of its use in the United States. Arch Surg 117:1036–1040, 1982.

50. Surr JH, Ibrahim SZ, Faber RG: The efficacy of graduated compression stocking in the prevention of deep vein thrombosis. Br J Surg 64:371–373, 1977.

51. Allenby F, Boardman L, Pflug JJ: Effects of external pneumatic intermittent compression on fibrinolysis in man. Lancet 2:1412–1414, 1976.

52. Salzman EW, Ploet J, Bettlemann M: Intraoperative external pneumatic calf compression to afford long-term prophylaxis against deep vein thrombosis in urological patients. Surgery 87:239–242, 1980.

53. Nicolaides AN, Fernandes E, Fernandes J, Pollock AV: Intermittent sequential pneumatic compression of the legs in the prevention of venous stasis and postoperative deep venous thrombosis. Surgery 87:69–76, 1980.

54. Clarke-Pearson DL, Synan IS, Hinshaw W, Coleman RE, Creasman WT: Prevention of postoperative venous thromboembolism by external pneumatic calf compression in patients with gynecologic malignancy. Obstet Gynecol 63:92–98, 1984.

55. Clarke-Pearson DL, Creasman WT, Coleman RE, Hinshaw W, Synan I: Perioperative external pneumatic calf compression as thromboembolism prophylaxis in gynecologic oncology: Report of a randomized controlled trial. Gynecol Oncol 18:226–232, 1984.

56. Salzman EW, Davies GC: Prophylaxis of venous thromboembolism: Analysis of cost effectiveness. Ann Surg 191:207–218, 1980.

57. Haegger K: Problems of acute deep vein thrombosis. Angiology 20:219, 1969.

58. Palko PA, Namson EM, Fedonik SO: The early detection of deep venous thrombosis using ^{131}I-tagged fibrinogen. Can J Surg 7:215, 1974.

59. Athanasoulis CA: Phlebography for the diagnosis of deep leg vein thrombosis, prophylactic therapy of deep venous thrombosis and pulmonary embolism. DHEW publication no. (NIH) 76–866 1975.

60. Wheeler HB, O'Donnell JA, Anderson FA: Occlusive cuff impedance phlebography: A diagnostic procedure for venous thrombosis and pulmonary embolism. Prog Cardiovasc Dis 17:199, 1974.

61. Clarke-Pearson DL, Creasman WT: Diagnosis of deep vein thrombosis in obstetrics and gynecology by impedance phlebography. Obstet Gynecol 58:52, 1981.

62. Yao JST, Gourmos C, Hobbs JT: Detection of proximal vein thrombosis by Doppler ultrasound flow-detection method. Lancet 1:1, 1972.

63. Anthonie WA, Lensing MD, Paolo P: Detection of deep-vein thrombosis by real-time B-mode ultrasonography. N Engl J Med 320:342–345, 1989.

64. Mintz MC, Levy DW, Axel L: Puerperal ovarian vein thrombosis: MR diagnosis. AJR 149:1273, 1987.

65. Clarke-Pearson DL, Synan IS, Creasman WT: Anticoagulation therapy for venous thromboembolism in patients with gynecologic malignancy. Am J Obstet Gynecol 147:369–375, 1983.

66. Moser KM, Fedullo PR: Venous thromboembolism: Three simple decisions. Chest 83:256–260, 1983.

67. Hull RD, Raskob GE, Rosenbloom D, Panju AA, Brill-Edwards P: Heparin for 5 days as compared with 10 days in the initial treatment of proximal venous thrombosis. N Engl J Med 322:1260–1264, 1990.

68. Bell WR, Royal RM: Heparin induced thrombocytopenia: A comparison of three heparin regimens. N Engl J Med 303:902–906, 1980.

69. Goldhaber SZ, Morpurgo M: Diagnosis, treatment, and prevention of pulmonary embolism. JAMA 268:1727–1733, 1992.

70. Mansour M, Chang AE, Sindelar WF: Interruption of the inferior vena cava for the prevention of recurrent pulmonary embolism. Am Surg 51:375–380, 1985.

Complications in Gynecologic Surgery: Prevention, Recognition, and Management,
edited by James W. Orr, Jr., and Hugh M. Shingleton.
J. B. Lippincott Company, Philadelphia, © 1994.

Chapter 4

Gastrointestinal Tract

Thomas W. Burke
Charles Levenback

The general gynecologist often approaches the gastrointestinal tract with trepidation. Much of this fear can be traced to a poor understanding of bowel anatomy and function, lack of experience in performing bowel surgery, limited exposure to the management of intestinal complications, and a healthy respect for the morbidity associated with significant gastrointestinal injuries. The accomplished pelvic surgeon must develop a working knowledge of gastrointestinal surgery for a number of reasons: (1) operative management of some of the more challenging gynecologic problems such as endometriosis, pelvic inflammatory disease, ovarian cancer, and irradiation injury frequently requires an intestinal procedure; (2) the symptoms of gastrointestinal pathology can occasionally mimic those associated with common gynecologic problems, leading to an erroneous or uncertain preoperative diagnosis; (3) preoperative identification of patients at high risk for gastrointestinal involvement by gynecologic disease may direct additional diagnostic studies and allow for adequate preoperative bowel preparation; (4) a detailed knowledge of intestinal anatomy and careful attention to surgical technique can reduce the incidence of bowel injury; and (5) appropriate management of injuries, when they occur, will minimize their morbidity.

Major gastrointestinal complications can have profound implications for the patient. Bowel obstruction, necrosis, perforation, and fistula formation are distressing and can be life-threatening. Successful resolution of major complications requires prompt diagnosis and correctly timed intervention, as well as selection and meticulous performance of an appropriate corrective procedure. Failure to follow this sequence frequently leads to a spiral of increasingly severe and morbid consequences. The gynecologist should focus attention on minimizing the risk of complication or on promptly diagnosing them, should complications occur. The management of significant bowel injuries can be complex and is best directed by a surgeon with experience. A neglected complication never resolves; appropriate consultation must be obtained early.

In this chapter we provide an overview of anatomy and function, review the diagnostic evaluation of the gastrointestinal tract, and outline preoperative and postoperative care of the intestine. We also discuss gynecologic procedures associated with bowel injury and identify the common sites of these injuries. A large section of the chapter is devoted to the recognition, evaluation, and management of immediate and delayed complications. The treatment of most gastrointestinal injuries is well defined and straightforward. Proper assessment of the problem and institution of an appropriate course of corrective action usually result in an acceptable outcome.

Normal Function and Anatomy

Delivery of optimal preoperative and postoperative care and the making of sound intraoperative decisions require a firm foundation in the structure and function of the alimentary tract.

Upper Tract

The foregut consists of the stomach, duodenum, pancreas, spleen, and liver, which receive their blood supply from the celiac trunk. This structure is very short and quickly divides into phrenic, gastric, hepatic, and splenic branches. The proper hepatic artery, portal vein, and common bile duct form the hepatoduodenal ligament (portal triad), which is one of the boundaries of the epiploic foramen of Winslow. The opening to the lesser peritoneal sac is a site of occult peritoneal metastases from gynecologic cancers. The retroperitoneal structures of the upper abdomen are rarely seen in any pelvic procedure. The celiac trunk in particular is in one of the most inaccessible sites in the abdomen.

Each surgeon should develop a systematic approach to exploration of the upper abdomen. We use a clockwise rotation starting with the right kidney, then proceeding to the gallbladder, right lobe of the liver, left lobe of the liver, stomach, spleen, and left kidney. The pancreas is in a fixed, retroperitoneal position, making palpation more difficult. The base of the transverse mesocolon runs over the head and inferior border of the pancreas. Lifting the transverse colon with one hand while placing the other hand at the base permits palpation of the body of the pancreas. The colon is then released and the operator's hand is placed over the pyloric junction to gently palpate the head of the pancreas. Palpation of the upper abdomen should be performed to the extent permitted by the incision. Carelessness in exploration of the upper abdomen can result in traction injuries to the liver or spleen. Caution should always be used in palpating these structures.

The volume of gastrointestinal secretion is related to the amount and type of food ingested (Table 4–1). If a patient is fasting, the quantity is small. An individual who eats three meals delivers about 8 L of fluid to the proximal small bowel, including 2 L of gastric, 1 L of biliary, and 2 L of pancreatic secretions.[1,2] Only 1 or 2 L will reach the colon.[3] Owing to the low pH of the gastric contents and powerful proteolytic qualities of pancreatic secretions, leakage of either of these materials results in major complications.

Small Bowel

The duodenum is entirely retroperitoneal and conforms to the head of the pancreas. It serves as a conduit for all the upper abdominal secretions since the stomach, bile duct, and pancreatic duct all terminate here. Little if any absorption occurs in the duodenum. The mean length of the small intestine is 350 cm, or approximately 12 feet.[3] The jejunum makes up the upper two fifths of the small intestine. It is characterized by a slightly red hue, thick wall, and absence of fat at the junction of the bowel and mesentery. The jejunum is a major site of absorption of water, electrolytes, fats, proteins, carbohydrates, and certain minerals.[4] The jejunum is part of the midgut and derives its blood supply from the superior mesenteric artery. An extensive arcade of anastomosing vessels distributes the blood to the bowel. Vascular occlusion of the superior mesenteric artery is catastrophic, whereas occlusion of a distal vessel will result in only a minor injury. The root of the small bowel mesentery runs at a 40-de-

TABLE 4–1. **Normal Volume and Composition of Gastrointestinal Secretions**

Site	Volume (L/day)	Electrolyte Composition (mEq/L)			
		Na^+	K^+	Cl^-	HCO_3^-
Salivary glands	≈ 1	20–80	10–20	20–40	20–160
Stomach	1–2	20–100	5–10	120–160	—
Liver	≈ 1	150–250	5–10	40–60	20–60
Pancreas	1–2	120	5–10	10–60	80–120
Small bowel	1–2	140	5	Varies	Varies

Modified from Lowery SF, Brennan MF: Life threatening electrolyte abnormalities. In Wilmore DW, Brennan MF, Harken AH, Holcroft JW, Meakens JL (eds): Care of the Surgical Patient, p 13. New York: Scientific American, 1991.

TABLE 4–2. **Identifying Characteristics of Small and Large Bowel**

	Jejunum	Ileum	Colon
Gross characteristics	Wide caliber Left upper quadrant Thick wall Reddish hue	Narrow caliber Fills pelvis Thin wall Pale	Teniae coli Abdominal periphery Thick wall Pale Appendices epiploicae
Blood supply	Superior mesenteric	Superior mesenteric	Superior and inferior mesenteric
Mesentery	Thin	Thick	Thick, variable

gree angle diagonally from left upper to right lower quadrant. For this reason, the jejunum is found in the left upper quadrant and is not seen through standard pelvic incisions unless the intestine is completely examined. The jejunum is usually not involved in adhesions from prior pelvic operations. Jejunal contents have very low bacterial counts except in patients with stasis from ileus or obstruction and those with bacterial overgrowth in the foregut.[5]

The ileum composes the distal three fifths of the small intestine. It is characterized by a thin wall, narrow caliber, pale hue, and fat at the bowel–mesentery junction. There is no clear boundary between the jejunum and ileum. The ileum is a minor site for absorption of water, electrolytes, proteins, carbohydrates, and minerals, although it does have a great reserve potential and can compensate for loss of a major portion of the jejunum. The terminal ileum is the unique site for absorption of bile salts, vitamin B_{12}, and fat-soluble vitamins. Resection of more than 100 cm of the terminal ileum will result in vitamin B_{12} deficiency, steatorrhea, and gallstones.[6] The blood supply to the ileum is also provided by the superior mesenteric artery, and a similarly rich collateral network is present. The ileum ends at the ileocecal valve, an important structure that helps control passage of liquid small bowel contents to the colon. Loss of the ileocecal valve will shorten transit times and exacerbate malabsorption symptoms due to small bowel resection. Reflux from the cecum to the ileum is not uncommon, so the terminal ileum usually has low levels of coliform bacteria. If an ileal resection or injury is anticipated, mechanical and antibiotic bowel preparation is recommended. Identifying characteristics of the various intestinal levels are summarized in Table 4–2. Sites of nutrient absorption from the small intestine are listed in Table 4–3.

TABLE 4–3. **Small Bowel: Sites of Absorption**

Nutrient Absorbed	Duodenum	Jejunum	Ileum
Water and electrolytes	1+	3+	2+
Fats	2+	3+	1+
Proteins	2+	3+	1+
Carbohydrates	2+	3+	1+
Bile salts	0	0	3+
Fat-soluble vitamins	1+	3+	1+
Water-soluble vitamins			
Vitamin B_{12}	0	0	3+
Folate	1+	3+	2+
Vitamin C		1+	3+
Minerals			
Fe	3+	2+	0
Ca	2+	3+	1+
Mg	1+	2+	2+
Zn	0	1+	2+

Colon

The colon is characterized by teniae coli running longitudinally along its wall and by fat appendages from the bowel, called appendices epiploicae. The right colon and proximal transverse colon share their blood supply with the rest of the midgut from the superior mesenteric artery. The middle colic artery is an important branch that is found in the mesentery of the transverse colon. Accidental injury during infracolic omentectomy can result in ischemia of the transverse colon. The hindgut, from the midtransverse colon to the rectum, receives its blood supply from the inferior mesenteric artery, which arises from the aorta at the level of L3 and can be injured during a retroperitoneal dissection or in patients with dense adhesions.

The colonic mesentery varies widely during its course and from patient to patient. The cecum can be fixed, with virtually no mesentery, or freely mobile to the degree that volvulus is possible. The hepatic flexure is fixed. The transverse colon mesentery can be quite long, easily reaching the pelvis. The pelvic surgeon should, therefore, be careful when operating in this area. The colon is also fixed at the splenic flexure, and the left colon is similarly immobile. The most common orientation of the sigmoid colon is as a loop that fills the left pelvis. Variations include a short, straight sigmoid, a longer sigmoid with a loop into the right pelvis, and a long sigmoid that ascends high into the abdomen and is vulnerable to torsion.[7] The rectum is retroperitoneal. Usually the peritoneal reflection is approximately 12 cm from the anus. Because the rectum is not always imaged well on barium enema examination, sigmoidoscopy is considered a superior method of evaluation.

The appendix is identified by the confluence of the teniae coli. It may be found in a variety of positions, but most commonly it is intraperitoneal in the right lower quandrant. Its variable position is a major reason why appendicitis can be difficult to diagnose and frequently mimics gynecologic conditions.

The major function of the colon is absorption of water and electrolytes, leaving formed stool. The colon normally absorbs 1 L/day but can increase daily absorption to as much as 6 L.[8] When the amount of fluid and solution entering the colon exceeds its absorptive capacity, diarrhea results. The absorptive capacity of the colon is reduced by irradiation or any procedure that shortens the colon, particularly if the ileocecal valve is removed or bypassed.

Evaluation of the Gastrointestinal Tract

Most gastrointestinal problems related to gynecologic surgery involve the small or large intestine, so we will focus on the diagnostic evaluation of these two areas. Many acute bowel injuries are obvious on gross inspection. Assessment of the intestine should, therefore, begin in the operating room. A careful and systematic examination of sites of injury should be performed at the completion of any pelvic operation. This examination should be particularly detailed if the operation involves lysis of adhesions, difficult dissection, or frequent intestinal manipulation. When detected, acute injuries should be corrected in the operating room.

Postoperative problems may become evident shortly after surgery or following a prolonged period of apparently normal function. Initial evaluation in the latter instance should consist of a history and physical examination. Additional diagnostic studies can then be considered to confirm or establish a precise diagnosis.

Plain Radiography

Radiographic evaluation of the abdomen typically includes a film taken with the patient lying supine, followed by a second film in which the abdominal contents are subjected to the effects of gravity (upright or right or left lateral decubitus positions). The flat plate film provides an overview of the abdominal cavity and is used to evaluate the general intestinal gas pattern. Large fluid collections, nephrolithiasis or cholelithiasis, and foreign bodies may also be detected.

The gravity-aided film permits an evaluation of intestinal gas–fluid interfaces and is most helpful in diagnosing bowel obstruction. The classic radiographic picture of multiple, stair-stepped, distended bowel loops is the hallmark of small bowel obstruction (Fig. 4–1*A* and *B*). Gas is usually absent in the large bowel and rectum. Occasionally, a fairly precise location for the site of obstruction can be predicted from radiographic findings. In many patients with mechanical obstructions, partial obstruction, or ileus, the film pattern may be more subtle. Clinical judgment and a careful evaluation of response to initial conservative therapy is essential in all cases. Serial radiographic examination is useful for monitoring the resolution of partial obstructions and ileus so that surgery can be avoided in patients who are responding to more conservative treatment.

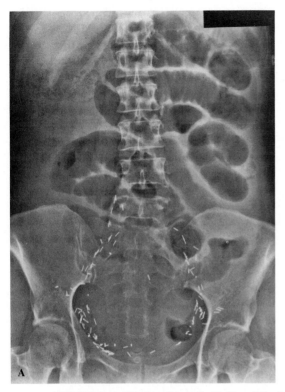 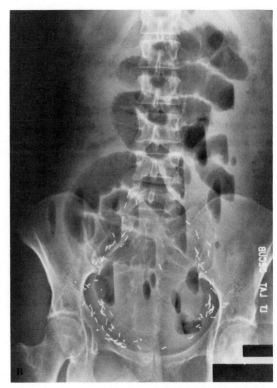

FIGURE 4–1. A. Classic radiographic findings of distal small bowel obstruction include multiple dilated loops of intestine arranged in a stair-stepped pattern. Little or no bowel gas can be seen in the colon and rectum. **B.** Air–fluid levels are evident on the lateral decubitus film. The patient was admitted with nausea and vomiting 1 month after radical hysterectomy for early cervical cancer. Obstruction was caused by an adhesive band entrapping a single loop of distal ileum.

Distention of the large bowel can also be readily determined on abdominal plain films. Large bowel obstruction or postoperative paralysis (Ogilvie's syndrome) is characterized by a prominent large bowel gas pattern (Fig. 4–2).[9] Typically there is little or no rectal air. The air–fluid levels seen in small bowel obstruction are absent or minimally evident because the ileocecal valve tends to limit the accumulation of gas and fluid to the large intestine.

The upright or decubitus film may also show extraluminal gas collecting in the less dependent portions of the peritoneal cavity (Fig. 4–3). Common locations of extraluminal gas include the undersurface of the diaphragm, adjacent to the liver edge, or immediately beneath the abdominal wall. Beyond the immediate postoperative period, this finding of "free air" suggests hollow viscus rupture or perforation and requires emergency intervention. Films obtained in patients with obstructive symptoms and findings, those undergoing a trial of conservative therapy, and those who develop acute symptoms should always be evaluated for the presence of extraluminal gas.

Small Bowel Study

Oral ingestion of barium or other contrast agent followed by fluoroscopy and plain radiography provides an outline of the esophagus, stomach, and small intestine and can distinguish between profound ileus and obstruction. Oral contrast studies have typically been avoided in patients with suspected obstruction because of fear of perforation and leakage of contrast medium into the peritoneal cavity. However, in appropriately selected patients, this risk is negligible. Water-soluble contrast medium affords inadequate visualization of the distal small bowel and should be avoided.[10,11] A decision to surgically correct small bowel obstruction can usually be made on the basis of clinical findings and plain radiographs without the use of contrast medium. Small bowel contrast studies are more

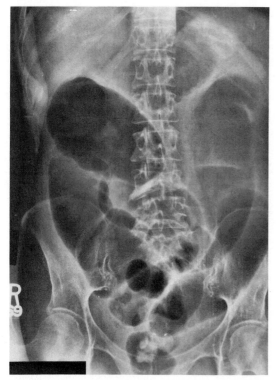

FIGURE 4–2. Massive dilation of the large bowel is demonstrated in this film from a patient with cervical cancer who sustained a stenotic, postirradiation sigmoid colon injury. Although bowel gas is seen in the rectum, complete obstruction of the midsigmoid was confirmed by barium enema examination. The obstruction was relieved by an end-descending colostomy with resection of the stenotic segment of sigmoid colon.

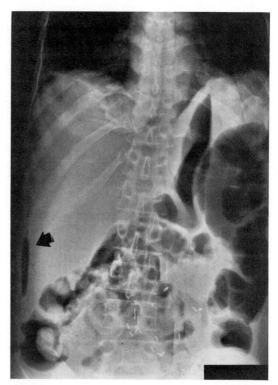

FIGURE 4–3. A small pocket of free air can be seen adjacent to the liver edge in this lateral decubitus film (*arrow*). The patient had ignored obstructive symptoms for several days and presented with an acute abdomen. At laparotomy, a small ileal perforation was noted proximal to an adhesive obstruction of the distal ileum.

helpful in the patient with atypical obstructive symptoms and findings or the patient with known or suspected small bowel fistula. Many small intestinal fistulas are complex and involve more than one bowel segment. They may also involve other pelvic organs such as the bladder, vagina, or large intestine. A preoperative small bowel study can identify the tracts of these complex fistulas, allowing the surgeon to better plan an appropriate corrective procedure.

Small bowel studies may also suggest a diagnosis of inflammatory bowel disease, extensive adhesions, or severe irradiation injury. The location and extent of injury can usually be established. If surgical intervention is indicated, contrast-enhanced studies may assist in developing operative plans.

Barium Enema Examination

Rectal instillation of barium contrast medium can be performed as a single-column barium enema that fills and distends the large bowel or as an air-con-

trast barium enema, which allows better evaluation of mucosal anatomy. The air-contrast study is preferred when intrinsic large bowel lesions are suspected. The single-column study can be used to confirm a diagnosis of large bowel obstruction or fistula. In these situations, the contrast medium will outline the abnormality, and an accurate assessment of the level of large bowel obstruction can be made. In patients with large bowel fistulas, contrast medium will spill into the bladder or vagina, outlining these organs. All patients with small bowel fistulas should undergo barium enema examination to exclude a large bowel component to a complex fistula. A large bowel study may also provide information about extrinsic displacement (Fig. 4–4), fixation from adhesions or tumor, and stenosis from chronic irradiation effect. When both large and small bowel studies are planned, the large bowel study should be performed initially; otherwise the large bowel study cannot be done until the contrast medium in the small intestine has cleared the entire bowel.

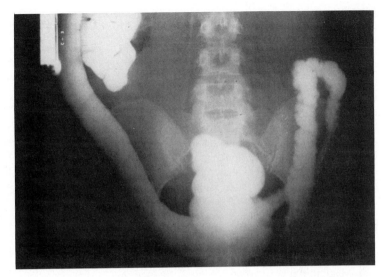

FIGURE 4–4. Bowel contrast studies occasionally provide information about the presence and magnitude of extrinsic disease. Impressive lateral displacement of the bowel is seen in this barium enema study of a patient who had a 26-kg dermoid cyst arising in the retroperitoneal space. Note the inferior displacement of the transverse colon and the lateral location of the distal ileum, which has filled with refluxing contrast material from the cecum.

Gastrointestinal contrast media may also be introduced into colostomies, mucous fistulas, or spontaneous fistulas to outline the course of the adjacent bowel segment or fistula tract. These are generally specialized studies ordered as part of the preoperative evaluation of patients with an existing bowel problem in whom additional therapy is planned. They are usually not needed as a part of the routine evaluation of postoperative intestinal problems. In cases where communication with the peritoneal cavity is suspected, Gastrografin may be preferable to barium sulfate as the contrast medium since it is less likely to cause chemical peritonitis.

Endoscopy

Upper gastrointestinal endoscopy allows direct visualization and biopsy of the esophagus, stomach, and duodenum. It is most commonly used as a diagnostic tool or to provide treatment for a primary gastrointestinal problem. Because benign gynecologic operations are normally limited to the pelvis, direct injuries to these upper abdominal organs are rare. In the gynecology patient, postoperative upper endoscopy is most often employed to diagnose or evaluate upper abdominal pain or bleeding not directly attributable to an operative complication.

In contrast, endoscopic visualization of the large intestine is often required to assess large bowel injuries, as many benign and malignant diseases of the female reproductive tract involve the large intestine. Because of its adjacent pelvic location, the rectosigmoid colon is at greatest risk. Intrinsic mucosal lesions, sites of obstruction, and fistula openings can be readily visualized. Diagnostic biopsies

should be performed when necessary. For most problems related to gynecologic procedures, proctoscopy or proctosigmoidoscopy is adequate. Cases that are more complex, those with suspected large bowel pathology, and assessment of bleeding may require a complete colonoscopy. Endoscopic decompression of the colon is also therapeutic in patients with Ogilvie's syndrome.[12]

Function Studies

Most patients who develop postoperative fistulas of the small intestine have drainage of obvious small bowel contents from an area of skin breakdown or through the vagina. Irritation from exposure to acid and enzymes quickly causes an intense local inflammatory response. Small fistulas, particularly those developing in an area of preexisting wound disruption, may be difficult to diagnose because the small volume of effluent through the tract does not produce the typical clinical findings. Drainage through small fistulas may be intermittent or may intermix with other local secretions, making an accurate clinical diagnosis impossible. In such cases, oral ingestion of a marker substance may be tried to confirm that the observed drainage originates in the small intestine. We have employed a simple and inexpensive bedside method using either activated charcoal slurry or brilliant green dye for this purpose. Black or green coloration of the drainage confirms the presence of a fistula. More sophisticated studies may then be necessary to completely define the abnormality.

Some surgeons recommend that patients with prior anorectal sphincter injuries that have been repaired and protected by diverting colostomy should undergo a test of anal continence prior to colostomy takedown. This can be accomplished by mixing a smooth, semisolid slurry of oatmeal and instilling it into the anorectal pouch. If the patient can maintain continence of this solution, reanastomosis of the large intestine can be undertaken. Patients who fail the continence test may be incontinent if the colostomy is taken down. An alternative approach is to measure rectal and anal sphincter tone with a manometer, which can also provide useful information about the strength of the sphincter, before subjecting the patient to a major surgical intervention.

Preoperative Bowel Preparation

Preoperative bowel preparation decreases the morbidity and mortality of colon surgery.[13] Reductions in the incidence of wound infection and other septic complications have been well documented.[14,15] Histopathologic examination of colon anastomoses in laboratory animals that underwent preoperative bowel preparation has shown improved healing of the anastomosis; presumably, similar effects occur in humans. Any gynecologic patient undergoing a planned colon operation or judged to be at significant risk for large bowel injury should undergo bowel preparation (Table 4–4).

Most infections following large bowel surgery are caused by the endogenous bacterial flora, primarily anaerobic gram-negative rods (*Bacteroides*) and aerobic coliforms (especially *Escherichia coli*). Less common pathogens include *Staphylococcus, Proteus, Pseudomonas,* and *Clostridium* organisms. Although it is probably impossible to sterilize the colonic lumen, reduction and alteration of bacterial content are feasible. In the normally functioning intestine, the small bowel contents do not contain a significant bacterial load.

Techniques for preoperative bowel preparation combine mechanical cleansing of the colon followed by oral antibiotics. Mechanical cleansing reduces total bacterial counts by removing fecal mass. Bacterial concentration (number of organisms per gram of feces) and composition (types of organisms) are unchanged. Oral antibiotics reduce bacterial concentration and alter composition.[16,17] The combination of mechanical cleansing followed by oral antibiotics is more effective than either component used alone. Oral neomycin sulfate and erythromycin base are the most commonly used antibiotic combination. Fecal antibiotic concentration is increased when the antibiotic is given after the mechanical portion of the bowel preparation. By design, these antibiotics are poorly absorbed; their action is largely confined to the intestinal lumen. Their use as a component of bowel preparation does not provide a significant systemic effect. Additional intravenous therapy should be employed for procedures requiring antibiotic prophylaxis. Short-term treatment (<24 hours) with a first- or second-generation cephalosporin has been recommended for gynecologic procedures in which prophylaxis has been shown to be beneficial.

Effective mechanical preparation can be achieved using a standard 3-day regimen (Table 4–5) or a "whole-gut lavage" with Golytely solution (Table 4–6). Whole-gut lavage has the advantages of shorter duration, reduced risk of dehydra-

TABLE 4–4. **Indications for Bowel Preparation**

Fixation of pelvic organs detected on examination
Endometriosis
Pelvic inflammatory disease
Undiagnosed pelvic mass
Known ovarian carcinoma
Pelvic exenteration
Bowel fistula repair
Planned colostomy or colostomy takedown
Extensive bowel adhesions expected
Exploration for radiation bowel injury
Planned bowel resection or bypass

TABLE 4–5. **Standard 3-Day Bowel Preparation**

Day 1:
 Low-residue diet
 Bisacodyl, 1 capsule PO at 1800 hr

Day 2:
 Low-residue diet
 Magnesium sulfate, 30 mL (50% solution), at 1000, 1400, 1800 hr
 Saline enemas until clear return at bedtime
 A completely absorbed high-calorie enteral feeding solution can be started via enteral feeding tube infusion in patients with caloric depletion

Day 3:
 Clear liquid diet, IV hydration as needed
 Magnesium sulfate, 30 mL (50% solution), at 1000, 1400 hr
 Neomycin sulfate, 1 g PO at 1300, 1400, 2300 hr
 Erythromycin base, 1 g PO at 1300, 1400, 2300 hr

Day of surgery:
 Fleet's enema at 0630
 Operation scheduled for 0800 hr

TABLE 4–6. **Whole-Gut Lavage
with Golytely Solution**

Golytely solution to be mixed in bulk by pharmacy:

Constituent	Concentration
NaCl	25 mM/L
Na$_2$SO$_4$	40 mM/L
KCl	10 mM/L
NaHCO$_3$	20 mM/L
Polyethylene glycol	80 mM/L

Day prior to operation:
Clear liquid diet
Begin chilled Golytely PO at 1200 hr (infused by nasogastric
   tube if patient unable to tolerate PO) (rate of ingestion,
   1–2 L/hr; total, 3–8 L)
Golytely ingestion discontinued when clear fluid passed per
   rectum (usually 3–6 hr)
Neomycin sulfate, 1 g PO at 1300, 1400, 2300 hr
Erythromycin base, 1 g PO at 1300, 1400, 2300 hr

Day of surgery:
Fleet's enema at 0630 hr
Operation scheduled for 0800 hr

tion and electrolyte imbalance, less interference with preoperative caloric intake, and higher patient acceptance.[18–21] We use this technique exclusively for the preoperative preparation of our patients. In most cases, adequate bowel preparation can be performed on an outpatient basis.

Complications of Bowel Preparation

Fluid and electrolyte imbalances can occur with any preparation technique but are more common with the 3-day regimen or lavage solutions, which do not contain an intraluminal osmotic agent (polyethylene glycol). The mechanical cleansing portion of the 3-day preparation can result in significant losses of water, sodium, potassium, calcium, magnesium, and phosphorus. Serum electrolytes must be monitored, and intravenous fluid and electrolyte supplementation is frequently necessary in debilitated patients. Lavage solutions that do not contain an osmotically active component can cause substantial absorption of water and electrolytes and must be used with care in patients with cardiac or renal disease. Addition of the intraluminal osmotic agent minimizes this risk.

Interference with oral caloric intake is a potential problem for patients undergoing bowel preparation, particularly when the operation has been preceded by a series of diagnostic tests also requiring colon cleansing. Weight loss and negative nitrogen bal-

ance are commonly observed. Because of its shorter duration, the lavage preparation causes less interference with caloric intake. A regular diet can be ingested until the day before operation. Perioperative parenteral nutritional support should be considered in any patient with an altered nutritional status.

Overgrowth of antibiotic-resistant colonic organisms (primarily *staphylococci* and yeast) can occur. This risk is minimized by the short duration of antibiotic exposure. The development of bacterial resistance to antibiotics is a theoretical risk that has not been a significant clinical problem. Pseudomembranous enterocolitis rarely occurs after bowel preparation. Patients who develop the characteristic watery diarrhea require appropriate diagnostic workup and treatment.

Special Problems

Patients with intestinal stomas who are scheduled for revision or reanastomosis procedures should undergo lavage preparation of the proximal bowel segment. Although the isolated distal bowel segment should not contain fecal material, cellular debris and mucus are present. This segment also contains the usual colonic bacteria. Adequate preparation of the distal colon can be achieved by lavage through a mucous fistula or by enema into a Hartmann pouch using normal saline or Golytely solution containing 1 g of neomycin sulfate and 1 g of erythromycin base per liter. Enemas can be given in the usual manner, but care should be taken not to overdistend the colon. Lavage through a mucous fistula can be accomplished by irrigating the distal segment using a bulb syringe or by using gravity infusion through a Foley catheter that has been placed into the mucous fistula.

Patients with intestinal obstruction or who require acute surgical intervention cannot undergo preoperative bowel preparation. When gastrointestinal stasis has been present, bacterial colonization of the small bowel contents is likely. Systemic antibiotic therapy (Table 4–7) will reduce infectious complications in these situations. To be effective, tissue antibiotic levels must be obtained prior to bacterial contamination. The addition of a topical antibiotic (neomycin sulfate or polymixin and bacitracin) into the surgical wound may reduce the incidence of postoperative wound infection.[22] Meticulous surgical technique and avoidance of gross fecal contamination of the peritoneal cavity are of prime importance when operating on unprepared bowel.

TABLE 4–7. Systemic Antibiotic Prophylaxis for Emergency Colon Surgery

1–2 hr before operation:
  Aqueous penicillin G, 4 million units IV q 6 h (substitute erythromycin, 500 mg IV, if penicillin allergy)
  Gentamicin sulfate, 1 mg/kg IV q 8 h
  Clindamycin, 300 mg IV q 6 h
Continue systemic prophylaxis for 24–28 hr

Bowel Injury During Surgery

Bowel injury can occur at any point during a gynecologic procedure. These injuries are rare, occurring in less than 0.5% of benign cases.[23] Intraoperative intestinal injuries can be divided into two broad categories: those related to adhesions from prior surgery that resulted in fixation of the intestine, and injuries related to pelvic pathology that distorts normal anatomy and fixes intestine in the pelvis. Preventing these injuries requires attention to the time-honored principles of surgery: knowledge of anatomy and disease, adequate exposure and lighting, and dissection using traction and countertraction. Adherence to these simple guidelines, coupled with adequate surgical experience, will allow the surgeon to anticipate and avoid most situations that put the intestine at risk.

Abdominal Surgery

Enterotomy is a potential complication of every abdominal entry. This risk is increased when operating through a previous scar. In patients with a previous vertical incision, opening the abdomen a few centimeters above the old scar usually allows easy entry into a free space. Emphasis is usually placed on extending the incision cephalad to achieve adequate exposure. In fact, adequate caudal exposure is required for good pelvic exposure. The skin and fascia must be incised to the symphysis and the rectus muscle separated to the same level. Extending the incision a few centimeters lower often results in dramatically improved pelvic exposure with no adverse cosmetic effect, since this portion will be in the pubic hair. The incision through the peritoneum should always be made with gentle sharp dissection. If the peritoneal cavity is not entered when anticipated, the presence of adherent bowel is likely. Persistent dissection under these circumstances should be avoided. Instead, the surgeon should attempt entry at a different level of the incision. Once the peritoneal cavity is entered, bowel adherent to the anterior abdominal wall is still at risk if the intestine is fixed on either side of the incision. Vigorous fascial traction can easily tear these fixed loops of bowel. Bowel adhesions must be taken down sequentially as the incision is extended. Many techniques to take down adhesions have been described. All share the principles of gentle traction, countertraction, and identification of a plane between structures, the so-called "white line." Most surgeons prefer using Metzenbaum scissors for this purpose. Blunt dissection should be avoided.

Once the abdomen is opened with an incision that will provide adequate exposure for the planned procedure, exploration should be performed. All abdominal and retroperitoneal structures should be gently palpated. Attention is then turned to the pelvic pathology. If adhesions obscure normal anatomic relationships, they must be removed. If the intestines are agglutinated, the surgeon must use patience and skill to lyse the adhesions and avoid enterotomy. Following individual bowel loops is helpful. However, when a difficult junction is encountered the field of operative focus should change. Excessive traction against dense pelvic adhesions will always result in bowel injury. The ileum is the most common site of small bowel injury in gynecologic surgery. Any adhesive process—inflammation, tumor, irradiation, or prior surgery—can lead to dense adhesions between the ileum and surrounding structures. The ileum can be partially twisted, folded back, curled, or kinked in numerous variations that make each dissection a challenge. Loops adherent deep in the cul-de-sac are particularly difficult to extract without enterotomy. Patients who have previously undergone a hysterectomy commonly have small intestine deep in the pelvis, even adherent to the vaginal cuff. Careless dissection of adherent loops from the pelvic side walls places the major vessels and ureter at risk. Although enterotomy is to be avoided, an accidental incision can be used to the surgeon's advantage, for it allows insertion of a finger into the lumen to guide further dissection. If closure is deferred, marking the injury site with a suture allows later recognition. If bowel resection appears inevitable, it is better to do this and preserve the integrity of the bowel than to struggle and create multiple enterotomies.

The wall of the colon is thicker and less prone to enterotomy, but serosal tears are common. Not all serosal tears require oversewing. However, if the mucosa is herniated, we prefer serosal repair. A redundant sigmoid or transverse colon is especially prone to injury since either may be located in unanticipated places (i.e., transverse colon adhesions to the uterine fundus). The sigmoid is frequently adherent to the left adnexa or left pelvic side wall. These adhesions must be lysed to permit packing of the sigmoid out of the pelvis. Always use moistened laparotomy packs when packing to avoid serosal abrasions. Self-retaining retractors should be placed with care to avoid pressure or traction injuries.

With the bowel packed, intestinal injury during abdominal hysterectomy most commonly occurs in the cul-de-sac. Patients with an obliterated cul-de-sac from any cause are at particular risk. During a difficult procedure, the operator may focus so much energy on avoiding ureteral injury that danger to the rectum may be overlooked. In this situation it becomes imperative to identify vital structures. This is best accomplished using a retroperitoneal approach. A useful technique in this situation is to develop the rectovaginal space, a potential space usually spared from the pathologic process obliterating the peritoneal cavity. Small, unrecognized injuries to the rectum can result in rectovaginal fistula. If any question about the integrity of the rectum exists, fill the pelvis with water. Beginning distal to the rectum, gently compress the colon and bring the hand down toward the rectum in a "milking" fashion. Leaks can then be identified by noting gas bubbles. If the patient is in Allen stirrups, an Asepto syringe or sigmoidoscope can be used to introduce air into the rectum.

Closing the abdomen presents another risk to the intestine. Incorporating bowel into the abdominal wall closure can result in obstruction or enterocutaneous fistula. This complication is preventable with careful technique. Adequate fascial margins should be present to allow closure. We usually close the abdomen using either a running[24,25] or interrupted mass closure. The final sutures are not tied down until all have been placed so that bowel cannot be inadvertently incorporated into the closure.

Vaginal Surgery

Entry into the peritoneal cavity via the cul-de-sac is a blind procedure and direct entry into any adherent structure is possible. If the loop of intestine can be mobilized and the enterotomy site clearly identified, it can be repaired.[26] If vaginal repair is not safe, laparotomy is indicated. The rectum is also vulnerable during vaginal hysterectomy. However, the enterotomy is, by definition, below the peritoneal reflection, and repair is best performed transvaginally. A layered closure that includes the va-

gina will help prevent fistulization. Vaginal evisceration is a rare complication following vaginal hysterectomy and can be repaired from below.[27]

Laparoscopic Surgery

As more gynecologic procedures are performed using operative endoscopy, bowel injuries are bound to occur. Two major kinds of bowel injury may occur during laparoscopy: trocar injuries and electrocautery injuries. Care must always be taken during placement of the Verres needle to insufflate the abdominal cavity. Standard precautions, such as checking proper needle function, aspiration through the Verres needle after placement, and ensuring high flow at low pressure, should be routine. Aspiration of bowel contents indicates injury. Although the procedure may be completed endoscopically, the site of the injury must be visualized and repaired.[28] Even if the needle is placed successfully, the bowel may be injured by subsequent trocar insertion. Such injuries are more likely to be complex, requiring laparotomy to repair. The risk of all insertion injuries is increased by previous surgery or any other adhesive process; however, prior surgery is not a contraindication to laparoscopy. Another way to minimize enterotomy is to use an open technique with the Hassan cannula.

Cautery injuries are a major concern as coagulation necrosis can extend beyond the visible burn. If simple oversewing of the visible burn is performed, delayed perforation can occur.[29] Several deaths associated with monopolar cautery bowel injuries were reported following sterilization procedures during the early 1980s.[30] For this reason, monopolar cautery was abandoned by most gynecologists. Subsequent investigators have suggested that the bowel injuries were in fact primarily traumatic and not a result of cautery.[31] Currently, monopolar cautery is commonly used in general surgical procedures with what is reported to be excellent safety.[32]

Regardless of the type of cautery used, several precautions must be employed. Only instruments with adequate insulation should be used. The tip of the cautery instrument must be under direct visualization at all times. Adequate pneumoperitoneum to maintain visualization of the cautery tip is mandatory. The operator should keep in mind that depth perception and peripheral vision are both diminished and contribute to difficulty in keeping the cautery tip away from other structures. Holding the laparoscope close to the operative field will improve visualization but decrease visualization of adjacent structures. Accidental discharge of the cautery must be avoided. Should a bowel injury occur, the full extent of the injury may not be apparent. Laparotomy is indicated to assess and repair the damage. This is especially important because patients undergoing traumatic bowel perforation usually become symptomatic within 12 to 48 hours, whereas electrocautery injuries may not become apparent until 4 to 10 days later, presumably owing to delayed bowel wall necrosis.

Routine Postoperative Care

Any surgical procedure that exposes the peritoneal cavity, especially in conjunction with general anesthesia, can interfere with bowel function. For minor outpatient procedures such as diagnostic laparoscopy, there is no need to restrict the patient's postoperative diet. For patients who undergo uncomplicated laparotomy, we keep the patient on an NPO diet on the day of surgery. If a nasogastric tube has been placed intraoperatively, we remove it in the operating room. These patients rarely develop ileus. When bowel sounds are present, we advance the diet to clear liquids. Occasionally a patient on a clear liquid diet develops distention and decreased bowel sounds, in which case the patient is again placed on an NPO diet. Continuing to feed a patient with an ileus is more likely to lengthen rather than decrease the duration of the ileus. When an ileus occurs, we usually do not place a nasogastric tube unless the patient vomits.

If a patient tolerates clear liquids for 24 hours and has a soft, nondistended abdomen and normoactive bowel sounds, a regular diet is ordered. Passage of flatus is not mandatory before starting a regular diet; however, it is prudent to document passage of flatus prior to discharge. With this strategy, a young, healthy patient may be discharged 3 or 4 days after uncomplicated abdominal surgery.

We are more cautious in patients who have undergone prolonged procedures, who are advanced in age, or who have undergone extensive intraoperative bowel manipulation. Although nasogastric tubes are not mandatory in these situations, many surgeons feel it is an appropriate precaution. We use the same general strategy as described above, except that we anticipate a longer postoperative hospitalization (5 or 6 days). It usually takes these patients an extra day or two to establish bowel sounds. We usually do not advance diet through full liquids and soft food; rather, we go directly to regular diet and allow the patient to select the diet she wants.

If a patient undergoes enterotomy, bowel resection, bypass, or colostomy, then we routinely place a nasogastric tube. An incidental appendectomy is not an indication for nasogastric compression. The management of the tube depends largely on the extent of surgery. For bowel resection, we usually remove the nasogastric tube after passage of flatus.

Management of Nasogastric Tubes

Appropriate care of a nasogastric tube is important to a patient's postoperative comfort. It is vital that the physician closely supervise management of the tube to prevent complications. The selection of the tube is usually made in the operating room. We usually use a 16 French tube, and we always use a sump tube. The sump mechanism permits the use of continuous suction while preventing entrapment of the gastric mucosa in the distal opening of the tube.[33] Nonsumping tubes require intermittent suction to accomplish the same goal. It is best to avoid a small-caliber tube since it may clog easily. If the tube is placed intraoperatively, we manually check for correct gastric positioning. The tip should reach about three fourths the distance from the gastroesophageal junction to the pylorus and lie along the greater curvature. If the tube is placed postoperatively, injecting air through the tube should produce characteristic bubbling sounds over the stomach. In most patients the second black mark on a Salem sump tube will be at the nares when the tube is well positioned in the stomach. Many techniques exist for taping the tube in place. We find that tape on the bridge of the nose and forehead is tolerated much better than on the cheeks or upper lip. The tube should be fixed loosely because the nares are surprisingly vulnerable to pressure necrosis.

With the tube in the correct position, the drainage in the first 24 hours is usually of small volume and is clear. The tube should be irrigated regularly, usually once per shift, to ensure proper function. As time progresses, the drainage will become darker, consistent with old blood. Although the material will be guaiac positive, the amount of bleeding is usually quite small. Bilious drainage suggests ileus. Our usual postoperative fluid replacement is dextrose 5½ in normal saline with 20 mEq of potassium chloride. In patients with a low nasogastric output, the rate can be adjusted accordingly. If output is high, other fluids may be appropriate. Pancreatic and biliary secretions have high sodium concentrations, and suction can thus result in hyponatremia associated with hypovolemia. The treatment is aggressive fluid replacement with normal saline. This type of hyponatremia must be distinguished from dilutional hyponatremia, which is treated with fluid restriction. Gastric secretions contain high concentrations of chloride and potassium and should be replaced accordingly with normal saline and potassium supplement.

The volume of drainage is a poor guide to the timing of tube removal. Some patients with ileus have very little reflux into the stomach, and the tube simply prevents entry of more air and secretions into the small bowel. Other patients with resumption of bowel function will drain over 1 to 2 L/day from a nasogastric tube. In patients with high volumes, clamping the tube for 4 to 8 hours and checking the residual volume may help to determine whether the small intestine can handle these secretions.

Prevention of Stress Ulcers

Patients who are NPO for long periods are at increased risk for stress ulcers. Although the acidity of gastric contents is not increased, the protective mucosal barriers are diminished. Patients with a history of peptic ulcer disease, gastritis, smoking, and use of aspirin or nonsteroidal anti-inflammatory drugs are at risk. Prophylaxis against ulcers should be considered. A variety of histamine receptor blockers are now available and will be successful in most patients. To keep the pH above 6,[34] antacids can be given via the nasogastric tube up to every 2 hours with 30-minute dwell time. Sucralfate is used in the treatment of ulcers and is believed to act locally at the mucosal surface. It is not used for prophylaxis.

Nutritional Support

Some patients cannot eat for extended periods before or after surgery. A well-nourished patient can tolerate up to 10 days of intravenous 5% dextrose fluids without signs or malnutrition. The simplest definition of malnutrition is a greater than 10% weight loss from baseline. Nutritional support is indicated in malnourished patients even if the NPO period is brief. Although the data are conflicting, we use 10 to 14 days of preoperative feedings in malnourished patients scheduled for major gynecologic surgery.[35,36]

Several routes of feeding are possible. One route is peripheral parenteral nutrition, which requires simple venipuncture and routine nursing care. Hyperosmotic peripheral solutions cause thrombophlebitis, so a large volume of fluid must be given. This will limit the number of calories some patients can receive.[37] A second option, total parenteral nutrition, must be given by central venous access. The major complications of this method relate to infection and insertion of the venous catheter. A third option, enteral feedings, prevents the gastrointestinal mucosa atrophy associated with starvation.[38–40] If the gastrointestinal tract is in suitable condition, we prefer enteral nutrition. If enteral feeding is anticipated during surgery, a feeding gastrostomy or jejunostomy can be placed. Pre- or postoperatively, a soft nasogastric or nasal duodenal tube can be used; however, these tubes can irritate the airways and esophagus. Percutaneous placement of a gastrostomy tube is appropriate when an extended period of enteral feeding is anticipated.[41] As a general rule, enteral feeding provides equal nutritional support and is more cost-effective than total parenteral nutrition.[42]

Immediate Complications: Intraoperative Repairs

No matter how meticulous and experienced a surgeon is, complications will occur. If an intestinal complication is identified at the time of gynecologic surgery, the extent of the injury and the timing of repair should be assessed.

Upper Abdominal Injuries

Fortunately, upper abdominal injuries are rare in gynecologic surgery. The liver and spleen are vulnerable to traction injuries, especially in patients with tumor adhesions that fix structures and tempt the surgeon to exert excess traction. At M. D. Anderson, one third of splenectomies performed were due to traction injuries occurring during omentectomy.[43] Traction injuries to the spleen that rupture the capsule usually require splenectomy, although recently surgeons have been attempting splenic repair to preserve this organ and prevent long-term infectious complications.[44,45] If a hemorrhagic injury to the liver or spleen occurs, the first step is to obtain adequate access to the upper abdomen by extending the incision to the xiphoid. The gynecologist can do this while awaiting the arrival of an appropriate consultant. Liver lacerations are usually repaired with 0 gauge chromic sutures on a special rounded, blunt needle. Hemostatic materials such as Gelfoam or Surgicel may be sutured into the laceration to aid in hemostasis. Bleeding from smaller injuries may be controlled with the cautery set on high, arcing the current so that the Bovie tip does not stick to the liver parenchyma. If it is available, an argon beam coagulator can be used for this purpose.

Gastric injuries are also rare. If the stomach is filled with air during intubation, then the risk of such an injury is increased. Placement of a nasal or oral gastric tube before making an extensive vertical incision is a reasonable precaution. Gastric injuries are repaired with a two-layer closure of delayed absorbable material, as described later. If the injury is extensive or the conditions less than ideal, a gastrostomy tube may be placed for prolonged drainage.

Pancreatic injuries are also unusual. The pancreas is entirely retroperitoneal and therefore is not seen or palpated by most gynecologic surgeons. If an injury does occur, appropriate intraoperative management is vital, since serious complications such as abscess formation, pseudocyst, and pancreatic-cutaneous fistula may result. It is vital to place a drain if a pancreatic injury occurs.

Small Bowel Injuries

The normal position of the duodenum is approximately 5 cm above the bifurcation of the aorta, in between the superior and inferior mesenteric arteries, making operative injuries unusual. Enterotomy can occur during para-aortic lymph node sampling, especially if the duodenum is low-lying or adherent to para-aortic nodes (Fig. 4–5). Repair is similar to what will be described for the jejunum and ileum.

Enterotomy to the jejunum or ileum is treated by first dissecting the enterotomy away from surrounding structures to make closure possible. Because the bowel tears easily, it should be handled with care. The surgical principles involved in suturing the small bowel include maintaining an adequate blood supply, using small-gauge absorbable suture material, using full-thickness pedicles, creating a watertight seal, and preserving the lumen.[46] Careful inspection for mesenteric injuries, which may compromise blood supply to the damaged portion, is paramount. Signs of vascular insufficiency include cyanosis, absence of peristalsis, and absence of bleeding from the cut edges. The closure is aligned so as to not narrow the caliber of the intestine and is usually achieved by closing the enterotomy perpendicular to the axis of the bowel. Once the site and orientation of the repair have been determined, stay sutures are placed at each angle.

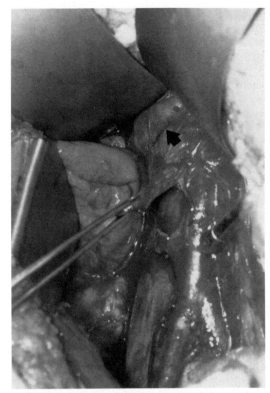

FIGURE 4–5. Injury to the upper gastrointestinal tract is rare during gynecologic procedures because the foregut is anatomically distant from the pelvis. An exception is the third portion of the duodenum, which crosses the vena cava in the midabdomen, as seen in this operative dissection (*arrow*). Inadvertent duodenal injury is a potential complication of right-sided para-aortic node biopsy.

Vascular pickups are used. Our preference is a single-layer closure with full-thickness bites using 3-0 polyglycolic delayed absorbable suture material. The sutures are placed approximately 3 mm apart, with the knots tied on the outside. If a second layer can be placed without compromising the diameter of the lumen, this is done with interrupted 3-0 suture (Fig. 4–6). The integrity of the seal is tested by milking gas and liquid past the repair site while observing for leakage. The adequacy of the lumen is confirmed by inching the bowel along the axis of the gut. A 1-cm diameter is adequate. Failure to recognize and repair an enterotomy can be catastrophic. Leakage of bowel contents will result first in localized and then in generalized peritonitis. In a postoperative patient, these events can proceed so rapidly that septic shock may be the presenting clinical situation. A repair can leak for several reasons: failure to close the entire injury, sutures

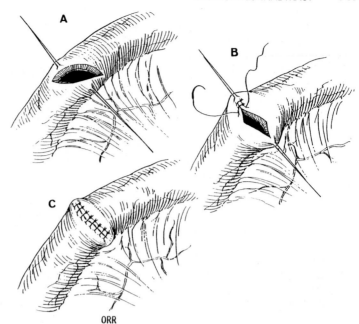

FIGURE 4–6. A small enterotomy can be easily repaired with a single-layer closure. **A.** Stay sutures are placed to orient the bowel wall defect so that it is perpendicular to the path of the bowel contents. **B.** Full-thickness, simple interrupted stitches of 000 delayed absorbable suture material are placed at 3-mm intervals. **C.** The completed closure should be watertight and result in no compromise of the luminal diameter.

placed too far apart, delayed necrosis from sutures placed too close together, inadequate blood supply, excessive tension, or distal obstruction with increased intraluminal pressure. Previous irradiation, preexisting peritonitis, small vessel diseases such as hypertension and diabetes, and intraabdominal tumor increase the risk of poor healing and breakdown. Resection should be performed if necessary to avoid these circumstances. If a leak develops, generalized peritonitis may ensue, but often the leak is small and the site is walled off by adhesions and omentum, resulting in abscess formation. As is the case with all abscesses, purulence will seek the route of least resistance to drain. In postoperative patients, that route is frequently the abdominal or vaginal incision. When the abscess drains, a fistulous path is left between the gut and the draining site.

Other circumstances arise in which a simple repair is not adequate and small bowel resection is necessary. Vascular insufficiency and multiple or extensive trauma to a loop, especially an irradiated segment, are indications for resection. A cyanotic loop should be carefully inspected to demarcate the extent of compromise and to look for signs of reperfusion. Reperfusion can occur after lysis of a dense, fibrotic band. The mesentery of the small bowel can be transilluminated and the likely compromised vessel identified. Viable resection margins with good blood supply are similarly identified. Gastrointestinal stapling devices have made a

small bowel resection quick and reliable, so if the viability of a segment of small intestine is in doubt, resection is recommended.[47–50]

Most small bowel injuries do not require additional antibiotic coverage beyond routine surgical prophylaxis with a first- or second-generation cephalosporin. If other factors are present that increase the risk of bacterial overgrowth in the small gut, such as ileus or obstruction, then we extend the antibiotic coverage in terms of drugs and duration.

Large Bowel Injuries

Large bowel injuries always raise the possibility of colostomy. In general, repair of the colon is safe in patients with good mechanical and antibiotic bowel preparation and favorable local conditions in the pelvis. In patients who have had good bowel preparation and limited injury, two-layer closure done in a similar fashion to that described for the small bowel without colostomy is appropriate. A second layer is always added except in the rare circumstance of a very narrow sigmoid. The second layer is interrupted, with the sutures 3 mm apart. In patients with a simple injury, unprepared bowel, and gross peritoneal contamination with stool, diverting colostomy and repair should be considered. A simple loop colostomy usually accomplishes diversion of the fecal stream and may be reversed without an additional laparotomy.

Previous irradiation, extensive injury, vascular

insufficiency, and adjacent tumor are all indications for resection. Resection can be accomplished with gastrointestinal stapling devices in a similar fashion as with the small bowel. After the damaged segment is resected, the likelihood of successful reanastomosis is assessed. Reanastomosis requires a tumor-free site, adequate mobility, and adequate blood supply. A side-to-side functional end-to-end reanastomosis performed with gastrointestinal stapling devices results in minimal spillage of bowel contents. A major advance in operative technology has been the introduction of end-to-end anastomotic stapling devices. These instruments are placed in the rectum and permit anastomosis to be performed deep in the pelvis much more quickly than with hand-sutured techniques. Several authors have reported that good results can be obtained in patients with pelvic tumors and prior radiation therapy, provided that there is no tension on the anastomosis, the bowel was adequately prepared, and there is no active infection. If a low anastomosis is necessary and these conditions cannot be met, a loop colostomy should be employed to divert the fecal stream for 6 to 8 weeks until the anastomosis can heal. It is our routine to place patients who undergo large bowel repair on broad-spectrum antibiotic coverage for at least 72 hours. It is our impression that with modern antibiotics and surgical techniques, the indications for colostomy following large bowel injury incurred during surgery for benign gynecologic conditions are very few.

The rectum can be entered during difficult pelvic dissectons. In a patient with an empty rectum, leakage of air or bowel contents will not be seen, complicating recognition of the injury. When such an injury is missed during hysterectomy, a rectovaginal fistula is the likely result. Injuries that occur below the peritoneal reflection are also repaired with the two-layer closure technique. Testing the integrity of the distal repairs can be very difficult. A useful technique is to fill the pelvis with water and insert a small amount of air into the rectum with an Asepto syringe and look for bubbles in the pelvic pool. This is only possible with the patient in lithotomy or Allen stirrups. If a difficult dissection is anticipated deep in the pelvis, especially in cases of endometriosis or severe pelvic inflammatory disease, placement of the patient in Allen stirrups can be a major asset to the surgeon. Rectovaginal fistula can still occur following repair, owing to delayed necrosis. Partially mobilizing the omentum and inserting the mobilized portion between the rectum and vagina may help by providing new blood supply to an extensively inflamed cul-de-sac. This omental pedicle graft may help prevent recurrent fistula formation.

Immediate Postoperative Complications

Perforation

Not all intestinal trauma is detected at the time of laparotomy. Other perforations may be delayed, such as those occurring after laparoscopy. The clinical manifestations of perforation vary widely, and the clinician must maintain a high index of suspicion. The classic signs and symptoms of peritonitis include pain, distention, fever, and leukocytosis. Unfortunately, free air under the diaphragm is not pathognomonic of perforation in the first 72 postoperative hours. These classic symptoms may not be present in patients with immunosuppression or prior radiation therapy. In fact, the amount of pus present in the peritoneal cavity in the absence of the usual signs and symptoms of peritonitis is sometimes remarkable. In a patient with peritonitis and in whom perforation is part of the differential diagnosis, a period of antibiotics and observation can be considered. During this time, vital signs and input and output must be carefully monitored. If the situation does not improve within 12 to 24 hours, or worsens, immediate exploration is indicated. Subtle early signs of sepsis such as mild hypotension, tachycardia, fluid retention, and change in mental status must be taken very seriously. Premature exploration with negative findings is preferable to catastrophic delay. It is important to avoid operating on a patient in septic shock, for the morbidity and mortality in this setting are excessive. If perforation is the true diagnosis, surgery is the only curative treatment.

Ileus

Some degree of adynamic ileus occurs after any abdominal procedure. There is no clear correlation between extent of the procedure and severity of the ileus.[51] Bowel function in uncomplicated cases returns in the first 2 or 3 postoperative days. Signs and symptoms of ileus are nausea, vomiting, and distention with absent bowel sounds. The patient should be placed on an NPO diet. If a patient vomits, the best approach is to place a nasogastric tube, since it will immediately stop the vomiting and associated discomfort. Abdominal radiographs will help distinguish ileus from obstruction. At least two views of the abdomen should be obtained, a supine view and an upright view. A lateral view can substitute for the upright view in patients who cannot stand. The common radiographic findings in patients with ileus are dilated loops of bowel with gas throughout the intestines. Because it is sometimes difficult to distinguish an early obstruction from ileus, repeat films are sometimes indicated. A patient with ileus needs time to recover bowel function. We find that a gentle enema or suppository does help some patients, but only those with clinical signs of improvement such as increasing bowel sounds or decreased distention. Patience on the part of the clinician is usually the best approach. There is a tendency to try to withhold narcotics that inhibit intestinal motility; however, this must be weighed against the need to maintain the patient's NPO status and to treat incisional pain. An uncomplicated ileus will resolve on its own schedule. The clinician should also keep in mind that ileus can be associated with other postoperative complications, including abscess, hematoma, pyelonephritis, urinary leaks, and peritonitis. These should always be considered, especially in patients who develop ileus that is more severe than anticipated or who develop ileus after initial recovery of intestinal function.

Obstruction

Intestinal obstruction is usually a delayed event. Physical examination will usually demonstrate a distended, tympanitic, nontender abdomen (Table 4–8). Abdominal radiographs will show the patterns associated with obstruction described earlier. In some patients the obstructive symptoms will be intermittent, giving the clinician hope for recovery of function. However, if the abdominal radiographs are consistent with complete obstruction, return of bowel function is unlikely. As in the case of ileus, consideration should be given to other complications as the underlying cause. However, the most common reason is rapid adhesion formation. Typically, a single band or kink is responsible for the obstruction. A rare cause of obstruction is a mechanical error, such as suturing the intestine into the abdominal wall closure. Some patients with a partial obstruction may respond to conservative measures and resume bowel function. If conservative therapy is going to be successful, signs of improvement become apparent within the first day of observation.[52] Once the diagnosis of complete obstruction is established, exploratory laparotomy should be performed.[53] In debilitated patients who are otherwise stable, surgery may be delayed. Some surgeons prefer a mercury-filled balloon-tipped long tube (Cantor, Miller-Abbot) to a nasogastric tube in these relatively stable patients. It is hoped that peristalsis and gravity will carry the weighted tip distally, decompressing the intestine and relieving obstruction. Generally, the long tube will not pass the obstruction in patients with absent bowel sounds. There are patients who do respond to prolonged observation; however, this must be weighed against the additional time, cost, and risk of nosocomial infection.

Reexploration for Bowel Complications

Unfortunately, in some situations exploratory laparotomy is the only way to exclude the possibility of perforation or of infarcted or strangulated bowel (Fig. 4–7). Patients who have signs of progressing sepsis, whose condition is deteriorating on antibiotic therapy, and whose physical examination and laboratory findings have excluded other sources of infection should be considered for reexploration. Once the decision is made to reexplore, the patient should be quickly stabilized with necessary blood products and intravenous fluids and taken to the operating room. Usually the simplest corrective procedure is appropriate, even if this means a third operation in the future. At reexploration, the surgeon must be certain that all the pathology is addressed. Failure to adequately identify and treat a bowel injury at reexploration will usually result in death.

TABLE 4–8. **Signs and Symptoms of Acute Bowel Complications**

Sign or Symptom	Ileus	Obstruction	Perforation
Pain	Generalized discomfort	Crampy	Severe, localized, progressive
Nausea, vomiting	Present	Present	Variable
Fever	Absent	Absent	Present
Leukocytosis	Absent	Variable	Present
Bowel gas pattern	Nonspecific	Distended small bowel, air–fluid levels, colon empty	Nonspecific
Free air	Absent	Absent	Present

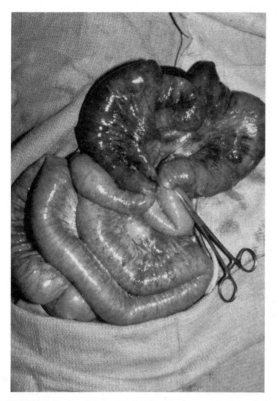

FIGURE 4–7. Small bowel infarction is characterized by dark red or black discoloration of the bowel segment with associated dilation and edema. The patient experienced acute pain in a long-standing incisional hernia. This loop of small intestine had become entrapped within the hernia sac and was sharply constricted by a fascial ring. Resection and reanastomosis were successfully accomplished.

Delayed Complications

Mechanical Small Bowel Obstruction

In the patient without cancer, most delayed small bowel obstructions result from intraperitoneal adhesions that have developed after surgery or other intraabdominal inflammatory events.[54] Several mechanisms for late bowel obstruction have been described: (1) "kinking" of a loop of small bowel that is tightly tethered by an adhesion, (2) torsion or volvulus of a loosely adhered loop of bowel about its mesentery, (3) internal herniation of a bowel loop through an adhesive ring, and (4) intussusception of a mobile proximal segment into a more fixed distal segment. Each of these mechanisms results in a discrete localized blockage of a relatively short segment of the small intestine.

Once the lumen is obstructed, intestinal fluids and gas accumulate. Initial efforts to propel luminal contents past the obstruction may lead to intense cramping and abdominal pain. Continued bowel contraction against the area of obstruction causes local irritation, inflammation, and edema, enhancing the degree of blockage. As obstruction progresses, abdominal distention increases and ultimately gives way to nausea and vomiting. In complete obstruction, vomiting becomes severe enough to preclude all oral intake. Fluid and electrolyte depletion within 2 to 3 days is common.

The patient with complete mechanical obstruction usually presents with a several-day history reflecting the events described. A medical history will often reveal a previous gynecologic operation. Illnesses known to involve peritoneal surfaces, such as endometriosis or pelvic inflammatory disease, increase the risk of adhesion formation. Any information regarding such disease should therefore be elicited. A review of available operative notes may indicate the degree and location of major bowel adhesions identified at prior surgeries. Often the patient has experienced similar, less severe episodes that resolved spontaneously.

Physical findings normally include a distended and tympanitic abdomen. Bowel sounds are absent or diminished. Vomiting of bilious or feculent material may be evident. Flat and upright abdominal films show multiple dilated loops of small intestine and air–fluid levels. The number and location of dilated bowel loops may provide radiographic clues to the level of obstruction. Blockage of the jejunum will produce only a few distended loops that are localized to the upper abdomen. An established obstruction of the terminal ileum is visualized as multiple dilated segments throughout the entire abdomen.

Although acute postoperative bowel obstruction can be difficult to delineate from ileus or partial obstruction, delayed small bowel obstruction almost always represents a mechanical problem. Once the diagnosis is determined, treatment should proceed quickly: (1) replace intravascular volume, (2) correct electrolyte abnormalities, (3) decompress the stomach and small bowel with nasogastric suction, and (4) explore the patient to relieve the obstruction. If the patient has a less classic presentation, a short period (24–48 hours) of bowel rest may be attempted to determine whether spontaneous resolution occurs. Patients undergoing a trial of conservative management must be monitored closely. The development of increased abdominal pain, rebound tenderness, fever, leukocytosis, or tachycardia is ominous. These may be the first signs of impending perforation or infarction,[55] and bowel rest should be abandoned in the presence of any significant adverse change in the patient's clinical status.[56] In our experience, patients with partial obstruction or symptoms from a cause other than obstruction will begin to improve within 24 hours.[57] Patients whose examination findings and symptoms persist after 24 hours of conservative management become candidates for exploration,[58–60] as chances that further conservative therapy will be successful are small and the risks of perforation and bowel necrosis become significant.[61]

Patients with small bowel obstruction should be explored through a midline vertical incision that can be modified to provide access to any point in the abdomen. The site and cause of small bowel obstruction are usually evident when the abdominal cavity is opened. The small intestine proximal to the site of blockage will be dilated and fluid-filled even if preoperative decompression by nasogastric tube has been instituted. Bowel distal to the obstruction is usually normal in caliber. The intestine should be examined to identify the cause of the obstruction. In most cases, lysis of a single adhesion or release of a trapped loop of bowel is all that is needed to relieve the obstruction. No attempt should be made to deflate dilated bowel or evacuate intraluminal fluid collections. The entire intestine should be carefully inspected to ensure viability as well as the absence of an occult perforation. Correct positioning of the nasogastric tube should be confirmed intraoperatively.

The postoperative management of patients with a bowel obstruction consists of continued decompression and bowel rest, along with fluid and electrolyte replacement. Continued careful monitoring for signs of an acute abdomen is important because bowel infarction, though rare, is a potentially fatal complication. The first clinical sign of resolution is a sudden drop in the volume of nasogastric suction output, indicating resumption of peristalsis and movement of fluid into the distal bowel. When objective evidence of returning bowel function is present—decreasing distention, active bowel sounds, passage of flatus or stool—decompression can be discontinued. We usually wait an additional 24 hours before instituting oral feedings, with the diet gradually advanced over 3 to 4 days.

Special Studies

The previous section provided an overview of the management of the patient with uncomplicated small bowel obstruction. Focal obstruction caused by limited adhesions is generally a straightforward surgical problem. Delayed small bowel obstruction in patients with massive adhesions, prior pelvic or abdominal irradiation, or active intra-abdominal cancer poses a more difficult management problem. Obstruction in these settings typically occurs months or years after initial surgery or diagnosis, and the history of the inciting event is well known. Many of these patients have a long history of gastrointestinal dysfunction and repeated episodes of partial obstruction. Management of these complicated blockages is a challenge for the skilled surgeon.

Massive abdominal adhesions develop in patients with diffuse or repeated inflammatory reactions within the peritoneal cavity. They may be expected in patients with extensive prior surgery, previous peritonitis or abdominal abscess, or prior intraperitoneal therapy with irritant agents (radioisotopes, chemotherapeutic drugs). Although obstruction in this situation can sometimes be localized to a single small bowel segment, it more commonly represents partial blockage of multiple bowel segments at multiple levels. A precise point of obstruction often is not discernible.

The patient should be prepared preoperatively as for any bowel obstruction. Once the abdomen is opened, adhesions should be lysed and the bowel mobilized. This is often a tedious process, and great care should be taken to avoid inadvertent enterotomy. When the entire small intestine has been cleared, it should be inspected for sites of irreparable injury or occult perforation. Although bowel resection and reanastomosis is not desirable in the obstructed patient, badly damaged segments should be excised.

Some surgeons attempt to manipulate the bowel so that future adhesions will fix the intestine in a position that minimizes the risk of subsequent obstruction. This can be accomplished by gently replacing the small intestine in wide, looping arcs within the abdominal cavity. The serosae of adjacent bowel segments are then sutured to each other using a technique originally described by Noble.[62] The goal is to provide smooth, sweeping turns within the small bowel so that acute angulation is unlikely as new adhesions form. An alternative approach is to thread a long intestinal tube, such as the Baker tube, throughout the entire length of the small intestine.[63] The tube is placed into the stomach through a gastrostomy and then manually advanced to the terminal ileum. When the small bowel is returned to the abdomen the tube serves as a stint and positions the small intestine in the same sweeping turns described for the Noble plication.

The Baker tube can be used for decompression, but we generally use a separate nasogastric tube for this purpose. We leave the tube in place for about 2 weeks to allow postoperative adhesion formation, and then gradually remove the tube over 12 to 24 hours.

Late bowel obstruction following pelvic or abdominal irradiation is a diagnostic and therapeutic dilemma. Because the terminal ileum attaches to the retroperitoneal portion of the right colon, it is relatively fixed and can receive a significant dose during external beam pelvic irradiation. The remaining small intestine is usually more mobile and migrates in and out of the pelvic field during the course of treatment, decreasing the total dose of any single segment. More proximal bowel loops adhered in the pelvis may also sustain significant radiation exposure and subsequent injury. These adhesions probably are the reason why patients with prior pelvic inflammatory disease or prior surgery are at greater risk for radiation bowel injury.[64,65]

Radiation bowel injury typically manifests as bowel obstruction 12 to 24 months after completion of therapy. Often the patient has been treated for multiple episodes of subacute obstruction. The late effects of irradiation include microvascular stenosis, mucosal ulceration, and fibrosis.[66] Macroscopically the bowel wall is pale and its mesentery is shortened and fibrotic. However, absence of these signs does not preclude the possibility of significant radiation effect. The terminal ileum demonstrates dense loop-to-loop adhesions and compromise of luminal diameter and wall motility.

Preoperative evaluation of obstructed bowel in an irradiated patient can be difficult, for the classic clinical and radiographic signs of obstruction are less likely to be present. The warning signs of impending perforation may be blunted by altered peritoneal function and host response. Because the hallmark of mucosal injury is surface breakdown and ulceration, the risk of progression to full-thickness injury is substantial. Reduced blood flow through the fibrotic mesentery further impedes the patient's ability to heal. Previous reviews of radiation injury have tended to emphasize repeated efforts at conservative management. Our current philosophy is that early and aggressive operative intervention is preferable and minimizes the risk of small bowel perforation.

The operation of choice for radiation injuries was formerly a bowel bypass procedure that left the injured segment in place.[67,68] Several recent reports have suggested that resection with reanastomosis is

an equivalent alternative that has the advantage of completely removing the damaged portion of the intestine.[69-71] Resection of both the terminal ileum and the cecum is recommended so that the reanastomosis involves nonirradiated bowel (Fig. 4–8).[72,73] We prefer resection for severe injuries, since this establishes intestinal continuity without risk of blind loop syndrome or later perforation. We have, however, performed bypass procedures in the unstable patient or when the morbidity of resection was considered excessive. The most pragmatic approach would seem to be individualizing the operative approach to the specific situation in a given patient.

Patients who have received extended field or whole-abdomen irradiation are at slightly greater risk of small bowel injury than those treated with

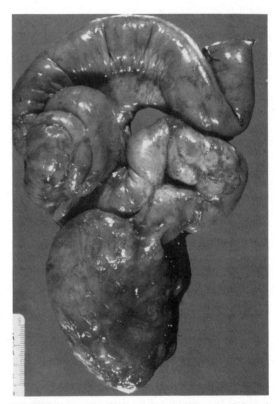

FIGURE 4–8. Irradiation injury to the small intestine frequently involves the terminal ileum since it is relatively fixed by its attachment to the cecum. A pale bowel surface, shortened mesentery, and multiple, dense, loop-to-loop adhesions are characteristic, as seen in this surgical specimen. In these cases, our preference is to attempt ileocecal resection with reanastomosis of the small bowel to the ascending colon when feasible. This allows construction of an anastomosis with nonirradiated bowel segments.

standard pelvic fields. This risk can be limited by adhering to dose tolerances that have been established for the larger treatment fields (approximately 45 Gy for extended fields and 30 Gy for the whole abdomen). When these patients develop obstruction, operative therapy must be carefully planned, for it is more difficult to limit reanastomosis to non-irradiated bowel segments.

Bowel obstruction in the patient with intraperitoneal metastatic gynecologic cancer usually is not surgically correctable. Many patients with ovarian epithelial or endometrial cancer have diffuse tumor spread refractory to standard therapy. Serosal involvement by tumor nodules prohibits effective peristalsis and frequently produces multiple sites of partial obstruction.[74] Patients usually present with protracted periods of bowel dysfunction, nausea, and vomiting. In the absence of effective systemic therapy, relief of these obstructions is not possible. Rare patients with an apparently localized recurrence may derive short-term benefit from surgical relief of the obstruction.[75] At exploration, virtually all patients have other sites of clinically occult disease that contribute to the obstructive symptoms.

Palliation can sometimes be achieved by percutaneous or operative placement of a gastrostomy tube. The tube can be opened to allow decompression and drainage during episodes of more severe symptomatology; it can be clamped to allow oral intake if symptoms temporarily abate. We teach the patient and her family members techniques for tube care and function and direct them to make day-to-day adjustments at home.

Large Bowel Obstruction

Delayed obstruction of the large intestine following gynecologic procedures is unusual. The large caliber, rich blood supply, and relatively fixed position of the colon render it relatively immune to the usual mechanisms of obstruction. Blockage of the large bowel can usually be attributed to irradiation injury or recurrent cancer. In each of these situations, the patient's history suggests the diagnosis. The pelvis is a frequent site of recurrence for any gynecologic cancer, and recurrences originating in the vaginal apex, at the pelvic wall, or in the cul-de-sac can easily grow to entrap the adjacent sigmoid colon at the level of the peritoneal reflection (Fig. 4–9). Stenotic irradiation injuries typically involve the sigmoid colon about 5 to 10 cm above the peritoneal reflection. This site corresponds to the level of the uterine tandem sources used for brachytherapy in patients with cervical or endometrial cancers.[76] Patients develop small vessel occlusion and fibrosis that ultimately results in loss of sigmoid luminal diameter and wall contractility. Often, obstruction is preceded by repeated bouts of proctitis. Volvulus is an unusual cause of obstruction that is seen in patients with redundancy of the sigmoid colon.

Patients with large bowel obstruction present with abdominal distention and cramping lower abdominal pain. Nausea and vomiting tend to be less

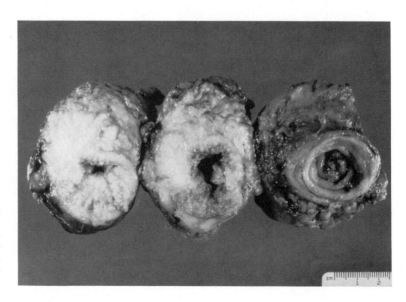

FIGURE 4–9. Extrinsic involvement by pelvic tumor can result in narrowing and occlusion of the distal colon. This specimen demonstrates tumor invasion of the sigmoid wall with virtually complete obstruction of the lumen.

prominent than in patients with small bowel obstruction. Typically, the patient reports a variable period of pain, difficulty with bowel movements, and reduced stool volume and caliber. The onset of symptoms is usually described as gradual. Rectal bleeding may be present. Often the patient has decreased her oral intake for a period of weeks in response to symptoms. Unsuccessful self-medication with stool softeners, laxatives, and enemas is commonly attempted.

Physical examination may demonstrate abdominal distention and tympany. Bowel sounds are usually decreased. Bimanual pelvic and rectal examinations should disclose a pelvic tumor mass or stenosis of the rectosigmoid. Plain radiographs show dilation of the large bowel. A barium enema study or proctoscopy can demonstrate the level and degree of obstruction (Fig. 4–10). It is important to study the large bowel before considering surgical intervention to diagnose recurrent cancer and to exclude the possibility of a new colonic cancer unrelated to previous tumor or treatment. In complex cases, simultaneous involvement of the small intestine should also be considered. The diagnostic evaluation should be tailored to the clinical findings.

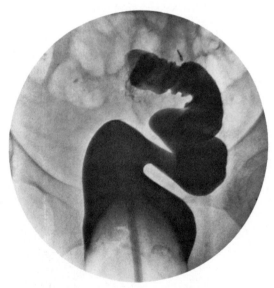

FIGURE 4–10. This spot film from a single-contrast barium enema examination shows complete obstruction of the sigmoid colon. The patient presented with a large pelvic recurrence of endometrial adenocarcinoma. The scalloped outline at the proximal sigmoid is indicative of serosal tumor implants and can be compared with the normal smooth colonic contour, seen distally. The patient described mild abdominal distention, cramping abdominal pain, and persistent nausea with minimal vomiting. Plain radiographs were not diagnostic. Palliative diverting colostomy was performed.

Stenotic large bowel obstruction from irradiation injury can be successfully treated by performing a diverting colostomy above the level of injury. If concomitant injury to the terminal ileum is absent or clinically insignificant, the patient can expect normal gastrointestinal function following diversion. Our preference is to resect the stenotic sigmoid segment to eliminate the potential for pain, infection, and bleeding. We then perform an end-descending colostomy using nonirradiated colon for the stoma, and close the rectum as a Hartmann pouch. Alternative approaches include a transverse loop colostomy or sigmoid resection with reanastomosis. The transverse loop procedure, while simple, potentially allows continuing stool passage into the stenotic distal limb and an ongoing risk of infection and perforation. We have approached reanastomosis with caution because the distal rectal segment has been heavily irradiated; its use in the anastomosis may hinder healing and lead to anastomotic disruption. Others, however, have reported acceptable results with reanastomosis using irradiated rectum.

Except for the rare patient with radically resectable local disease, the patient with large bowel obstruction from recurrent cancer is not curable. Candidates for palliative relief of obstruction must be chosen carefully. Unfortunately, failure to relieve obstruction will cause death from perforation, sepsis, or hemorrhage. Patients with limited life expectancy are best served by simple decompression employing a transverse loop colostomy or tube cecostomy. Both procedures are easy to perform and subject the patient to minimal risk. Patients with longer life expectancies (4 months or more) may be candidates for end-colostomy as described above. Occasionally we attempt resection of bulky pelvic recurrence at the time of diversion if the patient is symptomatic and resection is thought to be technically feasible with limited risk. It is important to avoid complex, high-risk operations when the surgical goal is palliation of an incurable disease.

Small Bowel Fistula

The late development of small intestinal fistulas generally represents an acute event superimposed on chronic bowel injury. The segment of small intestine forming the fistula is often compromised by a long-standing process such as dense adhesions, irradiation, infection, chronic obstruction, or tumor invasion (Fig. 4–11). Normal repair of apparently minor acute insults to the bowel wall or mucosa is impaired, and integrity of the bowel wall is lost.

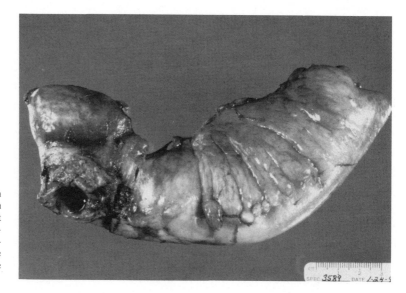

FIGURE 4–11. This loop of ileum formed an enterovaginal fistula when it became entrapped by recurrent cervical cancer. Resection and reanastomosis of the small bowel were performed to eliminate irritating drainage of small bowel contents through the vagina and onto the perineum.

Leakage of intestinal contents initiates an intense local inflammatory response as the body attempts to wall off the area of injury. Although often initially successful at containing small amounts of intestinal fluid, the continuing inflammatory response ultimately results in adjacent tissue breakdown. The accumulated bowel contents then exit the abdominal cavity through the area of tissue breakdown. Over time, a chronic draining tract is established, creating the fistula.

The fistula tract usually drains through the nearest adjacent structure, which can be the abdominal wall or another pelvic organ such as the bladder, vagina, or large bowel. The presence of foreign bodies, such as synthetic mesh, may also enhance the potential for fistula formation by promoting small bowel adhesions. When a significant background injury is present, multiple or complex fistulas can occur. Complex fistulas are more common when large segments of small intestine have been severely compromised. Rather than a single tract connecting a damaged loop of small intestine to the outside, these complex fistulas can interconnect multiple bowel loops or organs. Processes that involve adjacent pelvic structures in addition to the small bowel are also more likely to result in complex fistula formation. A diligent study of adjacent organs should be undertaken in all patients with small bowel fistulas. A surgical approach that fails to address all components of a complex fistula will be unsuccessful.

Patients with small intestinal fistulas frequently have an impressive clinical presentation. Typically, external drainage of irritating small bowel effluent is preceded by several days or weeks of abdominal pain that corresponds to the initial internal leak and resulting inflammatory response. Breakdown of adjacent tissue and external drainage prompt the patient to seek medical care. Small bowel contents cause an intense reaction in the skin or mucosa at the exit point (Fig. 4–12); skin or mucosal breakdown and pain occur rapidly. Although some immediate postoperative fistulas can be difficult to detect (particularly when breakdown through a fresh incision occurs), most delayed fistulas break down through an intact external surface and produce obvious signs and symptoms.

Physical examination readily identifies a defect in the abdominal wall or vagina. Drainage of small bowel contents is usually apparent on visual inspection. If a small bowel source of the drainage is uncertain, oral ingestion of charcoal slurry or brilliant green dye can be employed, as discussed earlier. Intense inflammation consisting of erythema and superficial breakdown of adjoining mucosa or skin is commonly noted. Tenderness and pain are prominent.

The initial management of the patient with a small bowel fistula must proceed in several directions simultaneously: (1) the volume of effluent must be reduced, (2) adjacent tissues must be protected from further erosive effects while the existing injury is treated, and (3) the source, complexity, and cause of the fistula must be investigated. Only after these initial steps have been taken can a definitive therapeutic plan be developed.

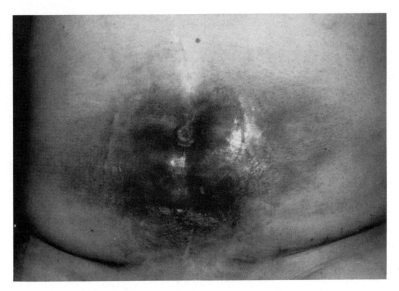

FIGURE 4–12. Small bowel contents cause intense inflammatory reactions in normal skin. Multiple cutaneous fistula tracts and chronic dermatitis are easily seen on the abdominal wall of this patient, who developed a complex enterocutaneous fistula after mesh repair of a large incisional hernia. The fistula had been present for several months at the time this photograph was taken. Symptomatic control of drainage had been attempted with an enterostomal appliance. After a 2-week period of bowel rest and intravenous nutritional support, the mesh graft was excised. Multiple small bowel loops adhering to mesh and forming the fistula were resected. A stapled small bowel reanastomosis was performed.

Effluent volume through the fistula tract, while somewhat dependent on the size of the fistula, can be substantially reduced by placing the bowel at complete rest. This is accomplished by using an NPO diet and nasogastric drainage. H_2-blocking drugs can be given to reduce gastric acidity. We begin total parenteral nutrition to support the patient calorically and promote healing.

Reducing or eliminating fistula drainage is the most important aspect of containing local injury. If continuing drainage is a problem, some attempt to minimize skin or mucosal contact should be employed. Enterostomal appliances can be placed over abdominal wall fistulas to collect effluent and protect the skin from further injury. Solid adhesive skin barriers may also be useful in limiting additional injury and promoting healing.[77] Containment of effluent through an enterovaginal fistula is more difficult. We have tried K-cup drainage via low suction in high-volume fistulas, but this is not completely satisfactory because drainage is usually incomplete, leakage around the cup is common, and the vaginal mucosa above the cup continues to be exposed to small bowel contents. Protection of perineal skin is also complicated. Adhesive barriers can be used but are difficult to maintain because of the many skin folds and movement during ambulation. Topical application of barrier ointments, such as aquafor or zinc oxide, may provide some limited protection. When drainage through the fistula is controlled, spontaneous healing of the local tissue injury occurs.

An appropriate diagnostic evaluation should be started. A small bowel contrast study will identify the location of the small bowel component to the fistula (Fig. 4–13). An effort must be made to identify additional tracts to other areas of the small bowel since many fistulas are complex. Barium enema examination should be performed in most cases to exclude large bowel involvement. Specialized contrast studies, such as vaginography, cystography, or fistulography, should be considered in cases not well visualized or evaluable on standard gastrointestinal studies.

Small-caliber fistulas in noncompromised patients may heal with conservative therapy consisting of bowel rest and parenteral nutritional support.[78–81] Spontaneous closure under these circumstances is more common in acute postoperative fistulas than those that occur after a prolonged time frame. In our experience, large-caliber fistulas or those originating in irradiated small bowel will rarely close spontaneously. Several recent reports have suggested that the use of somatostatin analogues may enhance fistula closure with conservative therapy.[82,83] Further experience with these agents, particularly in the high-risk setting, is needed. Fistulas caused by local tumor infiltration cannot be successfully managed conservatively.

The majority of patients with delayed small bowel fistulas require surgery. Our preference is to resect the involved bowel segment and fistula tract completely. Resection eliminates the potential for ongoing pain, necrosis, and drainage.[84] We then

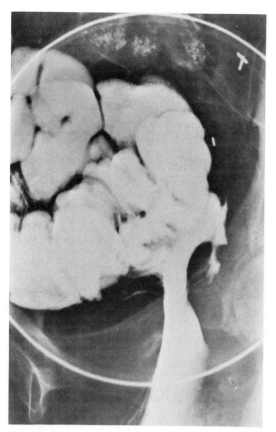

FIGURE 4–13. Barium contrast material from a small bowel study drains through a large ileovaginal fistula, providing a complete outline of the vaginal canal. This patient, who had cervical cancer, had a severe radiation bowel injury with multiple small bowel loops densely adhering to the pelvis. The fistula was corrected by excising the damaged bowel segment and performing a stapled reanastomosis.

perform small bowel anastomosis using segments not involved by chronic injury. Occasionally the fistulized bowel segment cannot be excised because of dense adhesive changes or patient instability. Bypass procedures or isolation of the segment can be performed in this situation. Often, mucous fistula formation can be avoided because the fistulous tract provides decompression of the isolated segment. When fistula formation is related to foreign material, this material should be removed if possible.

Postoperative bowel rest and nutritional support are continued until normal bowel function resumes. An oral diet can then be gradually instituted. Sometimes patients who have been subjected to prolonged bowel rest experience persistent nausea and vomiting when oral feeding is attempted. After ob-

struction has been excluded as a cause, enteral feeding with an elemental diet can be used to reestablish mucosal enzyme systems in the intestinal brush border.

Small intestinal fistulas in the patient with disseminated or recurrent cancer must be approached surgically. Major and potentially morbid operations are not desirable in these patients. Unfortunately, less aggressive approaches to symptom management are usually unacceptable. Surgical intervention should be limited to patients who have significant therapeutic options for their primary disease or those with a life expectancy long enough to warrant hospitalization for surgery and recovery. Nonsurgical palliative treatment should be provided for terminal care patients, even if symptom control is less than ideal.

Large Bowel Fistula

Perioperative rectovaginal fistulas are the result of a discrete surgical injury or postoperative infection. Repair can frequently be accomplished because the pelvic tissues are healthy and have maintained good blood supply.[85] Delayed large bowel fistulas are virtually always associated with a chronic precipitating injury, usually pelvic infection or abscess, irradiation, or tumor. Chronic infection of gynecologic or diverticular origin localized to the cul-de-sac can erode the rectosigmoidal wall at the level of the peritoneal reflection. Subsequent fistula formation most often involves the vagina but can include the uterus, bladder, or small intestine. Erosion and tissue breakdown from tumor or severe irradiation injury most often result in rectovaginal fistula formation.[86] Radiation damage typically involves the anterior sigmoidal wall adjacent to the tandem during brachytherapy placement for cervical cancer, or the lower rectal wall adjacent to needle implantation for vaginal tumors. Tumor destruction and fistulization most often involve the upper vagina and rectum. Many of these rectovaginal fistulas are accompanied by some component of large bowel obstruction, with fistula formation occurring proximal to the point of blockage.

Patients presenting with rectovaginal fistulas describe the onset of stool passage through the vagina. This has usually been preceded by a variable period of episodic obstructive symptoms and lower abdominal pain. Patients find the odor and hygiene problems associated with stool passage offensive. However, formed stool is much less irritating than small bowel contents, so mucosal and skin irritation is minimal. Patients with an infectious etiology will have signs and symptoms of infection or abscess formation. Patients with prior irradiation or active tumor growth will have an appropriate history or obvious findings on the physical examination.

Speculum examination confirms the presence of stool in the vaginal vault. Digital examination will often permit palpation of the fistulous opening. As described for small bowel fistulas, additional diagnostic studies should be performed to exclude a complex fistula that involves pelvic organs.

A staged repair can be considered for rectovaginal fistulas resulting from chronic infectious injury. The principles of correction are the same as those outlined for repair of acute perioperative rectovaginal fistulas. Active infection should be treated and the pelvic inflammatory response should be resolved before repair is attempted. This may require placement of a diverting colostomy prior to repair of the fistula. A layered fistula closure is performed. If possible, new blood supply is brought to the area of the closure, usually in the form of an omental pedicle graft or Martius flap.[87,88] The colostomy is left in place to protect the repair and then taken down as a third procedure when healing is complete.

We do not attempt repair of rectovaginal fistulas in cases of severe irradiation injury or active tumor. Even when the irradiated bowel segment can be excised, a large bowel anastomosis must still be created using one segment that has also been heavily irradiated. Anastomotic leak, abscess formation, and re-creation of the fistula are common outcomes. In addition, a traditional layered closure of the tract is virtually impossible to perform in an irradiated field with dense fibrosis, further enhancing the potential for failure. Although some investigators have reported successful staged repair of radiation-induced rectovaginal fistulas,[89–91] most experience suggests an exorbitantly high failure rate. We perform end-descending colostomy and Hartmann pouch formation as permanent therapy for most postirradiation rectovaginal defects.

Most rectovaginal fistulas caused by direct tumor invasion should be treated nonsurgically with symptom management. Palliative diversion can be considered in patients with legitimate therapeutic options or a life expectancy long enough to warrant operative intervention. If surgical diversion is considered, the most rapid and simple approach should be employed. The temptation to proceed with simultaneous tumor reduction should be resisted. A prolonged and morbid bowel procedure is a disservice to the patient with terminal cancer.

References

1. Gray GM: Acute diarrhea. In Wilmore DW, Brennan MF, Harken AH, Holcroft JW, Meakens JL (eds): Care of the Surgical Patient, chap 4, p 2. New York: Scientific American, 1989.
2. Philips SF: Diarrhea: A current view of pathophysiology. Gastroenterology 63: 495, 1972.
3. Dudrick SJ, Latifi R, Fosnocht DE: Management of short bowel syndrome. Surg Clin North Am 71:625, 1991.
4. Allard JP, Jeejeebhoy KN: Nutritional support therapy in short bowel syndrome. Gastroenterol Clin North Am 18:589, 1989.
5. Isaacs PET, Kim YS: The contaminated small bowel syndrome. Am J Med 67:1049, 1979.
6. Hofmann AF, Poley JR: Role of the bile acid malabsorption in pathogenesis of diarrhea and steatorrhea in patients with ileal resection. Gastroenterology 62:918, 1972.
7. Netter FH: Atlas of Human Anatomy, p. 268. Summit, NJ: CIBA-GEIGY, 1989.
8. Debongnie JC, Phillips SF: Capacity of the human colon to absorb fluid. Gastroenterology 74:698, 1978.
9. Vanek VW, Al-Salti M: Acute pseudo-obstruction of the colon (Ogilvie's syndrome): An analysis of 400 cases. Dis Colon Rectum 29:203, 1986.
10. Nelson SW, Christoforidis AJ, Roenigk WJ: Dangers and fallibilities of iodinated radiopaque media in obstruction of the small bowel. Am J Surg 109:546, 1965.
11. Goldberg HI, Dodds WJ: Roentgen evaluation of small-bowel obstruction. Dig Dis Sci 24:245, 1979.
12. Starling JR: Treatment of nontoxic megacolon by colonoscopy. Surgery 94:677, 1983.
13. Nichols RL, Condon RE: Preoperative preparation of the colon. Surg Gynecol Obstet 132:323, 1971.
14. Coppa GF, Eng K, Gouge TH, Ranson JH, Localio SA: Parenteral and oral antibiotics in elective colon and rectal surgery: A prospective, randomized trial. Am J Surg 145:62, 1983.
15. Condon RE: Bowel preparation for colorectal operations. Arch Surg 117:265, 1982.
16. Clarke JS, Condon RE, Bartlett JG, Gorbach SL, Nichols RL, Ochi S: Preoperative oral antibiotics reduce septic complications of colon operations. Ann Surg 186:251, 1977.
17. Playforth MJ, Smith GMR, Evans M, Pollock AV: Antimicrobial bowel preparation: Oral, parenteral, or both? Dis Colon Rectum 31:90, 1988.
18. Hewitt J, Reeve J, Rigby J, Cox AG: Whole gut irrigation in preparation for large bowel surgery. Lancet 2:337, 1973.
19. Davis GR, Santa Ana CA, Morawski SG, Fordtran JS: Development of a lavage solution associated with minimal water and electrolyte absorption or secretion. Gastroenterology 78:991, 1980.
20. Fleites RA, Marshall JB, Eckhauser ML, Mansour EG, Imbembo AL, McCullough AJ: The efficacy of polyethylene glycol–electrolyte lavage solution versus traditional mechanical bowel preparation for elective colonic surgery: A randomized, prospective blinded clinical trial. Surgery 98:708, 1985.
21. Bowden TA Jr, DiPiro JT, Michael KA: Polyethylene glycol electrolyte lavage solution (PEG-ELS). Am Surg 53:34, 1987.
22. Miyazawa K, Hernandez E, Dillon MB: Prophylactic topical cefamandole in radical hysterectomy. Int J Gynaecol Obstet 25:133, 1989.
23. Dicker RC, Greenspan JR, Strauss LT, et al: Complications

of abdominal and vaginal hysterectomy among women of reproductive age in the United States: The collaborative review of sterilization. Am J Obstet Gynecol 144:841, 1982.

24. Gallup DG, Talledo EO, King LA: Primary mass closure of midline incisions with a continuous running monofilament suture in gynecologic patients. Obstet Gynecol 73:675, 1989.

25. Shepherd JH, Cavanagh D, Riggs D, Praphat H, Wisniewski BJ: Abdominal wound closure using a nonabsorbable single-layer technique. Obstet Gynecol 61:248, 1983.

26. Pratt JH: Common complications of vaginal hysterectomy: Thoughts regarding their prevention and management. Clin Obstet Gynecol 19:645, 1976.

27. Hall BD, Phelan JP, Pruyn SC, Gallup DG: Vaginal evisceration during coitus: A case review. Am J Obstet Gynecol 131:115, 1978.

28. Bailey RW: Complications of laparoscopic general surgery. In Zucker KA: Surgical Laparoscopy, pp 311–329. St. Louis: Quality Medical Publishing, 1991.

29. Wheeless CR Jr: Gastrointestinal injuries associated with laparoscopy. In Phillips JM (ed): Endoscopy in Gynecology, pp 317–329. Downey, Calif: American Association of Gynecological Laparoscopists, 1978.

30. Deaths following female sterilization with unipolar electrocoagulating devices. MMWR 30:149, 1981.

31. Soderstrom RM, Levy BS: Bowel injuries during laparoscopy: Causes and medicolegal questions. Contin Obstet Gynecol 27:41, 1986.

32. Soper NJ, Barteau JA, Clayman RV, Becich MJ: Safety and efficacy of laparoscopic cholecystectomy using monopolar electrocautery in the porcine model. Surg Laparosc Endosc (in press).

33. Dennis C: The gastrointestinal sump tube. Surgery 66:309, 1969.

34. Zinner MJ, Zuidema GD, Smith PL, Mignosa M: The prevention of upper gastrointestinal tract bleeding in patients in an intensive care unit. Surg Gynecol Obstet 153:214, 1981.

35. Veterans Affairs Total Parenteral Nutrition Cooperative Study Group: Perioperative total parenteral nutrition in surgical patients. N Engl J Med 325:525, 1991.

36. Haydock DA, Hill GL: Improved wound healing response in surgical patients receiving intravenous nutrition. Br J Surg 74:320, 1987.

37. Rombeau JL, Rolandelli RH, Wilmore DW: Nutritional support. In Wilmore DW, Brennan MF, Harken AH, Holcroft JW, Meakens JL (eds): Care of the Surgical Patient, pp 1–40. New York: Scientific American, 1989.

38. Hwang TL, O'Dwyer ST, Smith RJ, Wilmore DW: Preservation of small bowel mucosa using glutamine-enriched parenteral nutrition. Surg Forum 37:56, 1986.

39. Adibi SA, Allen ER: Impaired jejunal absorption rates of essential amino acids induced by either dietary caloric or protein deprivation in man. Gastroenterology 59:404, 1970.

40. Raul F, Noriega R, Doffoel M, Grenier JF, Haffen K: Modifications of brush border enzyme activities during starvation in the jejunum and ileum of adult rats. Enzyme 28:328, 1982.

41. Ponsky JL, Gauderer MW, Stellato TA, Aszodi A: Percutaneous approaches to enteral alimentation. Am J Surg 149:102, 1985.

42. Bower RH, Talamini MA, Sax HC, Hamilton F, Fischer JE: Postoperative enteral vs. parenteral nutrition: A randomized controlled trial. Arch Surg 121:1040, 1986.

43. Morris M, Gershenson DM, Burke TW, Wharton JT, Copeland LJ, Rutledge FN: Splenectomy in gynecologic oncology: Indications, complications, and technique. Gynecol Oncol 43:118, 1991.

44. Feliciano DV, Bitondo CG, Mattox KL, Rumisek JD, Burch JM, Jordan GL: A four-year experience with splenectomy versus splenorrhaphy. Ann Surg 201:568, 1985.

45. Rappaport W, McIntyre KEJ, Carmona R: The management of splenic trauma in the adult patient with blunt multiple injuries. Surg Gynecol Obstet 170:204, 1990.

46. Gambee LP, Garnjobst W, Hardwick CE: Ten years' experience with a single layer anastomosis in colon surgery. Am J Surg 92:222, 1956.

47. Chassin JL, Rifkind KM, Sussman B, et al: The stapled gastrointestinal tract anastomosis: Incidence of postoperative complications compared with the sutured anastomosis. Ann Surg 188:689, 1978.

48. Lowdon IMR, Gear MWL, Kilby JO: Stapling instruments in upper gastrointestinal surgery: A retrospective study of 362 cases. Br J Surg 69:333, 1982.

49. Reiling RB, Reiling WA Jr, Bernie WA, Huffer AB, Perkins NC, Elliott DW: Prospective controlled study of gastrointestinal stapled anastomoses. Am J Surg 139:147, 1980.

50. Delgado G: The automatic staple versus the conventional gastrointestinal anastomosis in gynecological malignancies. Gynecol Oncol 12:302, 1981.

51. Graber JN, Schulte WJ, Condon RE, Cowles VE: Relationship of duration of postoperative ileus to extent and site of operative dissection. Surgery 92:87, 1982.

52. Peetz DJ, Gamelli RL, Pilcher DB: Intestinal intubation in acute, mechanical small-bowel obstruction. Arch Surg 117:334, 1982.

53. Playforth RH, Holloway JB, Griffen WO Jr: Mechanical small bowel obstruction: A plea for earlier surgical intervention. Ann Surg 171:783, 1970.

54. Bizer LS, Liebling RW, Delany HM, Gliedman ML: Small bowel obstruction: The role of nonoperative treatment in simple intestinal obstruction and predictive criteria for strangulation obstruction. Surgery 89:407, 1981.

55. Sarr MG, Bulkley GB, Zuidema GD: Preoperative recognition of intestinal strangulation obstruction: Prospective evaluation of diagnostic capability. Am J Surg 145:176, 1983.

56. Leffall LD, Spyhax B: Clinical aids in strangulation intestinal obstruction. Am J Surg 120:756, 1970.

57. Brolin RE: The role of gastrointestinal tube decompression in the treatment of mechanical intestinal obstruction. Am Surg 49:131, 1983.

58. Davis SE, Sperling L: Obstruction of the small intestine. Arch Surg 99:424, 1969.

59. Hofstetter SR: Acute adhesive obstruction of the small intestine. Surg Gynecol Obstet 152:141, 1981.

60. Brolin RE: Partial small bowel obstruction. Surgery 95:145, 1984.

61. Smith GA, Perry JF Jr, Yonehiro EG: Mechanical intestinal obstructions: A study of 1,252 cases. Surg Gynecol Oncol 100:651, 1955.

62. Noble TB Jr: Plication of small intestine as prophylaxis against adhesions. Am J Surg 35:31, 1937.

63. Baker JW: Stitchless plication for recurring obstruction of the small bowel. Am J Surg 116:316, 1968.

64. Potish RA: Prediction of radiation-related small-bowel injury. Radiology 135:219, 1980.

65. Weiser EB, Bundy BN, Hoskins WJ, et al: Extraperitoneal versus transperitoneal selective para-aortic lymphadenectomy in the pretreatment surgical staging of advanced cervical carcinoma. (A Gynecologic Oncology Group Study.) Gynecol Oncol 33:283, 1989.

66. Kinsella TJ, Bloomer WD: Tolerance of the intestine to radiation therapy. Surg Gynecol Obstet 151:273, 1980.

67. Russell JC, Welch JP: Operative management of radiation injuries of the intestinal tract. Am J Surg 137:433, 1979.
68. Lillemoe KD, Brigham RA, Harmon JW, Feaster MM, Saunders JR, d'Avis JA: Surgical management of small-bowel radiation enteritis. Arch Surg 118:905, 1983.
69. Localio SA, Stone A, Friedman M: Surgical aspects of radiation enteritis. Surg Gynecol Obstet 129:1163, 1969.
70. Schmitt EH III, Symmonds RE: Surgical treatment of radiation induced injuries of the intestine. Surg Gynecol Obstet 153:896, 1981.
71. Haddad GK, Grodsinsky C, Allen H: The spectrum of radiation enteritis: Surgical considerations. Dis Colon Rectum 26:590, 1983.
72. DeCosse JJ, Rhodes RS, Wentz WB, Reagan JW, Dworken JH, Holden WD: The natural history and management of radiation induced injury of the gastrointestinal tract. Ann Surg 170:369, 1969.
73. Hoskins WJ, Burke TW, Weiser EB, Heller PB, Grayson J, Park RC: Right hemicolectomy and ileal resection with primary anastomosis for radiation injury to the terminal ileum. Gynecol Oncol 26:215, 1987.
74. Osteen RT, Guyton S, Steele G Jr, Wilson RE: Malignant intestinal obstruction. Surgery 87:611, 1980.
75. Ketcham AS, Hoye RC, Pilch YH, Morton DL: Delayed intestinal obstruction following treatment for cancer. Cancer 25:408, 1970.
76. Chau PM, Fletcher GH, Rutledge FN, Dodd GD Jr: Complications in high dose whole pelvis irradiation in female pelvic cancer. Am J Roentgenol Radium Ther Nucl Med 87:22, 1962.
77. Eakin M: Fistulas: A nursing challenge. Dimensions Oncol Nurs 5(3):26, 1991.
78. MacFayden BV Jr, Dudrick SJ, Ruberg RL: Management of gastrointestinal fistulas with parenteral hyperalimentation. Surgery 74:100, 1973.
79. Graham JA: Conservative treatment of gastrointestinal fistulas. Surg Gynecol Obstet 144:512, 1977.
80. Halasz NA: Changing patterns in the management of small bowel fistulas. Am J Surg 136:61, 1978.
81. Soeters PB, Ebeid AM, Fischer JE: Review of 404 patients with gastrointestinal fistulas: Impact of parenteral nutrition. Ann Surg 190:189, 1979.
82. Nubiola P, Badia JM, Martinez-Rodenas F, et al: Treatment of 27 postoperative enterocutaneous fistulas with long half-life somatostatin analogue SMS 201–995. Ann Surg 210:56, 1989.
83. Curtin JP, Burt LL: Successful treatment of small intestine fistula with somatostatin analog. Gynecol Oncol 39:225, 1990.
84. Aguirre A, Fischer JE, Welch CE: The role of surgery and hyperalimentation in therapy of gastrointestinal-cutaneous fistulae. Ann Surg 180:393, 1974.
85. Wise WE Jr, Aguilar PS, Padmanabhan A, Meesig DM, Arnold MW, Stewart WRC: Surgical treatment of low rectovaginal fistulas. Dis Colon Rectum 34:271, 1991.
86. Anseline PF, Lavery IC, Fazio VW, Jagelman DG, Weakley FL: Radiation injury of the rectum: Evaluation of surgical treatment. Ann Surg 194:716, 1981.
87. Aartsen EJ, Sindram IS: Repair of the radiation induced rectovaginal fistulas without or with interposition of the bulbocavernosus muscle (Martius procedure). Eur J Surg Oncol 14:171, 1988.
88. Elkins TE, DeLancey JOL, McGuire EJ: The use of modified Martius graft as an adjunctive technique in vesicovaginal and rectovaginal fistula repair. Obstet Gynecol 75:727, 1990.
89. Harris WJ, Wheeless CR Jr: Use of the end-to-end anastomosis stapling device in low colorectal anastomosis associated with radical gynecologic surgery. Gynecol Oncol 23:350, 1986.
90. Allen-Mersh TG, Wilson EJ, Hope-Stone HF, Mann CV: The management of late radiation-induced rectal injury after treatment of carcinoma of the uterus. Surg Gynecol Oncol 164:521, 1987.
91. Wheeless CR Jr: Incidence of fecal incontinence after coloproctostomy below five centimeters in the rectum. Gynecol Oncol 27:373, 1987.

Complications in Gynecologic Surgery: Prevention, Recognition, and Management,
edited by James W. Orr, Jr., and Hugh M. Shingleton.
J. B. Lippincott Company, Philadelphia, © 1994.

Chapter 5

Urologic Complications

Robert L. Holley
Larry C. Kilgore

T he anatomic proximity of the genital and urinary tracts suggests that a thorough understanding of pelvic anatomy is the cornerstone
for gynecologic surgery. Familiarity with normal
urinary tract anatomy and the various anomalies encountered in clinical practice will help prevent urinary tract injury, an unwelcome complication for
patients and a common cause of medicolegal actions against gynecologic surgeons.

Anatomy of the Urinary Tract

Lower Urinary Tract Anatomy

The paired retroperitoneal kidneys are located beneath the diaphragm, bordered by the psoas muscles.
The renal blood supply originates from the aorta,
passes through a series of afferent interlobar arteries and arcuate arterioles, and ends in the important
glomerular capillary network located in the renal
cortex (Fig. 5–1). Efferent blood flow is more complex, as cortex vessels supply proximal and distal
tubules, portions of the loops of Henle, and collecting ducts before leaving the kidney. Juxtamedullary
efferents also give rise to the vasa recta, specialized
vessels that provide a rich oxygen supply to the
loop of Henle.[1] The kidney's collecting system begins at Bowman's capsule, where it interfaces with
the glomerular capillary bed. Bowman's capsule
connects, in order, the proximal tubule, the loop of
Henle, the distal convoluted tubule, and the collecting ducts. The collecting ducts then coalesce in the
medullary portion of the kidney to form the calyces
and then the renal pelvis.

Ureter

The ureteral wall is composed of three layers: an
external adventitia, a smooth muscle layer, and an
inner mucous membrane.[2] The outer loose connective tissue sheath contains the blood vessels that
supply the ureter; they anastomose freely with one
another (Fig. 5–2). Damage to these vessels by
overly aggressive ureteral or periureteral dissection
can result in ureteral wall ischemia, subsequent necrosis, and even rupture.[3]

The ureter is about 25 to 30 cm long and has approximately equal abdominal and pelvic components. In the abdomen, the ureter passes along the
anterior aspect of the psoas muscle to the pelvic
inlet and crosses the iliac vessel at the bifurcation of
the common iliac.[4] The pelvic ureter passes along
the posterior lateral pelvic wall, anterior to the
internal iliac artery, and proceeds lateral to the
uterosacral ligaments to enter the base of the broad
ligament. It courses beneath the uterine artery approximately 1.5 cm lateral to the cervix at the level
of the internal cervical os (Fig. 5–3). The ureter
then passes medially over the anterior fornix of the
vagina before entering the vesical trigone.

The ureteral blood supply is from multiple
sources. The renal pelvis and upper ureter receive
arterial blood supply from the renal and ovarian
vessels, the middle ureter derives its blood supply
from the aorta and common iliac artery, and the pel-

131

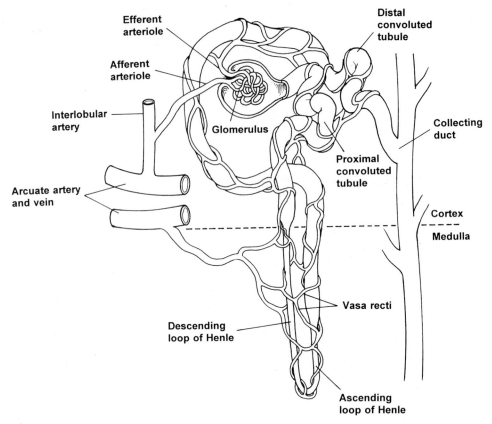

FIGURE 5–1. Renal nephron.

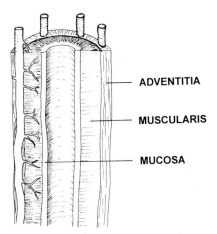

FIGURE 5–2. Sagittal section of the human ureter showing adventitial sheath, muscularis, and mucosa. (Redrawn from Bright TC, Peters PC. Ureteral injuries secondary to operative procedures. Urol 1977; IX:22.)

vic ureter receives branches from the inferior and superior vesical, uterine, vaginal, and middle hemorrhoidal arteries (Fig. 5–4).[2,3] All these vessels anastomose freely with each other in the adventitial layer.

The blood supply to the abdominal portion of the ureter approaches from the medial side; therefore, ureteral incision or stenting in this portion should be performed along its lateral margin. In contrast, the pelvic ureter derives the majority of its blood supply from lateral sources; thus a medial dissection would incur the least risk of damage.[3] The pelvic ureter may be mobilized extensively along its course, as in radical hysterectomy for cervical carcinoma, as long as the adventitial blood supply is not interrupted.[5]

Bladder

The urinary bladder serves as a reservoir for urine and aids in its excretion through the urethra by contraction of the detrusor muscle. Anteriorly the blad-

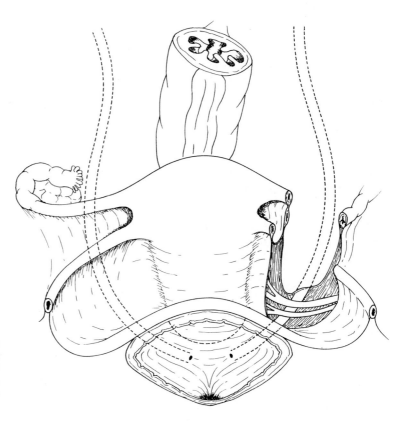

FIGURE 5–3. Course of the pelvic ureter. (Redrawn with permission from Thompson JD, Rock JA (eds): Te Linde's Operative Gynecology, p 753. Philadelphia: JB Lippincott, 1992.)

der lies against the lower abdominal wall, covered on its superior surface by peritoneum. Inferiorly the bladder rests on the pelvic diaphragm and, in the genital hiatus, on the urogenital diaphragm. Posteriorly it lies adjacent to the vagina and cervix. The bladder is enveloped in endopelvic fascia.[4]

The bladder wall consists of coarse, smooth muscle bundles lined with a transitional epithelial mucosa, loosely attached to the muscular layer by a submucosa.[6] It has traditionally been stated that the bladder musculature is arranged in three layers—inner longitudinal, middle circular, and outer longitudinal[7]; however, Woodburne[8] suggests that the muscular wall of the bladder is a meshwork consisting of muscle fascicles running in many directions, crisscrossing and decussating.

Functionally the bladder may be divided into two portions, the dome and the base.[9] As the bladder fills, the musculature of the dome thins considerably as filling progresses and the bladder assumes a spherical or ovoid shape. The detrusor muscle relaxes receptively and, except in pathological conditions, the intravesical filling pressure does not rise

above 15 to 20 cm H_2O until the bladder capacity is reached. The bladder base consists of the vesical trigone, vesicourethral junction, and the detrusor loop. Its muscular wall is thicker and varies less with distention. The triangular vesical trigone is composed of small-diameter muscle bundles arising from the intramural ureters, bordered by the ureteral orifices and the intervening ureteric ridge and the proximal urethra (Fig. 5–5).[10] No circular vesical sphincter has been identified in the region of the vesical neck.[8,11]

The majority of bladder innervation is cholinergic, derived from the parasympathetic fibers that arise from the second through fourth segments of the sacral spinal cord. Parasympathetic stimulation results in detrusor muscle contraction and bladder emptying. Sympathetic bladder innervation is derived from the T11–12 and L1–2 segments of the spinal cord.

The bladder's arterial blood supply is derived from the superior and inferior vesical arteries, both of which originate from the anterior division of the internal iliac artery.[4]

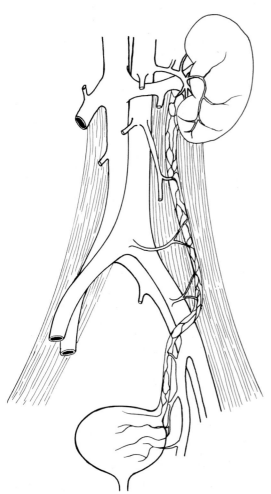

FIGURE 5–4. Blood supply of the ureter. (Redrawn with permission from Thompson JD, Rock JA (eds): Te Linde's Operative Gynecology, p 755. Philadelphia: JB Lippincott, 1992.)

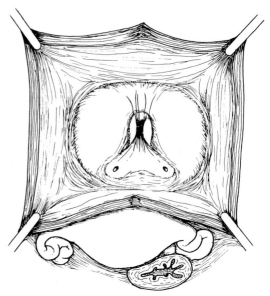

FIGURE 5–5. Vesical trigone and bladder base. (Redrawn with permission from Thompson JD, Rock JA (eds): Te Linde's Operative Gynecology, p 44. Philadelphia: JB Lippincott, 1992.)

Urethra

The muscular-walled urethra serves as a conduit to convey urine from the bladder to the environment. Approximately 3 to 4 cm long in normal adult women, it extends from the vesicourethral junction portion of the trigone to the external urethral meatus. The distal urethra is lined by stratified squamous epithelium; the demarcation between transitional epithelium, as found in the bladder, and squamous epithelium is variable, depending on the individual's hormonal status.[6]

The urethral wall consists of a series of layers, a prominent inner longitudinal layer and a thinner outer circular layer.[12] The poorly developed outer circular layer may contribute minimally to resting intraurethral pressure. The longitudinal layer may

function to shorten and funnel the urethra during micturition; its parasympathetic innervation tends to corroborate this role.[10,12]

The striated urogenital sphincter consists of an upper sphincter portion and a lower, archlike pair of muscular bands, the urethrovaginal sphincter and the compressor urethrae.[6] These muscles occupy from 20% to 80% of the urethral length when measured from the urethrovesical junction.[12] The circular fibers of the striated sphincter insert ventrally into the trigonal plate and surround the urethral lumen for approximately 20% to 60% of its length. The distal portion of the striated sphincter, lying adjacent to the urethral lumen for much of its length, consists of two bands of muscle that arc over the ventral surface of the urethra in such a way as to close off the urethra by compression (Fig. 5–6). All three portions of the striated urogenital sphincter function as a single unit. Controversy exists as to whether their innervation is somatic or autonomic.[6]

A rich vascular plexus lies between the urethral mucosa and muscular layers throughout the entire urethral length.[13] These venous channels are capable of marked distention and form a corpus spongiosum composed of erectile tissue; this vascular plexus aids in the formation of a watertight closure of the mucosa. Rud et al.[14] showed that one third of the resting intraurethral pressure is due to the urethral submucosal vascular bed; the striated

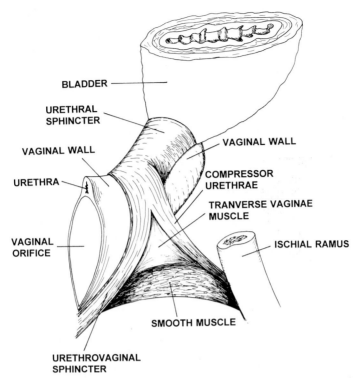

FIGURE 5–6. The striated urogenital sphincter in relation to the vagina and bladder. Pubic bones and the perineal membrane have been removed. (Redrawn with permission from Ostergard DR, Bent AE (eds): Urogynecology and Urodynamics, p 9. Baltimore: Williams & Wilkins, 1991.)

urogenital sphincter contributes one third and the smooth muscles one third.

The urethral blood supply is derived from the inferior vesical and vaginal branches of the anterior division of the internal iliac vessels.[4] Urethral and lower vaginal support is provided by a fascial attachment of the paravaginal and paraurethral tissues to the arcus tendineus fasciae pelvis and by muscular attachment of the same tissues to the medial aspect of the levator ani. It is postulated that these attachments maintain the normal position of the vesical neck at rest, aided by the normal resting tone of the levator ani.[12] When the levator relaxes at the onset of micturition, the vesical neck rotates inferiorly to the limits of the elasticity of the fascial attachments. Contraction of the levator at the end of micturition restores the vesical neck to its usual position.

The pubovesical muscles are extensions of the detrusor muscle, bilateral symmetrical slips of muscle that terminate in the retropubic connective tissue and thereby gain traction on the pubis.[8] They are believed to assist in vesical neck opening during micturition.[15,16]

Prevalence of Urinary Tract Abnormalities

Various authors[17–19] report that congenital abnormalities of the urinary tract occur in 3.3% to 11.1% of the population. Urinary tract anomalies account for approximately 50% of all congenital malformations.[18,19] Many urinary tract abnormalities such as ureteral duplication are minor, asymptomatic, and never reported. Barakat and Drougas[19] reported an overall prevalence of urinary tract anomalies in 4.6% of 13,775 autopsies conducted from 1928 to 1986. In this study, urethral abnormalities were found in 0.25% of autopsies; most commonly noted were absence/hypoplasia, hypospadia, epispadia, and posterior urethral valves. Bladder abnormalities were found in 0.23% of autopsies, absent or hypoplastic bladder occurred in 13 per 10,000 autopsies, bladder exstrophy in 4, and other bladder abnormalities in 6 per 10,000 autopsies. Ureteral abnormalities occurred in 1.35% of autopsies and included absence/hypoplasia, duplication, hydroureter, and stenosis, in order of decreasing frequency. Over 85% of all abnormalities were seen in

TABLE 5–1. **Hemodynamics and Flow Rates**

Parameter	Rate
Cardiac output	5,000 mL/min
Renal blood flow rate	1,250 mL/min
Glomerular filtration rate	125 mL/min
Urine flow rate	2 mL/min

the upper urinary tract. Overall, kidney abnormalities were present in 2.07% of autopsies. Most commonly discovered was renal dysplasia, followed in decreasing order of frequency by horseshoe kidney, agenesis, hypoplasia, hydronephrosis, and infantile and adult polycystic disease.[19] Renal vascular anomalies were found in 0.57% of autopsies.

Renal Physiology

For centuries, astute physicians and surgeons have measured urine output in the hope of assessing the condition of patients with a variety of illnesses. In a sense, urine formation and output represent the summation of a number of complex physiologic mechanisms. Nonetheless, the ability to monitor acute changes in renal function during the perioperative period is limited. Deterioration in renal function may easily go unrecognized, resulting in compromised postoperative care or permanent alterations.[20] Therefore, an understanding of renal physiology and pharmacology in relation to surgery and anesthesia is imperative for the pelvic surgeon.

In the healthy woman, renal blood flow (RBF) accounts for 20% to 25% of cardiac output, or about 1,250 mL/min. Ninety percent of RBF is directed to the renal cortex and the glomerular apparatus. Approximately 10% of RBF (125 mL/min) is filtered by the kidney. This volume is recognized as the glomerular filtration rate (GFR). The majority of the GFR is reabsorbed, resulting in a urine flow rate of 2 mL/min (Table 5–1). Therefore, in a 24-hour period, over 180 L of fluid is filtered, resulting in the excretion of only 1 to 2 L of urine.[21]

The renal system has three primary functions: filtration, reabsorption, and secretion. Central to renal physiology are control mechanisms affecting sodium and water filtration and reabsorption. The renal system filters roughly 65,000 mEq of sodium daily. Sixty-five percent of this filtrate is reabsorbed in the proximal renal tubule and 25% is reabsorbed in the ascending loop of Henle. The remaining 10% is presented to the distal tubule, where, under the influence of aldosterone, the majority is reabsorbed. Only 1% to 2% of filtered sodium is secreted daily, regulated by changes in volume status and a number of complex neurohumoral mechanisms (Table 5–2).

Water filtration and reabsorption in the proximal tubule are similar to that for sodium. In the loop of Henle, however, water is absorbed to a lesser extent. Variable rates of water reabsorption then occur in the distal tubules and collecting ducts under the primary influence of antidiuretic hormone (ADH). Surgery, anesthesia, and trauma may affect renal function by altering filtration and reabsorption.[22]

Neurohormonal Regulation of Renal Function

Renin–Angiotensin–Aldosterone System

The renin–angiotensin–aldosterone (RAS) system is a complex, highly integrated regulator of cardiovascular and renal physiology controlling blood

TABLE 5–2. **Sodium, Water, and Osmolar Excretion**

	Flow Rate (mL/min^{-1})	Na$^+$ (mEq/L^{-1})	Osmolality (mOsm/kg^{-1})
Plasma	750	140	290
Filtrate	125	140	290
Final urine			
Euvolemic young adult	2	100	300
Maximal aldosterone secretion	2	1	100
Minimal ADH secretion	20	10	50
Maximal ADH secretion	0.2	300	1,400
"Average" perioperative patient	0.5	20	800

Reproduced with permission from Prough DS, Foreman AS: Anesthesia and the renal system. In Barash PG, Cullen BF, Stoelting RK (ed): Clinical Anesthesia, 2nd ed, p 1125. Philadelphia: JB Lippincott, 1992.

pressure (especially during stress) and blood volume. Renin is secreted from the kidney in response to changes in blood volume, sodium concentrations, and the sympathetic nervous system. Circulating renin enzymatically cleaves angiotensinogen to angiotensin I, which in turn is converted to angiotensin II, primarily in the lung. Angiotensin II, a potent vasopressor, also stimulates the release of aldosterone from the adrenal cortex. Acting primarily on the distal tubule and collecting ducts, aldosterone promotes sodium retention and potassium loss. This cascade of events is frequently activated by surgery and anesthesia.[23]

Antidiuretic Hormone

Antidiuretic hormone is produced by the posterior pituitary in response to changes in intravascular volume and blood osmolarity. Increased osmolarity promotes release of ADH through hypothalamic receptors, while atrial baroreceptors, detecting increases in intravascular volume, inhibit its release. Typically, during periods of high ADH production, the kidneys release concentrated urine of low volume. ADH may result in dramatic changes in urine output. Acting primarily on the cortical tubules, ADH dramatically increases water reabsorption. Surgery with its concomitant blood loss, and anesthesia with its associated decrease in cardiac output and vasodilation, frequently result in higher circulating levels of ADH.[22]

Prostaglandins

Prostaglandins are also involved in sodium and water metabolism and are produced in large quantities in the kidneys. Many prostaglandins are potent vasodilators in the kidney and may increase RBF during periods of blood loss or hypovolemia. The use of prostaglandin inhibitors (nonsteroidal antiinflammatory agents) should be avoided during periods of hypovolemia as they may result in detrimental effects to the renal system.[20]

Diuretics

It is an understatement that pelvic surgeons and anesthesiologists should be familiar with commonly used diuretics, the most commonly prescribed medication in the United States.[23] Preoperatively, many patients with a coexisting illness, including hypertension and heart disease, are taking regular doses of diuretics. The thiazide diuretics act primarily on the distal convoluted tubule and affect sodium reabsorption, whereas the more potent loop diuretics act on the ascending loop. Potential problems for patients taking either kind of diuretic include changes in overall volume status or electrolyte abnormalities. Patients presenting with contracted intravascular volumes may be more susceptible to significant complications when exposed to additional volume loss. Associated hypokalemia poses additional perioperative problems. Arrhythmias in the perioperative period are more common when potassium stores are depleted, and hypokalemic patients who suffer perioperative myocardial infarction may be at increased risk for fatal ventricular arrhythmias.[20] Data from the Multiple Risk Factor Intervention Trial also identified a specific subset of patients with an unusual risk. Diuretic use by patients with preoperative or baseline electrocardiographic (ECG) abnormalities increases the risk for sudden coronary death in the perioperative period. Patients with normal baseline ECGs are not at such risk.[24]

Tests of Renal Function

Many patients experience altered renal function during the perioperative period. Usually these changes go undetected. Measurements of urine output, serum creatinine, and blood urea nitrogen (BUN) form the basis of routine postoperative management. Tests of RBF, GFR, and tubular function are not routine but are available and may be necessary to fully assess the renal effect of anesthesia and surgery (Table 5–3).

Creatinine

Creatinine, a product of muscle metabolism, is usually released into the circulation at a constant rate. Urine output and serum creatinine levels frequently are the only parameters of renal function measured in the postoperative period. Generally, measurements of serum creatinine correlate well with GFR and renal function.[20] However, significant losses in renal function may occur before serum creatinine levels rise. In fact, only 30% of kidney function is

TABLE 5–3. **Perioperative Tests of Renal Function**

Serum creatinine
Serum blood urea nitrogen
Creatinine clearance rate
Urine/plasma creatinine ratio
Urine sodium concentration

necessary to maintain normal serum creatinine levels. Additionally, specific situations such as crush injuries cause muscle trauma, which may elevate circulating levels of creatinine and falsify evaluations of renal function.[24]

Blood Urea Nitrogen

The BUN correlates poorly with renal function although it is frequently measured for this purpose. Dehydration from any source, gastrointestinal bleeding, and high levels of protein administration can falsely elevate BUN.[25]

Creatinine Clearance

Measurement of the creatinine clearance rate is the most frequently used test of GFR. Because a portion of creatinine is secreted by the tubules, the creatinine clearance time may slightly overestimate GFR. Short-duration collection times (1–2 hours) can produce reliable measurements of creatinine clearance and allow rapid assessment of changing renal function.[24]

Urine to Plasma Creatinine Ratio

This test of tubular function specifically represents the function of the distal convoluted tubule. Urine to plasma creatinine ratios of 30 or greater are reassuring and represent adequate tubular function.[26]

Urine Sodium Concentration

Urine sodium concentrations of less than 20 mEq/L represent normal renal function during episodes of hypovolemia. With loss of renal function, values will be elevated despite low-volume states.

Renal Effects of Anesthetic Agents

Anesthetic agents may directly or indirectly alter renal function.[27] The predominant indirect effects include changes in the circulatory system and the sympathetic nervous system; direct effects include alterations in tubular transport and reabsorption.[28] Some authors have likened the effects of anesthetics on renal function to those of sleep, with concomitant changes in circulatory physiology and neurohormonal regulation.[29] Nevertheless, few clinical studies have thoroughly evaluated the isolated effects of anesthetic agents secondary to the multiplicity of factors associated with the perioperative management of the surgical patient.[29] In addition to the nature and duration of surgery, important associated factors include the patient's preoperative medical status and volume status in relation to preoperative preparation or intraoperative blood loss.

Most general anesthetic agents are myocardial depressants.[30,31] Their effect on the renal circulatory system depends primarily on compensatory vasoconstrictive mechanisms that maintain arterial blood pressure.[32] These forces may decrease RBF and depress renal function.

A number of studies have demonstrated changes in the kidney's ability to autoregulate RBF secondary to anesthetic agents. Despite compensatory maintenance of arterial blood pressure in these studies, RBF decreased by as much as 30% to 70%.[33–36] The kidney's ability to vasodilate in the face of blood loss may be compromised in the presence of anesthetics.[1] In the clinical setting, blood loss with associated hypotension may variably affect renal blood flow and function, depending on the anesthetic agent chosen.[27]

Some have suggested that GFR is not affected by anesthetic agents; however, many authors have reported 30% to 50% decreases in GFR with inhaled and spinal anesthetics.[35–38] Mazze et al.[35] and Barry et al.[39] reported more dramatic alterations in GFR if intravascular volume was depleted. Anesthetics also appear to independently alter neurohormonal mechanisms. Some consider the activation of the renin–angiotensin system to be the most important effect.[40,41] Anesthesia-mediated ADH release and catecholamine release have been demonstrated.[42,43] These hormonal effects of anesthetics may augment similar compensatory mechanisms produced by surgery.

Direct effects of anesthetic agents on the kidney are less compelling. Alterations in sodium transport have been demonstrated in the laboratory.[28] Additionally, the inhaled anesthetic agent methoxyflurane, which is biotransformed into fluoride, has caused nephrotoxicity in some clinical settings.[44–46]

Renal Effects of Anesthesia and Surgery

Although anesthetic agents may independently alter renal function, the combined effect of surgery and anesthesia poses the greatest risk to renal function. Although usually reversible and undetected, acute renal insufficiency develops in as many as 10% of patients who undergo major elective surgical procedures.[47,48] A higher percentage of patients will have less dramatic changes but additional insults to the renal system could be disastrous.[49]

Pringle et al.[50] studied eight patients undergoing surgery and ether anesthesia and reported changes in renal function. Before surgery, urine output averaged 50 mL/h, but it decreased progressively toward 1.2 mL/h during surgery and returned to 17 mL/h in the first 24 postoperative hours. Subsequent studies have elucidated a predictable pattern of renal function during surgery. General anesthesia produces a temporary reduction in all measured renal functions, including RBF, GFR, sodium excretion, and urine flow rate.[34] Regional anesthetics and surgery may produce comparable effects, depending on the level of sympathetic block.[51] Depressed renal function resolves quickly after short, uncomplicated procedures. However, prolonged exposure to anesthetics and surgery activates neurohormonal systems, with resultant alterations in sodium and water metabolism. These changes may last for several days following the procedure despite normalization of hemodynamics.[52] In addition to activation of neuroendocrine systems, exposure to anesthetics and surgery produces changes in intravascular and extracellular volume. The end result is a decrease in the excretion of sodium and water in urine.

The renal cortex is innervated by a rich supply of sympathetic nerve fibers derived from spinal segments T4 to L1. Regional anesthesia affects the sympathetic nervous system and may alter the kidney's ability to vasoconstrict and autoregulate.[26] As the level of spinal and epidural anesthesia increases, the effect on RBF may be more dramatic.[53] Appropriate attention to intravascular volume and cardiovascular homeostasis minimizes problems with hypotension and decreased perfusion. Many clinicians favor carefully controlled regional anesthesia in patients with renal insufficiency.

Despite increases in aldosterone production, hyponatremia is a frequent problem in patients exposed to surgery and anesthesia. Many factors contribute to this apparent discrepancy, including the dominant effect of ADH and the liberal use of fluids low in sodium content.[54] Specific attention to preoperative hydration and the use of isotonic replacement fluids help minimize this problem.

The classic surgical "stress response" is associated with the production of catecholamines, ADH, cortisol, glucagon, and endorphins as well as activation of the RAS system. Surgery and anesthesia produce a similar pattern that in turn affects renal function.[55] Although these mechanisms are protective, undesirable effects including arrhythmias, cardiac stimulation, decreased RBF, and retention of salt and water can occur. These effects mandate that

the pelvic surgeon combine an understanding of altered perioperative renal function with careful perioperative management to minimize the risk of complications.

Postoperative Complications in Patients with Normal Renal Function

Oliguria: Diagnosis and Management

An adult ingesting a normal diet is obligated to excrete approximately 500 mOsm of solute daily.[56] Half of the excreted solutes are sodium and potassium salts; the other half are urea, the by-product of protein catabolism. With maximal concentration of the urine to 1,200 mOsm/kg H_2O, 400 to 500 mL/24 hr of urine is required to clear the body of nitrogenous wastes.[57,58] If the kidneys cannot concentrate the urine above 300 mOsm/kg H_2O, the osmolality of plasma, 1.67 L of urine would be required to excrete the same 500 mOsm of solute.[56] The ability to concentrate urine above plasma osmolality is one of the first properties lost in diseases of the kidney.

Oliguria, by convention, is defined as excretion of less than 400 mL/day of urine.[21] Azotemia refers to an increase in the serum concentrations of urea and creatinine that occurs as GFR falls. Acute renal failure is defined as a rapid deterioration in renal function sufficient to result in accumulation of nitrogenous wastes in the body.[59] In clinical situations, acute renal failure must be differentiated from chronic renal failure, which refers to permanent loss of nephrons with decreased functioning renal mass, leading to irreversible compromise of kidney function.[60]

Three conditions must be met for the kidneys to excrete the obligatory daily solute load: the kidneys must be adequately perfused, the kidneys must function, and the urine formed must be able to escape from the body. These conditions permit the clinical approach to oliguria to be separated into three areas: prerenal azotemia, postrenal or obstructive uropathy, and intrinsic renal disease (Table 5–4).

Prerenal Azotemia

Oliguria with avid renal salt and water retention has been considered the hallmark of reversible prerenal azotemia.[61] A decrease in the effective circulatory volume that occurs with dehydration, excessive blood loss, or third space sequestration leads to increased sympathetic tone with a resulting rise in

TABLE 5–4. Causes of Oliguria

Prerenal
  Decreased volume
    Dehydration
    Blood loss
    Third space sequestration
  Circulatory
    Septic shock
    Cardiogenic shock
  Vascular
    Renal artery stenosis
    Renal vein thrombosis

Postrenal
  Acute obstructive uropathy
    Ureteral obstruction
    Urethral obstruction
    Urinary extravasation

Intrinsic renal disease (see Table 5–6)

renal vascular resistance and a decrease in RBF.[61] Activation of renin-angiotensin II causes further renal vasoconstriction with a resulting fall in RBF and GFR.[56] In concert with increases in plasma concentrations of aldosterone and ADH, a decrease in glomerular capillary pressure and altered peritubular factors result in avid tubular reabsorption of salt and water with a decrease in urine flow.[62] Thus, patients with prerenal azotemia excrete an extremely concentrated urine with osmolality generally greater than 350 mOsm/kg H_2O and a urinary sodium concentration usually less than 20 mEq/L.[63]

Although the most common cause of prerenal azotemia is excessive loss of blood or body fluids, volumes may shift from one space to another, as occurs in the third space losses of ileus or ascites (Table 5–5). Likewise, gram-negative septicemia causes venodilation with an increase in venous capacitance resulting in decreased venous return and diminished cardiac output. In these clinical situations, vasodilatory drugs and anesthetics may expand the available vascular volume and lead to hypotension and renal hypoperfusion.

Patients must also be assessed for diminished cardiac output or renal vascular occlusion (arterial or venous) as causes of prerenal azotemia. Myocardial failure is associated with edema and an expanded extracellular fluid volume; however, RBF is decreased with pump failure.[56] Effective therapy for cardiac failure should restore cardiac output and RBF.

Renal vascular occlusion may be thrombotic, atherosclerotic, or may follow extensive retroperitoneal operative dissection.[64] Intravenous pyelography (IVP) and arteriography may be useful in determining the presence of vascular obstruction; however, caution should be exercised in patients with renal insufficiency because of the potential toxicity of the contrast medium.[65]

The diagnosis of prerenal oliguria can often be made clinically. Hypovolemic patients demonstrate tachycardia, poor skin turgor, low blood pressure, and dry mucous membranes. Systolic and diastolic blood pressures do not normally drop more than 20 mm Hg when a woman moves from the prone position to an upright position,[64] and thus measured orthostatic blood pressure changes can be a valuable clinical sign in the assessment of hypovolemia. However, elderly or extremely ill postoperative patients may be unable to cooperate. The clinical estimation of volume status in these situations can be inaccurate or confusing. An accurate assessment of volume status can be ascertained directly by measuring right atrial pressure (with a central venous catheter) and/or left atrial pressure (pulmonary capillary wedge pressure) with a Swan-Ganz catheter.[66,67]

Successful treatment of prerenal oliguria necessitates restoring renal perfusion by establishing an adequate blood volume. Whole blood or packed red cells are appropriate for volume restoration when significant blood loss has occurred. Isotonic fluids of the proper composition should be used to replace the loss of electrolyte-rich fluids. Sequestration of

TABLE 5–5. Sources of Perioperative Fluid Losses

Preoperative
  NPO
  Sweating
  Vomiting
  Nasogastric suction
  Enemas
  Diuretics
  Salt-losing nephropathy

Intraoperative
  Blood loss
  Evaporation; skin, exposed viscera, ventilation

Postoperative
  Wounds
  Damaged muscle
  Third space losses
    Ileus
    Ascites
    Concealed hemorrhage
    Pleural effusion

fluids from a postoperative ileus or ascites must be recognized and replaced by standard techniques. The presence of prerenal oliguria as a result of either congestive heart failure or cirrhosis implies severe disease and often a poor prognosis.

Postrenal Oliguria

Obstructive uropathy may manifest as anuria, oliguria, fluctuating oliguria and polyuria, or as non-oliguric renal failure.[61] Because of its frequency (2%–14%),[68,69] obstructive uropathy is a common and potentially reversible cause of acute renal failure.

Oliguria progresses to anuria with bilateral ureteral or urethral obstruction. The partially obstructed kidney is polyuric and loses concentrating ability; and sodium wasting occurs.[70] However, experimental[71] and clinical[72] studies suggest that urinary indices in early obstructive uropathy with minimal renal insufficiency may resemble those of prerenal azotemia. Urinary indices in obstructive uropathy depend on the duration and severity of obstruction.[63]

Ureteral obstruction may occur secondary to calculi, tumor invasion, endometriosis, arterial aneurysm, retroperitoneal fibrosis, or surgical trauma.[73,74] The diagnosis and management of ureteral obstruction are dealt with elsewhere. Bladder outlet obstruction may be caused by tumor invasion of the bladder or urethra, or by overzealous retropubic suspension for stress urinary incontinence. Obstruction at the bladder outlet is usually heralded by symptoms of hesitancy, dribbling, nocturia, and decreased caliber of the urinary stream. Urethral insertion of a Foley catheter remedies the obstructive symptoms and preserves kidney function. Anuria in any patient with a Foley catheter in place should prompt the surgeon to check for catheter patency. Blunt abdominal trauma or surgical accidents may lead to unrecognized perforation of the lower urinary tract with extravasation of urine, formation of a urinoma, and possible obstruction.

While the prerenal and renal causes of marked oliguria are being evaluated, obstructive uropathy should always be suspected. Urinalysis may be of little assistance; obstruction is associated with marked variability in urinary indices.[63] If the clinical situation warrants, hydronephrosis may be excluded with ultrasound, computed tomography, or retrograde catheterization. Unilateral ureteral obstruction is unlikely to produce oliguria or azotemia unless there is coexisting intrinsic disease of the contralateral kidney, ureter, or both.

Postrenal oliguria is treated by relieving the obstruction, which may be as simple as placing a Foley catheter. Transvesical placement of ureteral stents or percutaneous nephrostomy are the procedures of choice for temporarily relieving obstruction proximal to the bladder to preserve kidney function until more definitive therapy can be undertaken.[75] When bilateral obstruction is present, near-normal renal function can be achieved by diverting a single kidney; however, early stenting or diversion theoretically preserves more kidney function.

Profound diuresis with urine isosmotic with plasma often follows relief of obstruction. The urine potassium content is usually low and the serum levels are high. One-half isotonic saline may be used safely to replace losses. In the patient with edema and volume overload, postobstructive replacement fluids should be administered conservatively to allow the patient to reach her ideal weight in 48 to 72 hours.[56] In patients at ideal weight and with no evidence of volume excess, fluid replacement during diuresis should match urine output until renal function stabilizes. Occasionally postobstructive diuresis will be brisk and induce a severely hypovolemic state if fluids are not replaced adequately. In this instance, a central venous line may assist in monitoring volume status to allow adequate resuscitation.

Intrinsic Renal Disease

Acute parenchymal renal disease is diagnosed only when pre- and postrenal causes of oliguria and chronic renal insufficiency have been excluded. A variety of mechanisms including immunologic, toxic, ischemic, and allergic may cause acute parenchymal renal disease (Table 5–6).

Acute tubular necrosis (ATN) accounts for over 80% of the cases of acute renal failure seen in a general hospital[56] and is by far the most common cause of acute postoperative renal failure. In fact, ATN is generally referred to as acute renal failure[21]; prerenal and postrenal conditions are so designated. Acute renal failure occurs in 5% of all hospital admissions and in 10% to 20% of critically ill patients.[76] Despite the ready availability of dialysis, the mortality from acute renal failure remains above 50% in most surgical series.[64,77]

The two major mechanisms of renal insult that result in acute renal failure are ischemia and nephrotoxins.[78] Nephrotoxins account for 11% to 25% of all cases of acute renal failure.[79–81] Most notable have been the aminoglycosides[79,82] and cisplatin.[83,84] Other drugs causally related to acute renal failure include aspirin, captopril, methoxyflurane, amphotericin B, radiographic contrast me-

TABLE 5–6. **Intrinsic Renal Disease**

Acute glomerulonephritis
  Poststreptococcal
  Idiopathic
  Systemic lupus
Microvascular occlusion
  Scleroderma
  Wegener's granulomatosis
  Hemolytic-uremic syndrome
  Small vessel vasculitis
  Malignant hypertension
Acute interstitial nephritis
  Drugs
  Multiple myeloma
  Hypercalcemia
Intrarenal obstruction
  Calculi
  Bilateral papillary necrosis
  Uric acid nephropathy
Acute tubular necrosis
  Ischemia
  Toxic injury
    Endogenous toxins
      Heme pigments
      Gram-negative endotoxemia
    Exogenous toxins
      Aminoglycoside antibiotics
      Methoxyflurane
      Ethylene glycol
      Heavy metals
      Methanol
      Insecticides and herbicides
      Carbon tetrachloride
      Cisplatin
      Radiographic contrast medium

dium, nonsteroidal anti-inflammatory agents, and cyclosporin A.[61] Ischemic acute renal failure due to inadequate renal perfusion such as occurs in cardiac failure, sepsis, or hemorrhagic shock accounts for approximately 50% of all cases of acute renal failure.[79,82]

In oliguric acute renal failure, microscopic and chemical analysis of urine may be helpful. The kidney is unable to excrete a concentrated, low-sodium urine. Analysis finds the urine osmolality less than 400 mOsm/kg H_2O and the urine sodium concentration greater than 40 mEq/L.[63] Proteinuria is usually present, and the sediment contains red blood cells, white blood cells, renal tubular casts, amorphous debris, and a brown granular cast typical of ATN.[56]

Retrospective studies[85,86] indicate that nonoliguric renal failure may account for as many as 20% to 30% of all cases of acute renal failure. Anderson and Schrier[59] and Diamond and Yoburn[87] pointed out that nephrotoxic failure occurred more fre-

quently in nonoliguric than in oliguric subjects. Serum and urinary diagnostic indices suggest that the insult is less severe in nonoliguric than in oliguric acute renal failure.

Differentiation between prerenal states, acute renal failure, and other causes of acute oliguria depends heavily on the analysis of urinary electrolytes and osmolality. Useful diagnostic parameters are summarized in Table 5–7.

Initial Treatment of Oliguria

Fluid challenge is the fundamental therapeutic intervention in the management of acute oliguria. Since the most common cause of acute renal failure is prolonged renal hypoperfusion, oliguria usually indicates inadequate vascular volume. Patients with cardiac failure or cirrhosis may require central monitoring prior to a fluid challenge. In other patients, oliguria should prompt the infusion of isotonic fluids at a rate sufficient to restore vascular volume and renal perfusion. A long period is sometimes observed between fluid replacement and the onset of diuresis. In normal humans, an improvement in cortical blood flow following IV saline loading may require 48 hours to appear.[88]

If the urine output does not increase with an adequate volume challenge, placement of a central venous or pulmonary arterial line should be considered. If vascular volume is adequate and urine output remains low, a trial of furosemide or dopamine may be indicated. Diuresis should be attempted with caution, for if volume status is not carefully monitored, diuresis may further reduce intravascular volume. Furosemide in a dose of 1.5 to 6.0 mg/kg given every 2 to 4 hours by slow IV infusion may prove therapeutic.[89] Renal dopamine doses of 1.5 to 2.5 µg/kg/min cause vasodilation of the renal vessels and may provoke diuresis and solute excretion.[90] Continued oliguria following adequate volume replacement and a trial of furosemide and/or dopamine establishes the diagnosis of acute oliguric acute renal failure.

The indications for dialysis in patients with acute renal failure are volume expansion with congestive heart failure intractable to standard therapy, electrolyte abnormalities not controlled by more conservative means, severe acidosis, and actual or impending uremic symptoms.[56] Dialysis should be performed with sufficient frequency that the patient has no symptoms secondary to uremia. For hemodialysis, this generally means at least three times per week.

Recovery from acute renal failure may be her-

TABLE 5–7. **Urinary Indices in Acute Renal Failure**

	Prerenal Azotemia	Acute Glomerulonephritis	Acute Tubular Necrosis	Nonoliguric Acute Tubular Necrosis	Obstructive Uropathy
Urine osmolality, mOsm/kg H_2O	>350	>350	<400	<400	<400
Urine sodium, mEq/L	<20	<20	>40	>40	>30
Urine/plasma creatinine ratio	>40	>40	<20	<20	<20
Fractional excretion* of filtered sodium	<1	<1	>1	>1	>1
Urine sediment	Normal or occasional hyaline and granular casts	Red cells and red cell casts	Brown granular casts, cellular debris	Brown granular casts, cellular debris	Usually negative

* Measured as $\dfrac{\text{Urine Na/Serum Na}}{\text{Urine creat./Serum creat.}} \times 100$.

alded by a diuretic phase that begins in 10 to 14 days in 50% of patients and in 15 to 30 days in another 40% to 45%.[56] Renal biopsy should be considered if diuresis has not occurred after 30 days of oliguria.

Oliguria During Surgery or in the Recovery Room

Oliguria in the operating room or recovery room should be assumed to be secondary to hypovolemia until proven otherwise. Adequate intravascular volume and renal perfusion must be maintained despite the excessive blood loss. Vasopressor agents should not be administered unless adequate intravascular volume has been confirmed with invasive monitoring. In the presence of hypotension secondary to hemorrhage or third space losses, volume correction with isotonic fluids or red blood cells should be accomplished before vasopressors are given.

The prophylactic benefit of mannitol- or furosemide-induced perioperative diuresis in patients at risk for intraoperative acute renal failure has been suggested.[91] Prough and Zaloga[21] administered diuretics to patients at risk for renal failure: (1) in anticipation of an interval of fixed, complete renal ischemia (i.e., suprarenal cross-clamping), (2) in acute pigmenturia accompanying intravascular hemolysis or rhabdomyolysis, (3) in acute volume overload, and (4) if aggressive prerenal support is ineffective. In these cases, diuretics may limit renal damage.

General anesthetics may depress renal function, especially in volume-depleted patients.[64] Conduction anesthesia (spinal or epidural) may decrease RBF secondary to diminished cardiac preload related to sympathetic blockade. Extensive surgical blood loss or third space loss diminishes intravascular volume and renal perfusion. Manipulation of vessels with severe atherosclerotic changes may lead to multiple atheromatous emboli to the kidneys, compromising their function.

Late Postoperative Oliguria

Oliguria may appear several days after surgery. It may manifest as increasing azotemia with diminished urine output unresponsive to adequate volume replacement, or as declining renal parameters in the setting of adequate or increased output, as in partial obstructive uropathy. Late postoperative oliguria is most often related to volume depletion secondary to enteric fistulas, continuous nasogastric suction, or a third space collection such as ileus, ascites, or pleural effusions. The patient may be relatively asymptomatic, and clinical signs of volume depletion may not be obvious. Obstructive uropathy must be excluded. Adequate volume and appropriate electrolyte replacement should be instituted. A diligent search for third space sequestration of fluids should be undertaken. Nephrotoxic antibiotics and the use of radiopaque dyes or other drugs are also possible causes of late postoperative oliguria.

Urinary Tract Injury and Fistulas

Complications resulting from urinary tract injury have always been considered the more serious hazards of gynecologic surgery. Operative injury to the lower urinary tract is an infrequent complication of pelvic surgery but a constant reminder of the close anatomic proximity of the urinary and reproductive tracts. Despite this close association, operative urologic injury is uncommon—a credit to surgical skill as well as to the attention given to the urinary tract by gynecologic surgeons. Nonetheless, injuries to the urinary tract are the most common reason for medicolegal actions against gynecologic surgeons.

Incidence of Urologic Injury

The bladder is the most common site of urinary tract injury during pelvic surgery. When vesical injuries are recognized and immediately repaired, the potential complications are not life-threatening. In contrast, ureteral injuries, especially if unrecognized, may result in permanent kidney damage or loss of the renal unit. The great majority of ureteral injuries are associated with total abdominal hysterectomy performed for benign indications. Many ureteral and some bladder injuries are not recognized intraoperatively. Indeed, 70% to 95% of cases go undetected.[92-95] However, in one series reported from a major teaching hospital, 84% of injuries were recognized during the procedure, suggesting that even physicians in training can be taught to assess possible urologic injury during the operation.[96]

The exact incidence of accidental lower urinary tract injury during obstetric and gynecologic surgery is difficult to determine because most cases are unreported. Various authors[97-99] report an overall incidence of lower urinary tract injury of 0.2% to 2.5%. Bladder injuries are more common than ureteral injuries, with a ratio of 5.3:1[96] in a series of 5,517 major nonradical gynecologic procedures. Graber et al.[99] (1964) reported a 1.9% incidence of bladder injury in a series of 819 abdominal hysterectomies.

Ureteral injuries are more troublesome and potentially more morbid than vesical injuries. Thompson[100] stated that about 75% of ureteral injuries result from gynecologic procedures; of these, 75% follow abdominal operations and 25% follow vaginal operations. The highest frequency (1%–2%) occurred during extensive abdominal operations for invasive cancer of the cervix. The rate is higher for abdominal hysterectomy (0.5%–1%) than for vagi-

nal hysterectomy (0.1%). This difference in frequency is thought to be primarily due to the fact that patients with more extensive pelvic disease are most often approached by the abdominal route. Although information is still being compiled, it appears that the risk of ureteral injury is not necessarily decreased during laparoscopically assisted procedures.

Urethral Injuries

Urethral injuries resulting in fistulas are rare. Obstetric injury from protracted labor or a difficult forceps delivery was once the major cause of urethral injury in the United States and continues to be a major cause of urethral injuries in developing countries. Unintentional urethral damage more commonly results from faulty repair, infection, or hematoma following excision of a suburethral diverticulum.[97] Additionally, urethral injury may occur during anterior colporrhaphy and, if it is unrecognized at operation, a urethrovaginal fistula may follow. Traumatic catheterization may rarely cause fistula formation. Rigid catheters are especially hazardous.

Urethral injury when recognized at operation should be repaired. Proper mobilization of urethral and periurethral tissues and reapproximation with fine interrupted absorbable sutures is necessary. Urinary drainage by suprapubic tube or transurethral catheter aids in successful healing. The duration of catheter drainage depends on the extent of injury and the condition of the tissue at the time of repair.

The principles employed for urethrovaginal fistula repair are similar to those used for repair of a vesicovaginal fistula, which is discussed later in this chapter.

Bladder Injuries

Its proximity to the uterus, cervix, and anterior fornix of the vagina makes the bladder vulnerable to injury during hysterectomy. In fact, most iatrogenic bladder damage occurs during hysterectomy, and this operation has replaced obstetric injury as the leading cause of vesicovaginal fistulas. Bladder damage is generally not catastrophic if it is recognized and treated promptly. Conversely, if bladder damage is not recognized, it almost inevitably results in a postoperative vesicovaginal fistula. As Mengert[101] said, "It is no sin to cut the bladder. The sin is not to recognize it."

The appearance of fluid in the wound is usually the first indication that the bladder has been traumatized during abdominal or vaginal surgery. Instillation by Foley catheter of 400 to 600 mL of sterile milk or sterile water colored with methylene blue will confirm that injury has occurred but will not necessarily define the limits of the laceration. Direct inspection of the interior of the bladder may be performed at abdominal surgery to delineate the extent of injury, but cystoscopy may be necessary when the injury occurs during vaginal surgery. In either circumstance, ureteral catheter placement makes suture ligation of the ureters less likely during repair.

As a general rule, bladder injuries should be repaired when discovered. Everett and Mattingly[102] analyzed 77 cases of bladder injury recognized at surgery; none of these cases failed to heal when recognized and repaired at the time of the initial injury. However, Guerriero[103] argued that temporizing by insertion of a Foley catheter and awaiting spontaneous closure may be prudent when the patient is unstable, when the patient is a poor operative risk, when the injury is discovered during the secondary healing phase, 8 to 15 days postoperatively, or when an injury occurs in an already infected operative site.

Late recognition of bladder damage usually is associated with a vesicovaginal fistula that appears 3 to 12 days postoperatively with urine leaking through the vagina.

Bladder Damage During Abdominal Hysterectomy

Various circumstances and surgical maneuvers can lead to bladder damage during abdominal hysterectomy (Table 5–8). There are five critical points in the performance of abdominal hysterectomy where the bladder is at risk of injury (Fig. 5–7).[99]

1. *Incising the parietal peritoneum.* Failure to empty the bladder before surgery may increase the risk of injury, as the bladder is relatively resistant to injury when collapsed. Bladder drainage by indwelling catheter should be considered before cesarean section or abdominal or vaginal hysterectomy. Accidental bladder injury at the time of peritoneal entry usually occurs in the dome of the bladder. When such injuries occur, the bladder may be easily repaired after careful assessment of the extent of the injury. A continuous closure with 3–0 delayed absorbable suture on a small tapered needle is recommended. The first layer should invert and close the mucosa securely. A second layer of continuous or interrupted suture may be placed in the muscularis to imbricate and support the first layer.

TABLE 5–8. Causes of Bladder Damage During Abdominal Hysterectomy

Damage occurs most often when:
- Incising the parietal peritoneum

  Causes:
  Failure to catheterize bladder preoperatively
  Displacement of bladder by pelvic tumor, previous surgery
  Extensive adhesive disease

- Entering the vesicouterine fold

  Causes:
  Entering the vesicouterine fold too low
  Displacement of bladder by large tumors, myomas, or pelvic adhesions

- Separating the bladder from the uterine fundus, cervix, and upper vagina

  Causes:
  Dissection in the wrong plane
  Abnormal adhesions from previous cesarean section, endometriosis, previous irradiation

- Entering the vagina anteriorly

  Cause:
  Insufficient mobilization or retraction of the bladder

- Mobilizing or suturing the vaginal vault

  Causes:
  Grasping the bladder and vaginal vault with Kocher clamps
  Suturing the bladder into the vaginal vault

Bladder decompression for 7 to 10 days postoperatively is recommended. The repair of bladder dome injuries usually does not encroach on the ureters, and ureteral catheterization is unnecessary.

2. *Entering the vesicouterine fold.* If the fold is entered too low, the dome of the bladder may be unintentionally opened. The bladder may be elevated by anatomic distortion or by previous pelvic surgery. Bladder decompression by Foley catheter and careful inspection of the bladder should minimize this risk.

3. *Separating the bladder from the uterine fundus, cervix, or upper vagina.* Adhesions from previous cesarean section, endometriosis, pelvic inflammatory disease, or previous irradiation can cause abnormal adherence of the bladder base to the lower uterus and upper vagina. The major etiologic factor in this injury is overly aggressive blunt dissection in an incorrect surgical plane between the bladder base and the pubovesicocervical fascia. During abdominal or vaginal hysterectomy, the bladder base should be dissected from the cervix with sharp dissection. When using Metzenbaum

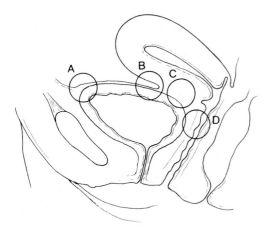

FIGURE 5–7. Usual sites of bladder entry and injury during abdominal hysterectomy. Injury to the dome of the bladder occurs when entering the parietal peritoneum (*A*) or the vesicouterine fold (*B*). Cervical injury many occur during dissection of the bladder from the uterus (*C*). Injury may also occur when entering the vagina anteriorly or suturing the vault (*D*).

scissors, the operator should direct the points of the scissors away from the bladder. An added measure of safety may be achieved by performing an intrafascial hysterectomy, as advocated by Richardson.[104] Injury at this level should be repaired as previously described.

4. *Entering the anterior vagina.* Bladder damage may occur during this phase of the operation if the bladder has been insufficiently mobilized or retracted prior to entering the anterior vaginal wall. Mobilization of the bladder may prove difficult in the presence of extensive adhesive disease, previous cesarean section, or prior irradiation therapy.

5. *Mobilizing or suturing the vaginal vault.* Many surgeons prefer to grasp the margins of the vaginal cuff with instruments after uterine removal and before placement of hemostatic vaginal angle sutures. These instruments may grasp the bladder if it is not retracted sufficiently, resulting in injury to the supratrigonal region. The bladder may also be injured during cuff closure or placement of hemostatic sutures along the vaginal cuff. Placement of these sutures in an anterior to posterior manner may decrease these risks.

The risk of bladder injury during abdominal hysterectomy can be minimized by certain surgical maneuvers and precautions, summarized in Table 5–9.

Bladder Damage During Vaginal Hysterectomy

Most bladder injuries during vaginal hysterectomy are in the supratrigonal portion of the bladder base or, rarely, in the area of the bladder trigone.[105] Failure to identify the correct anatomic plane between the bladder and the cervix may result in inability to locate and enter the vesicouterine peritoneal fold. Most gynecologic surgeons recognize this maneu-

ver—i.e., the ability to successfully enter the correct tissue plane between the bladder and cervix—as the crux of a successful vaginal hysterectomy. As with an abdominal hysterectomy, the bladder base should be dissected from the cervix using sharp dissection and without cutting beyond the area of clear visibility. Forceful, blunt dissection with a finger or a gauze sponge in the vesicocervical space is to be avoided. During bladder advancement, firm downward traction on the cervix should be maintained, with gentle countertraction of the bladder with a right-angled retractor (Fig. 5–8).

The correct plane between bladder and cervix is white and relatively avascular. Misdirected dissection in this area may invite troublesome bleeding, obscuring the operative field and causing the dissection to proceed in a superficial plane with possible bladder injury. When injury occurs, the operator

TABLE 5–9. **Avoiding Bladder Injury During Abdominal Hysterectomy**

- Open the parietal peritoneum high.
- Develop the bladder flap high.
- Use sharp rather than blunt dissection in developing the plane between the bladder and cervix.
- Free the bladder below the level of the cervix both centrally and laterally to avoid damage.
- Perform an intrafascial hysterectomy whenever possible (see Fig. 5–4).
- Avoid the use of right-angle clamps at the vaginal angles.
- Leave the vagina open and draining unless the vault area is dry.
- If the operative field is bloody, enter the vagina posteriorly.
- Suture the vaginal vault under direct vision with the bladder retracted.
- If bladder position is uncertain, use methylene blue in saline to inflate the bladder and locate its limits.

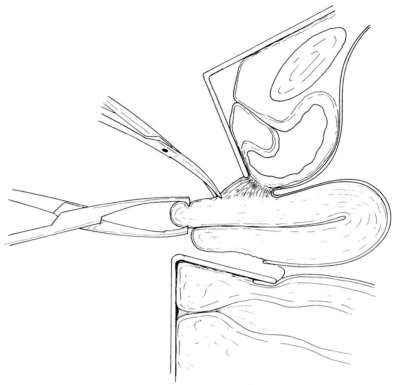

FIGURE 5–8. Dissecting the vesicouterine space during vaginal hysterectomy. Firm downward traction on the cervix with gentle bladder retraction facilitates sharp dissection with scissors. (Modified with permission from Thompson JD: Hysterectomy. In Thompson JD, Rock JA (eds): Te Linde's Operative Gynecology, p 711. Philadelphia: JB Lippincott, 1992.)

should verify the location and extent of injury. Cystoscopy may be helpful. If there is a concern of ureteral compromise, 5 mL of indigo carmine should be injected IV. In 5 to 7 minutes, blue dye will emerge from the ureteral orifices. Once ureteral patency is confirmed, the bladder repair may be completed transvaginally with a two- or three-layered continuous closure of 3-0 delayed absorbable suture. The suture line should be tested by distending the bladder with sterile milk, and additional sutures should be used to reinforce any areas that are not watertight in the repair. The dissection should then be continued in the proper plane. Continuous catheter drainage for 7 to 10 days postoperatively may be necessary; bladder distention should be avoided during the healing phase. After the bladder laceration has been repaired, there is no contraindication to proceeding with the vaginal hysterectomy and/or anterior colporrhaphy, if indicated. In some instances, bladder repair may be performed after completion of the hysterectomy.

Bladder injuries that occur during anterior col-porrhaphy usually result from misdirected dissection of the bladder from the underlying pubovesicocervical fascia and anterior vaginal wall. As before, sharp dissection of the bladder from the underlying fascia with small, curved scissors is preferable to blunt finger dissection or the use of instrument-held sponges. Injuries to the bladder during anterior colporrhaphy are frequently in the area of the trigone. Similar testing for ureteral integrity is essential before and after repair of a defect in this area. Surgical maneuvers to avoid bladder damage during vaginal hysterectomy are summarized in Table 5–10.

Injuries to the Bladder During Retropubic Procedures

Surgery performed to correct anatomic stress incontinence may be complicated by unintentional bladder damage. Performance of a retropubic urethropexy by either Burch[106] or Marshall-Marchetti-Krantz[107] techniques necessitates mobilizing the

TABLE 5–10. Avoiding Bladder Damage During Vaginal Hysterectomy

- Insert a Foley catheter into the bladder before dissecting in the vesicocervical space.
- Dissect cautiously when dividing the bladder pillars and developing the plane between bladder and uterus.
- Use sharp dissection with small curved scissors when advancing the bladder. Keep the points of the scissors directed away from the bladder. Avoid blunt dissection in this area.
- Verify the presence of bowel/omentum after opening the peritoneum of the vesicouterine fold. Do not proceed further without positive identification of bowel.
- Maintain gentle retraction on the bladder to keep it out of harm's way.
- When closing the vaginal cuff, suture cautiously to avoid penetrating the bladder.
- Use sharp dissection to dissect the bladder from pubovesicocervical fascia and the anterior vaginal wall during anterior colporrhaphy.

bladder and its associated fascia to allow bilateral suture placement in the pubovesicocervical fascia lateral to the bladder neck. Failure to mobilize the bladder or to expose the paraurethral fascia adequately may result in suture placement through the bladder wall into the lumen, with subsequent anchoring of the suture to Cooper's ligament or to the posterior aspect of the symphysis pubis. Permanent sutures within the bladder may act as a nidus for vesical calculi or may cause ischemic necrosis, leading to perforation and the development of cellulitis secondary to the accumulation of urine in the space of Retzius. The surgeon can identify the bladder margin with greater accuracy by inserting his fingers into the vagina and elevating the paraurethral fascia to aid in suture placement.

A Foley catheter with a 30-cc bulb is recommended for all retropubic and/or urethropexy procedures. The larger catheter bulb aids in identification of the bladder neck; when funneling of the bladder neck is present, a catheter with a 5- or 10-cc bulb may be pulled down into the proximal urethra, creating a false impression of the true location of the bladder neck and resulting in pathologic urethral kinking, urethral obstruction with prolonged catheter dependence, and detrusor instability.

When the anatomy in the space of Retzius is distorted by scarring from previous surgery, safe placement of urethropexy sutures without damaging the bladder or urethra may pose a special challenge. Under these circumstances, the bladder dome may be opened to allow placement of the bladder neck sutures under direct vision. Opening the bladder also allows direct observation of indigo carmine excretion from the ureteral orifices to confirm patency, facilitate passage of ureteral catheters if necessary, and allow placement of a suprapubic catheter under direct vision.

Injury to the bladder neck most commonly occurs during retropubic urethropexy in patients who have previously undergone operation for genuine stress incontinence.[105] In this situation, the proximal urethra and bladder neck may be densely adherent to the symphysis pubis, making sharp dissection exceedingly difficult. Exposure may be limited, and associated bleeding at the operative site further limits visibility. When laceration of the bladder neck occurs, immediate repair is prudent to avoid extension into the proximal urethra and urethrovesical junction. Closure using double layers of 3-0 delayed absorbable suture should be in the vertical axis to avoid funneling of the bladder neck. After repair and testing for suture-line leaking, the urethropexy may be completed. Postoperative bladder drainage for 7 to 10 days by urethral or suprapubic catheter is important for adequate healing. A Jackson-Pratt drain in the space of Retzius may assist in preventing hematoma formation.

Needle urethropexies such as the modified Pereyra procedure[107a] should be accompanied by water cystoscopy using an oblique lens to verify that no permanent suture has entered the bladder lumen. Any such suture should be removed immediately and replaced more laterally. Verification of ureteral patency using cystoscopy following IV instillation of 5 mL of indigo carmine should be considered after every urethropexy.

Bladder Damage During Laparoscopy

Bladder injuries may occur during the performance of laparoscopic procedures. Especially hazardous is the insertion of laparoscopic trocars in the presence of an incompletely drained bladder. Most laparoscopic bladder injuries occur in the dome of the bladder secondary to the insertion of lower abdominal trocars. Recognized injuries involving the bladder dome may be managed conservatively with urethral catheter drainage for 7 to 10 days. Water cystoscopy should be performed to verify the location and extent of damage. Unintentional bladder puncture with a 5 to 7 mm trocar will seal off promptly as long as the bladder is decompressed by catheter. However, large, 10 to 12 mm trocars pose a greater hazard. Suturing of the bladder injury during laparoscopy or at open laparotomy may be necessary if inspection reveals a large defect. Laceration through the dome of the bladder into the trigone is most unusual. In such cases, verification of ureteral integrity can be assessed with IV indigo carmine injection and/or passage of a ureteral stent.

The widespread use of laser, electrocautery, and thermal cautery at laparoscopy offers the potential for damage if these energy modes are misdirected. Recognized bladder damage with laser or cautery should be closely inspected at laparoscopy and water cystoscopy, followed by urethral catheter drainage for 7 to 10 days. Cases involving extensive dissection secondary to endometriosis or chronic pelvic inflammatory disease are more apt to result in unintentional penetration of the viscera with lasers or electrothermal energy.

Automated stapling devices such as are used in laparoscopically assisted hysterectomy may engender bladder injury when the broad ligaments are stapled and cut in the course of gaining access to the retroperitoneal space. The operator should identify the superior and lateral margins of the bladder before applying stapling devices, especially if the patient has previously undergone cesarean section or has chronic adhesive disease.

Vesicovaginal Fistulas

Although vesicovaginal fistulas from obstetric causes are still common in developing countries, the majority of such fistulas seen today result from total abdominal or vaginal hysterectomy for benign disease.[100] In a recent retrospective study of lower urinary tract fistulas, Tancer[108] reported that 91% of 151 fistulas followed gynecologic procedures; of these, 110 were vesicovaginal fistulas occurring in the vaginal vault, 92 after total abdominal hysterectomy and 18 after vaginal hysterectomy. Risk factors for fistula formation after hysterectomy included prior cesarean section, endometriosis, recent cold-knife conization, and previous irradiation therapy. Similarly, Lee et al.[109] reported on 156 patients with a vesicovaginal fistula evaluated at the Mayo Clinic between 1970 and 1985. Of these, 132 occurred after abdominal hysterectomy, 20 after vaginal hysterectomy, 4 after radical hysterectomy, 3 after vaginal repair, 5 after cesarean section, 6 after cesarean hysterectomy, 6 after trauma, and 6 after radiation therapy.

DIAGNOSIS OF VESICOVAGINAL FISTULAS. The usual patient with a vesicovaginal fistula experiences painless, constant leakage of urine through the vagina. Most vesicovaginal fistulas resulting

from gynecologic surgery manifest as urinary leakage through the vagina before the 12th postoperative day.[110]

The diagnosis may often be readily made by careful vaginal speculum examination. Filling the bladder with a dilute solution of methylene blue or sterile milk and inspecting the vaginal vault and anterior vaginal wall for leakage may be necessary. Cystoscopy with the patient in the knee–chest position is often helpful in determining the site and number of fistulas and assessing the condition of the tissue. The "flat tire" test may be helpful in discerning very small fistulas: the bladder is filled with carbon dioxide, the vagina with water, and the vaginal opening is identified from the location of rising bubbles.[111]

Occasionally, severe stress incontinence or bladder instability may cause continuous leakage and mimic a fistula. In this situation, the tampon test described by Moir[112] may be helpful. Three tampons are placed in the vagina in tandem. Methylene blue is placed in the bladder and the patient is allowed to walk for 10 to 15 minutes. The tampons are then removed and examined. If the upper tampon is blue, a vesicovaginal fistula is present; if it is wet and not blue, a ureterovaginal fistula is suspect. If the lowest tampon is blue, transurethral leakage is the likely cause. Staining of the middle tampon may indicate a fistula at the bladder neck or proximal urethra, depending on the position of the tampon in the vagina.

A ureterovaginal fistula may be diagnosed with IVP, retrograde pyelography, or IV injection of 5 mL of indigo carmine and observing blue dye in the vagina when the bladder has not been filled with methylene blue.[111]

TIMING OF VESICOVAGINAL FISTULA REPAIR. Previously, many physicians recommended delaying repair for 4 to 6 months after discovery to allow maturation of the fistula tract. With delayed repair, cure rates have averaged 90%.[100] However, delay creates a hardship for the patient, who is usually experiencing continuous leakage of urine, a chronic unpleasant urinous odor, and extreme vulvar irritation and excoriation.

Recent reports advocate "nondelay" with repair occurring 6 to 13 weeks after hysterectomy, with favorable results.[113–115] In Tancer's series,[108] 107 patients underwent surgical repair by the Latzko technique within 13 weeks of discovery; 98 patients were cured by the primary repair. Each of the nine patients in whom the first attempt failed underwent a repeat Latzko operation within 12 weeks of the failed procedure. All repeat operations were successful. Less favorable results have been reported with early repair in patients in whom fistulas resulted from irradiation or extensive surgery for pelvic malignancy.[100] Bresette and Patterson[111] recommended that repair be undertaken as soon as the bladder and vaginal site are nonfriable and free of edema, as judged from cystoscopy and inspection of the tissue per vagina.

Spontaneous healing with the use of continuous bladder drainage has been reported to occur in 15% to 20% of patients.[100] Spontaneous healing is unusual except for very small fistulas only a few millimeters in diameter. One recent study reported spontaneous healing within 13 weeks of hysterectomy in only three patients of 110 with vesicovaginal vault fistulas.[108]

SURGICAL REPAIR OF VESICOVAGINAL FISTULAS.
Most vesicovaginal fistulas that occur in the United States are small, simple fistulas in the vaginal vault that result from unrecognized bladder injury during pelvic surgery. Thus, this discussion will address the repair of small fistulas.

First described in 1913, the Latzko technique for partial colpocleisis has become the procedure of choice for repair of simple vesicovaginal fistulas in the supratrigonal region. Latzko[116] described the operation in detail in 1942 and reported cures in 29 of 31 cases. More recent series report success rates of 92% to 93% for primary repair by the Latzko technique.[108,117,118]

Important preoperative steps include catheter drainage of the urethra for 10 days to 2 weeks before the procedure, administration of appropriate antibiotics for known infection, the use of an estrogen-containing vaginal cream, and careful assessment of the vagina and bladder for resolution of edema and inflammation.[111]

The procedure (Fig. 5–9) requires complete denudation of the vaginal mucosa around the fistula. Infiltration of sterile saline beneath the vaginal mucosa around the fistula may facilitate dissection. If exposure is difficult, the incision may be brought down by placing a no. 8 Foley catheter into the fistula and inflated in the bladder. Latzko did not excise the fistulous tract. However, Thompson[100] recommended excision if the fistula appeared fresh,

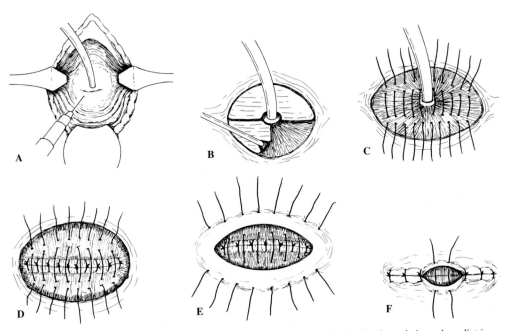

FIGURE 5–9. Closure of a simple posthysterectomy vesicovaginal fistula by the Latzko technique. **A,** pediatric Foley catheter is placed into the bladder through the fistula for traction. Normal saline is injected submucosally to aid dissection. **B,** the vaginal epithelium to be excised is marked off in quadrants and each quadrant is removed. **C,** a deep layer of no. 3-0 delayed absorbable suture is placed in a transverse axis. **D,** after removal of Foley catheter and tying of the first layer of sutures, a second layer is placed. **E,** a final layer of interrupted absorbable sutures is placed through the edges of the vaginal mucosa. **F,** vaginal closure is completed. (Redrawn with permission from Nichols DH, Randall CL: Vaginal Surgery, p 376. Baltimore: Williams & Wilkins, 1989.)

indurated, and necrotic. An older, scarred, and epithelialized tract may be left in situ. The partial colpocleisis is begun by approximating the bladder submucosa transversely with interrupted sutures of 3-0 delayed absorbable suture on a fine tapered needle. This first suture line should be tested by filling the bladder with 100 to 200 mL of sterile milk or methylene blue and noting any sites of leakage. If present, such points should be reinforced with additional sutures. A second and third layer of interrupted 3-0 absorbable suture should be placed, each inverting the previous line of suture and approximating the anterior and posterior vaginal walls (see Fig. 5–9E).

Depending on the operator's assessment of the size of the fistula and the health of the tissue, a suprapubic tube may be placed if drainage for 7 to 14 days is planned. If bladder drainage for only a few days is anticipated, a transurethral Foley catheter may be placed. A fistula in the area of the trigone may be approached by simple excision of the tract followed by closure. The ureter should be catheterized to prevent suture encirclement of a ureter. An incision is made about the fistulous opening and the vaginal mucosa is mobilized for a sufficient distance to allow a three-layered closure. The fistula tract should be excised followed by closure with continuous or interrupted 3-0 delayed absorbable sutures. These sutures should begin and end beyond the limits of the fistula. After the suture line has been tested for leaks with 100 to 200 mL of sterile milk or methylene blue instilled through a urethral catheter, a second and third layer of 3-0 delayed absorbable continuous or interrupted suture are placed, each layer inverting the preceding layer. The vaginal mucosa is trimmed and approximated without tension with 3-0 interrupted suture.

The vaginal approach may be contraindicated when excessive vaginal scarring from previous repairs is present, when the location is inaccessible by the vaginal route, for fistulas associated with radiation for gynecologic malignancy, and for complex fistulas involving the intestine, ureters, or uterus.[111] In these cases, a longer delay may be indicated before closure is attempted. Increasing the vascularity of the tissue by mobilizing omentum, the bulbocavernosus fat pad, or gracilis muscle from the inner thigh may be done. In some cases, a combined transabdominal-transvaginal approach may be required. For patients who have undergone several unsuccessful attempts at repair, a staged reconstruction may be used. The first stage consists of urinary diversion using a sigmoid or ileal conduit with transabdominal fistula repair. After the fis-

tula heals, the conduit is implanted into the dome of the bladder, restoring continuity of the urinary tract.

Ureteral Injuries

The anatomic proximity of the ureter to other pelvic structures makes it a prime structure for injury during gynecologic operations. It is noteworthy that ureteral injury is relatively rare, occurring in 0.4% to 2.5% of all gynecologic procedures.[119] Of all injuries to the urinary tract, those involving the ureter are the most difficult to recognize and produce the most serious complications. Untreated ureteral injuries may result in fistula formation or loss of kidney function. The gynecologic surgeon must be vigilant in every operative procedure to identify the location of the ureters and take the necessary steps to avoid iatrogenic injury.

Sites of Injury

Ureteral injuries associated with gynecologic surgery usually occur in one of four locations (Fig. 5–10)[105]: (1) at or above the infundibulopelvic ligament near the pelvic brim, (2) in the base of the broad ligament where the ureter passes beneath the uterine vessels, (3) along the lateral pelvic side wall just above the uterosacral ligaments, and (4) as the ureter passes through the cardinal ligament and turns anteriorly and medially to enter the bladder. Approximately 80% to 90% of all ureteral injuries occur in the distal portion of the ureter from the

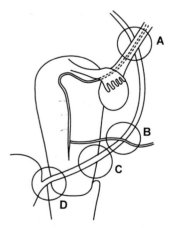

FIGURE 5–10. Common sites of ureteral injury associated with hysterectomy. **A,** infundibulopelvic ligament; **B,** junction of the uterine artery and ureter; **C,** uterosacral ligaments; **D,** cardinal ligament at the ureterovesical junction. (Redrawn with permission from Shingleton HM: Repairing injuries to the urinary tract. Contemp Ob/Gyn March 1984: 76.)

uterine artery to the ureterovesical junction.[105] The least frequent site is at or above the infundibulopelvic ligament at the pelvic brim.

Types of Ureteral Injury and Pelvic Conditions Predisposing to Injury

Six types of operative ureteral trauma have been described by Thompson[100]: (1) crushing injury from misapplication of surgical clamp(s), (2) ligation with suture, (3) transection (either partial or complete), (4) angulation with secondary partial or complete obstruction, (5) ischemia from stripping of the adventitia and depriving a segment of ureter of its blood supply, and (6) resection of a segment of ureter, either intentionally in radical surgery for malignancy or unintentionally. Ureteral injuries may be unilateral or, rarely, bilateral. Injury may result during extremely difficult dissections in the presence of grossly distorted anatomy or during seemingly routine procedures.

Certain pelvic conditions may predispose the ureter to injury:

1. *Lateral displacement of the cervix.* Extreme lateral displacement of the cervix brings the cervix very close to, even in contact with, the ureter. Displacement may be caused by adhesions that draw the uterus toward the same side of the pelvis, or by tumors such as large leiomyomas situated on one side of the uterus and pushing the cervix to the opposite side.

2. *Masses adherent to the pelvic peritoneum.* A mass may adhere to the peritoneum overlying the ureter. Such masses may include inflammatory, ovarian, tubal, or intestinal masses (Fig. 5–11). In

mobilizing masses before removal, the peritoneum and underlying ureter may be traumatized. In these clinical situations, the gynecologic surgeon should open the retroperitoneal space lateral to the mass, identify the ureter, and dissect the mass away from the ureter with the ureter under direct vision. Injuries may occur when the surgeon attempts to develop a plane between the mass and the parietal peritoneum without previously identifying and protecting the ureter. Blunt dissection in this clinical situation may not be prudent.

3. *Intraligamentary tumors.* Myomas or other tumors may develop between the folds of the broad ligament, causing lateral displacement and compression of the ureter (Fig. 5–12). The ureter may be mistaken for a blood vessel and ligated unintentionally. Again, identifying the ureter in its retroperitoneal location before resection will aid in avoiding injury.

4. *Inflammatory exudates in the base of the broad ligament.* The ureter is protected from a contiguous abscess or inflammatory exudate by its sheath, which becomes greatly thickened in these situations. However, the ureter may be injured during incision and drainage of an abscess in the broad ligament, whether approached abdominally or vaginally.

5. *Retroperitoneal tumors.* A tumor mass lateral to the ureter will displace the peritoneum with the attached ureter toward the midline. In the operative treatment of such a mass the ureter may be injured (Fig. 5–13).

6. *Cancer of the uterine cervix.* The parametrium is often involved by direct extension or metastasis of cervical carcinoma. Dissection of the ureter with

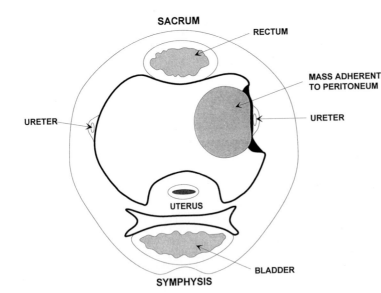

FIGURE 5–11. Mass adherent to the parietal peritoneum covering the ureter, the removal of which is associated with danger of ureteral injury. (Redrawn with permission from Sampson JA: Ureteral fistulae as sequelae of pelvic operations. Surg Gynecol Obstet 8:479, 1909.)

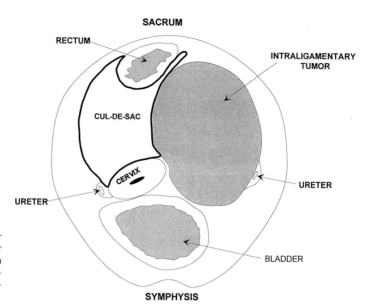

FIGURE 5–12. Intraligamentary tumor overlying the ureter. Removal of the tumor may engender ureteral injury. (Redrawn with permission from Sampson JA: Ureteral fistulae as sequelae of pelvic operations. Surg Gynecol Obstet 8:479, 1909.)

development of the uterovesical ligament and tumor resection may result in direct injury or devascularization.

Ureteral Injury
During Abdominal Operations

The abdominal or upper ureter may be injured during the course of colonic resection, aortic reconstruction, sympathectomy, laminectomy, pancreatic and duodenal resection, ureterolithotomy, and excision of retroperitoneal lymph nodes and tumors.

Causes of ureteral injury during abdominopelvic operations are summarized in Table 5–11. Injury occurs most frequently where the ureter crosses beneath the uterine artery lateral to the cervix.[120] This injury occurs in cases where the uterine vessels slip from the clamp or ligature and the operator attempts reclamping or oversewing in the face of profuse hemorrhage. Controlling the hemorrhage by direct pressure in the region of the uterine artery, followed by an attempt to identify and clamp the bleeding vessels under direct vision, is preferable to blind clamping or suturing in the base of the broad ligament. Failure to control the hemorrhage by

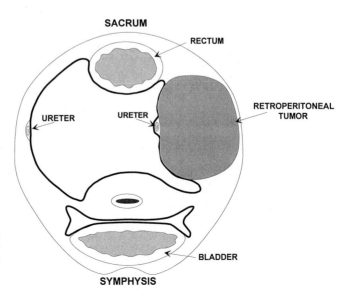

FIGURE 5–13. Retroperitoneal tumor lateral to the ureter. Attempted removal may cause ureteral injury. (Redrawn with permission from Sampson JA: Ureteral fistulae as sequelae of pelvic operations. Surg Gynecol Obstet 8:479, 1909.)

TABLE 5–11. **Injuries to the Pelvic Ureter During Abdominal Surgery**

Injuries occur more often during:
- Clamping the uterine vessels during abdominal hysterectomy
- Clamping and ligating the infundibulopelvic ligaments during adnexectomy
- Surgery for endometriosis, malignancy, pelvic inflammatory disease, adnexal disease, myomas
- Reperitonealization
- Cul-de-sac obliteration by the Moschcowitz technique
- Clamping and suturing the vaginal cuff
- Retropubic urethropexy—Burch or Marshall-Marchetti-Krantz procedure
- Wertheim hysterectomy for cervical carcinoma

pressure followed by accurate ligature placement should be followed by ligation of the anterior division of the hypogastric artery.[121]

When adnexectomy is performed, it is essential to identify the ureter before clamping and ligating the infundibulopelvic ligament. The ureter normally passes just medial to the ovarian vessels as they cross the iliac vessels at the pelvic brim. In the setting of extensive adnexal disease, pelvic infection, or endometriosis, the usual course of the pelvic ureter may be obscured from view, rendering it susceptible to injury. Insertion of urethral catheters (no. 6 or 7 French) during water cystoscopy may be done to more clearly delineate the position of the ureter. Alternately, cystotomy and passage of a Silastic stent (internal diameter 0.2 cm) may be necessary to evaluate for ureteral injury. Shingleton[122] argued against the routine placement of ureteral catheters during pelvic surgery, contending that excessive manipulation of a ureter containing a rigid catheter could cause damage. This opinion was corroborated by Spence and Boone.[123] Likewise, Mushlin and Thornbury[124] found that routine IVP before hysterectomy did not reduce the frequency of ureteral injury.

Should a ureteral orifice fail to spurt dye or a ureteral stent fail to pass a point of obstruction, the ureter should be approached retroperitoneally, the operator tracing it from the pelvic brim to the point of obstruction. In vaginal cases, exploration through the vagina may be difficult but sometimes is possible. Thompson and Benigno[125] recommended vaginal repair of ureteral injuries in selected cases. If the point of obstruction cannot be located, a ureteral catheter should be passed to the point of obstruction either during water cystoscopy or open cystotomy.

The point of obstruction can then be identified and the appropriate repair performed.

Ureteral injury during abdominal surgery may also occur during reperitonealization, during cul-de-sac obliteration by the Moschcowitz technique, during clamping or suturing of the vaginal cuff, and during retropubic urethropexy by the Marshall-Marchetti-Krantz or Burch techniques.[126]

A Wertheim hysterectomy has traditionally been responsible for the majority of injuries to the lower 4 to 6 cm of the ureter. Complete dissection of the terminal ureter may compromise its blood supply, causing ischemia, necrosis, and rupture of the ureteral wall and leading to urinoma formation followed by a ureterovaginal fistula.[3] However, Riss et al.[127] reported that improvements in operative technique had reduced the incidence of ureterovaginal fistulas from 6.4% (1898–1909) to 0.6% (1980–1986).

Ureteral Injury During Vaginal Operation

Ureteral injuries occur rarely during vaginal hysterectomy; van Nagell and Roddick[128] in 1972 reported ureteral complications from vaginal hysterectomy in 0.12% to 4.76% of cases. It is interesting to note the position of the ureter relative to the uterine artery when traction is applied to the uterus in abdominal versus vaginal hysterectomy (Fig. 5–14). In the figure, the dotted line represents the usual position of the uterus. As traction is applied during abdominal hysterectomy, the uterus is elevated, displacing the uterine artery superiorly and away from the ureter. As downward traction is applied to the cervix, the uterine vascular pedicle tends to pull the ureter downward, thus exposing the "knee" of the ureter to potential injury during clamping and suturing of the uterine vessels. Considering these anatomic changes, it is remarkable that more ureteral injuries do not occur during vaginal hysterectomy.

It is imperative when clamping the uterine vessels to place the clamp at a right angle to the vessel and as close to the uterus as possible; especially hazardous is blind clamping or suturing in the base of the broad ligament, should the uterine vessels escape from the clamp. Failure to adequately retract the bladder base and terminal ureter away from the cervix before clamping the uterine arteries may also result in ureteral ligation or transection.

Uterosacral ligament plication for the prevention of enterocele may engender ureteral injury because of the proximity of the ureters to the lateral margins of the uterosacral ligaments. During closure of the

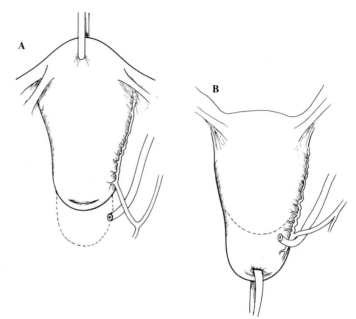

FIGURE 5–14. Relationship of the ureter to the uterine artery during hysterectomy. The usual position of the uterus is indicated by the *dotted line*. **A.** Upward traction as in abdominal hysterectomy displaces the uterine artery away from the ureter. **B.** Downward traction on the uterus as in vaginal hysterectomy causes the uterine vascular pedicle to pull the ureter downward, exposing its "knee" to potential injury. (Redrawn with permission from Nichols DH, Randall CL: Vaginal Surgery, p 376. Baltimore: Williams & Wilkins, 1989.)

peritoneum after removal of the uterus, the operator may incorporate a ureter in the purse-string suture if caution is not exercised in the vicinity of the uterosacral ligament.[96]

Ureteral injuries during anterior colporrhaphy occur more commonly when previous surgery has caused abnormal adherence of the bladder and terminal ureters to the underlying pubovesicocervical fascia and anterior vaginal wall. Sharp dissection should be employed, with the points of the scissors directed away from the bladder. Any question of ureteral injury should prompt the operator to inject 5 mL of indigo carmine IV, followed by water cystoscopy, to verify bilateral excretion of dye from the ureteral orifices.

Management of Ureteral Injuries Recognized at Operation

According to Zinman et al.,[93] only 20% to 30% of ureteral injuries are recognized at the time of operation. Symmonds[129] in 1976 stated that the methods of managing recognized ureteral injuries varied with the degree of trauma, location, and the condition for which the operation was performed, as well as the general condition of the patient.

TRAUMA TO THE URETERAL SHEATH. Injury to the ureteral sheath may compromise the important longitudinal adventitial vascular supply, leading to necrosis, perforation, and fistula formation. Masterson in 1957 demonstrated that all vascular sources of ureteral blood flow in the pelvis could be sacrificed during the pelvic dissection, provided that the longitudinal adventitial vessels were not destroyed. The ureteral sheath may be traumatized during dissection of adnexal masses adherent to the parietal peritoneum of the pelvic side walls, as seen in endometriosis or the sequelae of pelvic inflammatory disease. Damage involving a small segment of the sheath can be repaired with several interrupted 4-0 or 5-0 delayed absorbable sutures placed in the sheath, not through the muscularis. Damage to a larger segment of ureteral sheath should prompt the operator to consider placement of a ureteral catheter (double-J) for 7 to 10 days while revascularization of the ureter takes place.

CLAMP INJURY OR SUTURE LIGATION OF THE URETER. The most common ureteral injury in patients who develop ureterovaginal fistulas or anuria secondary to bilateral ureteral ligation is suture and clamp trauma.[129] If the ureter has been included in a clamp or ligature on the ovarian or uterine vessels, the clamp should be removed immediately, the vessel safely ligated above the site of injury, and the ureter inspected carefully. If the damage is slight, the area of injury should be drained extraperitoneally through an adjacent stab wound.[100] The peritoneum should be closed over the site so that any drainage will be extraperitoneal. A suture placed near (or even through) the ureter for a short time generally does little damage and should simply be removed.

If after removal of a clamp or ligature the tissues do not regain color and tone to the operator's satisfaction, ureteral catheterization for 7 to 10 days should be performed to allow revascularization.[97] This can be accomplished by water cystoscopy and retrograde catheterization of the ureter or by open cystotomy in the dome of the bladder and passage of a Silastic catheter (internal diameter 0.2 cm) past the point of injury into the renal pelvis. The stent may be brought out with a Foley catheter or left coiled in the bladder to be removed with a cystoscope.

TRANSECTED URETER. When the ureter has been partially or completely divided or so devitalized by suturing or clamping that necrosis occurs, more aggressive management is indicated. A partially transected ureter can be repaired with several interrupted sutures of 4-0 delayed absorbable suture; appropriate stenting and retroperitoneal drainage should be employed. The appropriate repair for a completely transected ureter depends on the level of the ureteral transection in the pelvis, the length of the segment traumatized or removed, the mobility of the ureter and bladder, the quality of the pelvic issues, the condition for which the operation is

being performed, and the general condition and anticipated lifetime of the patient.[129]

URETERONEOCYSTOSTOMY. There are various authors[93,100,129–131] who agree that injuries to the pelvic ureter within 5 cm of the vesicoureteral junction are best managed by ureteroneocystostomy. Direct reimplantation of the ureter is often successful, but the patient may experience vesicoureteral reflux. The submucosal tunnel technique as described by Politano and Leadbetter[132] in 1958 aims to achieve an antirefluxing anastomosis (Fig. 5–15).

When injury to the pelvic ureter is so extensive that the proximal ureter cannot be brought to the bladder without tension, several techniques are available to reduce the ureterovesical gap. The Boari bladder flap tube technique[133–135] has been widely employed for 10- to 15-cm defects, with a reported success rate of 50% to 80%.[136] However, this method has the inherent difficulties of any vascularized pedicle graft, and some authors[93,105] have found it less than satisfactory, owing to the high incidence of reflux and the frequent compromise in the blood supply at the anastomotic site.

The psoas muscle hitch, popularized by Harrow,[137] has been used successfully by others[138–142] for ureteral injuries more than 5 cm above the ureterovesical junction. Once it has been determined that the ureter will not reach the bladder without tension, a horizontal incision is made in the anterior

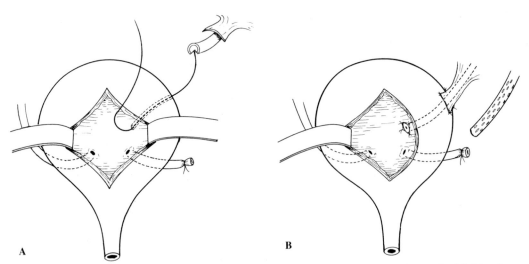

FIGURE 5–15. Submucosal tunnel ureteroneocystostomy. **A.** Ureter is spatulated for 0.5 cm and a 4-0 delayed absorbable suture is placed in the angle of the incision. Two 1-cm incisions approximately 1.5 cm apart are made, one on the exterior of the bladder, one within the lumen above the trigone. **B.** The submucosal tunnel is developed with scissors and a 1-0 traction suture is used to draw the ureter into the tunnel. 4-0 delayed absorbable sutures are used to suture the spatulated ureteral orifice to the bladder mucosa and to fix the adventitia of the ureter to the external wall of the bladder. (Modified with permission from Symmonds RE: Ureteral injuries associated with gynecologic surgery: Prevention and management. Clin Obstet Gynecol 19:623, 1976.)

bladder wall. The operator's finger within the bladder is used to elevate it to just above the pelvic brim. There it is sutured to the psoas muscle with 3-0 delayed absorbable suture (Fig. 5–16A). A ureteroneocystostomy is performed, preferably by the submucosal tunnel technique as previously described. The anastomotic site is reinforced by interrupted sutures of 4-0 delayed absorbable suture between the serosa of the bladder and the adventitia of the ureter. The horizontal incision in the bladder is then closed vertically. An indwelling Silastic stent is placed to the renal pelvis and coiled in the bladder for postoperative drainage. Extraperitoneal drainage with a Jackson-Pratt drain followed by closure of the peritoneum completes the anastomosis. Additional length can be obtained by mobilizing the kidney (Fig. 5–16B).[138] The surgeon's hand can be passed up and over the entire kidney and the kidney displaced down to a lower level; it may be temporarily maintained at the lower position by placing several 1-0 delayed absorbable sutures between the renal capsule and the psoas fascia.

URETEROURETEROSTOMY. If the ureter is transected above the pelvic brim, the preferred method of repair is ureteroureterostomy.[100,105,119,131] The site of obstruction or injury must first be identified; a no. 6 or 7 French ureteral catheter should be passed upward via cystoscopy to the level of obstruction to aid in identification. The ureter above and below the site of injury is mobilized, devitalized tissue is trimmed, and both ends of the ureter are spatulated for 5 mm (Fig. 5–17). A Silastic tube (internal diameter 0.2 cm) is passed through the lower ureter into the bladder and into the renal pelvis through the upper segment. The anastomosis is performed by drawing the ends of the ureter together over the Silastic tubing and approximating the seromuscular wall of the ureter with interrupted 4-0 delayed absorbable sutures, tied gently without undue tension. The Silastic stent or double-J stent may be left indwelling for 2 to 3 weeks and removed at cystoscopy.[100,129] Drainage is established extraperitoneally before the peritoneum is closed over the anastomosis. As an added precaution, a percutane-

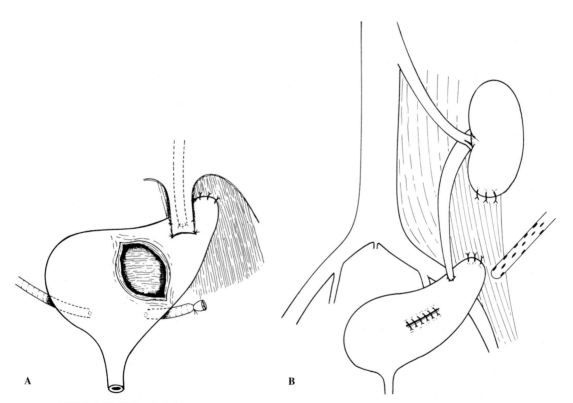

FIGURE 5–16. Utilization of the psoas muscle hitch for ureteroneocystostomy. **A.** A horizontal incision is made in the bladder to allow mobilization of the bladder to the pelvic brim, where it is sutured to the psoas muscle with 3-0 delayed absorbable suture. A ureteroneocystostomy is then performed. **B.** The kidney is mobilized caudally and sutured to the iliopsoas fascia. (Modified with permission from Symmonds RE: Ureteral injuries associated with gynecologic surgery: Prevention and management. Clin Obstet Gynecol 19:623, 1976.)

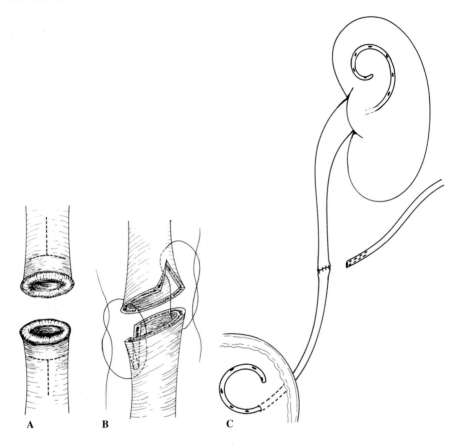

FIGURE 5–17. Ureteral end-to-end anastomosis. **A.** The cut ends are trimmed and the ureter is spatulated. **B.** 4-0 delayed absorbable suture is used to approximate the seromuscular wall. The sutures are tied without undue tension. **C.** The ureter is stented and drained retroperitoneally. (Modified with permission from Thompson JD: Operative injuries to the ureter: Prevention, recognition and management. In Thompson JD, Rock JA (eds): Te Linde's Operative Gynecology, p 773. Philadelphia: JB Lippincott, 1992.)

ous nephrostomy tube can be placed at the time of the procedure and brought out through the flank to allow urinary drainage if the stent should become occluded.

OTHER PROCEDURES. Transureteroureterostomy involves an anastomosis between the injured ureter and the recipient ureter on the opposite site. It is performed when a segment of ureter has been excised above the pelvic brim or as a secondary procedure when primary ureteroureterostomy has failed.[131] Great caution should be exercised with transureteroureterostomy since technical errors in performance may jeopardize both ureterorenal units. Ehrlich and Skinner[143] and Sandoz et al.[144] have reported on complications experienced with transureteroureterostomy.

In a patient who has extensive, irreparable ureteral injury and poor function of the contralateral kidney, renal autotransplantation may be successful if done by a skilled transplant surgeon.

In the event of ureteral injury where the medical condition of the patient is unstable, a cutaneous ureterostomy will maintain renal function in a patient who cannot tolerate a prolonged anastomotic procedure.[145] Obstruction of the ureteral ostium can be prevented by splaying the ureteral stoma and anchoring the ureter to the abdominal fascia and skin margins to prevent retraction.

Percutaneous nephrostomy can be used to maintain renal function temporarily when ureteral obstruction occurs. Performed under local anesthesia with computed tomographic guidance, percutaneous nephrostomy has become the procedure of choice for preserving kidney function while other therapy is planned.[75,146] Percutaneous nephrostomy also allows the passage of stents down the ureter and sometimes past the point of obstruction.

Nephrectomy should be performed seldom and only when normal contralateral renal function has been unequivocally established. Zinman et al.[93] stated that nephrectomy should be performed in the presence of an extensively destroyed ureter in elderly patients, patients at poor cardiovascular and pulmonary risk, patients with metastatic cancer, and patients with extensive pyelonephritis and intrarenal and perirenal abscesses. If a functioning nephrostomy tube is present, a 24-hour creatinine clearance time of more than 20 mL/min represents sufficient renal function to justify a reconstructive procedure.[93]

Management of Ureteral Injuries Unrecognized at Operation

Certain signs and symptoms will identify the patient who has an undiagnosed ureteral injury. The appearance of any of the signs or symptoms listed in Table 5–12 in any postoperative patient should provoke suspicion of ureteral injury, and IVP should be performed. Retrograde pyelography may be necessary to more accurately delineate the precise anatomy because a higher density of contrast medium is delivered to the injured site.[147] If the pyelogram shows unilateral obstruction or hydronephrosis, an attempt should be made via water cystoscopy to pass a ureteral catheter in retrograde fashion past the point of obstruction. If this is successful, the catheter should be left in place for 14 to 21 days to allow the ureter to heal without stricture formation. After stent removal, follow-up IVP should be performed at 4- to 6-week intervals to rule out stricture. If the ureteral catheter will not pass the obstruction, either immediate ureteral re-

TABLE 5–12. Symptoms and Signs of Postoperative Ureteral Injury

Flank pain, tenderness
Fever, sepsis
Ileus, abdominal distention
Unexplained hematuria
Urine leak
  Vaginal
  Cutaneous
Urinoma
Abnormal pyelogram
  Urine leak
  Obstruction
Oliguria or elevated serum creatinine
Anuria

pair or percutaneous nephrostomy should be done to preserve remaining renal function. When percutaneous nephrostomy is successful, definitive surgery may be deferred for 8 weeks, as many injuries will resolve with percutaneous nephrostomy alone.[146]

Controversy exists as to the management of ureteral obstruction secondary to ligation discovered in the immediate postoperative period (first 48–72 hours) or later (2–3 weeks and beyond). Early deligation is favored by many authors,[147–149] with the rationale that the sooner the reconstruction is attempted, the easier it is to find the tissue planes and restore continuity. The longer the delay, the more difficult is the dissection and the more dense the fibrosis, according to those who favor early treatment of ureteral injuries. Certainly, surgery should be delayed in a patient with significant pelvic infection, cellulitis, or abscess formation, or in any patient whose medical status is precarious and in whom definitive surgery for ureteral obstruction might pose a significant threat. In such patients, kidney drainage by percutaneous nephrostomy for 6 to 8 weeks followed by reparative surgery is preferable.

However, when unintentional ureteral ligation occurs during hysterectomy in a young, healthy woman with normal renal function, without pelvic infection or cellulitis, immediate repair consisting of ureteroneocystostomy may be considered and performed safely within 10 to 14 days following the original surgery. Hoch et al.[92] reported a 93% success rate with immediate ureteral repair in 19 patients whose injuries were first recognized 1 to 24 days following the original surgery.

Bilateral ureteral ligation is rare and is apparent when the patient is found to be anuric following surgery with no predisposing cause such as hypotension or hypovolemia. Estimates of how long an obstructed, uninfected kidney can survive without irreversible damage range from 7 days to 158 days.[75,150] IVP should be performed whenever ureteral ligation is suspected but is especially important in a woman with anuria and a rising serum creatinine level. If bilateral ligation is demonstrated, passage of ureteral catheters is attempted before the patient is taken to surgery. In the unlikely instance that both ureters can be catheterized and the obstruction relieved, the stents should be left in place for 14 to 21 days. When the condition cannot be relieved bilaterally by stenting, the earlier that deligation is performed, the better. If the patient is seriously ill from uremia or infection, bilateral percutaneous nephrostomies are preferable to performing surgery on an unstable patient. Definitive repair can then be delayed for 6 to 8 weeks.

Gynecologic surgeons should be able to prevent and recognize most, and repair many, urinary tract injuries. In every abdominal procedure, he or she should be able to expose the ureter in the retroperitoneal space and keep it out of harm's way. Intraoperative bladder lacerations should be recognized and repaired from the abdominal or vaginal approach. Ureteral injury should be recognized and ureteral catheterization performed via open cystotomy. The gynecologist should use water cystoscopy to determine the location and limits of bladder laceration and to test for ureteral patency by IV injection of indigo carmine. He or she should be able to repair a posthysterectomy vesicovaginal fistula by the Latzko or layered technique. However, the practicing gynecologist is wise to consult a skilled pelvic surgeon, urologist, or gynecologic oncologist in certain complicated situations. These include ureteral reimplantation with or without bladder hitches, bladder flap procedures, complex urologic fistulas, ureteral end-to-end anastomosis, or urinary diversions.

Anesthesia and Surgery in Individuals with Preexisting Renal Disease

Patients with chronic renal failure undergo frequent elective and emergency surgical procedures for common surgical problems as well as for problems that arise as a result of renal failure (Table 5–13). Regardless of the operative procedure, special precautions must be taken to compensate for the impaired ability of the kidneys to regulate fluid and electrolyte balance and excrete metabolic waste products. The incidence of complications is closely related to the GFR.[151] Thus, the GFR is an important surgical consideration, and preservation of residual GFR is vitally important.

Preoperative Assessment

Optimal preoperative preparation will help reduce the hazards of anesthesia and identify patients at increased surgical risk (Table 5–14). A careful and thorough history and physical examination should reveal the cause of chronic renal failure, the duration of chronic renal failure, the frequency of dialysis needed to maintain homeostasis, and the timing of the most recent dialysis. Physical examination should identify the spectrum of physical signs seen in chronic renal failure; of vital interest is the intravascular volume status. Clinical estimates of volume status may be inaccurate, especially in the el-

TABLE 5–13. Clinical Problems in Chronic Renal Failure

Cardiovascular
 Hypertension
 Pericardial disease
 Myocardial dysfunction
 Lipid abnormalities

Pulmonary
 Uremic lung
 Infection

Neuromuscular
 Muscular irritability
 Seizures
 Neuropathy

Hematopoietic
 Anemia
 Bleeding tendency

Gastrointestinal
 Nausea, vomiting, ileus
 Hyperacidity
 Hepatitis

Endocrine
 Hyperparathyroidism
 Uremic osteodystrophy
 Impaired glucose metabolism

Immune
 Lowered resistance to infection

Acid–base balance and electrolytes
 Metabolic acidosis
 Hyperkalemia
 Hypocalcemia

derly, chronically ill debilitated patient. In such cases the clinician should make accurate estimates of volume status by measuring central venous pressure or by placing a Swan-Ganz catheter to measure pulmonary capillary wedge pressure.[66]

Drugs commonly taken by patients with chronic renal failure include digitalis, which is excreted primarily by the kidney. Signs and symptoms of digitalis toxicity should be carefully monitored in uremic patients. Hypertensive patients are often receiving β-adrenergic blockers along with other antihypertensives, and these agents should be discontinued just prior to surgery. These drugs tend to reduce cardiac contractility and vascular reactivity.[151] Diuretics can result in hyponatremia and hypovolemia and should be used with great caution. Corticosteroids and immunosuppressive agents are usually administered to patients who have undergone renal transplantation; these drugs blunt the immune response and render the patient more susceptible to infection.

TABLE 5–14. **Preoperative Assessment in Chronic Renal Failure**

History and physical examination
 Duration of CRF
 Frequency of dialysis
 Intravascular volume status (signs of congestive heart failure)
 Hepatic congestion

Drugs that may influence anesthesia or surgery
 Digitalis
 Antihypertensives
 Diuretics
 Corticosteroids

Laboratory
 Electrolytes, blood urea nitrogen, serum creatinine, hemoglobin, hematocrit, acid–base status, bleeding time, prothrombin time, partial thromboplastin time

Laboratory determinations of serum electrolytes, BUN, and creatinine levels should be performed after the last dialysis before surgery. Electrolyte abnormalities, particularly hyperkalemia, should be corrected before surgery. Surgery is generally well tolerated in patients whose GFR remains over 25 to 30 mL/min (25% of normal); however, as the GFR approaches 10 to 15 mL/min, surgical morbidity approaches 55% to 60%.[152] The hemoglobin and hematocrit should be noted. Because most of these patients have long since adjusted to hematocrit levels of 20% to 30%, no attempt should be made to normalize the hematocrit by transfusion before surgery.[153] Acidosis should be corrected before surgery with sodium bicarbonate if mild or by dialysis if severe (pH < 7.25). Clotting abnormalities should be noted and, if significant, attempted correction with dialysis should be undertaken.[154]

Anesthetic Considerations

Regional Anesthesia

Regional anesthesia avoids the effects of narcotics, muscle relaxants, and volatile anesthetics and is a logical choice for patients with chronic renal failure. Intubation is avoided, decreasing the risk of associated pulmonary infection, and the risk of aspiration of gastric contents during intubation is largely eliminated.

The bleeding tendency of uremia can pose a problem with spinal or epidural anesthesia because of the potential for hematoma formation.[155,156] With adequate dialysis, the platelet dysfunction is reversed in most patients with chronic renal failure, and there should be no objection to the use of epidural or spinal anesthesia.[154,157] Sympathetic blockade with epidural or spinal anesthesia can result in a significant drop in blood pressure and GFR with a high block.[151] The use of epinephrine to prolong the duration of action of local anesthetics should be avoided in the hyperkalemic, acidotic patient because of the risk of precipitating a cardiac arrhythmia.

General Anesthesia

Sodium thiopental, given slowly and titrated carefully, is the induction agent of choice in patients with chronic renal failure.[151,156] Pentothal is 50% unbound in uremic patients compared to 28% in control patients; hence the need for a judicious reduction in dosage for the uremic individual.[158]

Narcotic analgesics may have a profound and prolonged effect in patients with chronic renal failure. The prolonged effect of morphine is due to accumulation of the drug and its metabolites as a result of abnormal renal function, continued metabolism, release of the drug and its metabolites from tissues, and enterohepatic circulation.[159,160] Even after hemodialysis, naloxone may be required to reverse the systemic effects of morphine.[160]

Fentanyl appears to be the narcotic of choice in chronic renal failure owing to its short half-life and minimal cardiovascular effects.[151,156] The use of droperidol and fentanyl for induction of anesthesia for major surgery has provided a stable cardiovascular system during maintenance of anesthesia and rapid recovery with minimal vomiting.[161]

Neuromuscular blocking drugs are often not required because of the relative reduction in muscle mass in many patients with chronic renal failure. Should muscle relaxation be required, succinylcholine (1 mg/kg) has been shown to be safe in renal failure.[162–164] However, succinylcholine is known to cause release of potassium from skeletal muscle during the process of depolarization.[156,165] Caution should be exercised with the use of succinylcholine in patients with chronic renal failure and a serum potassium concentration above 5.5 mEq/L.

Tubocurarine is the nondepolarizing muscle relaxant of choice in chronic renal failure in the opinion of various authors.[151,156,166] Generally only small doses are needed, and their effects can be reversed with the administration of atropine and neostigmine methyl sulfate. Although tubocurarine is mainly excreted through the kidneys, alternative excretion through the liver and biliary system has been shown. The neuromuscular blocking actions of *d-*

tubocurarine are potentiated by acidosis, and in such circumstances difficulty in reversing the drug's effects may be experienced.[142,167,168]

Inhalational agents are rapidly eliminated from the body, independent of renal function. They are definitely advantageous in controlling hypertension intraoperatively and in reducing the dosage of muscle relaxants. However, they may cause excessive depression of myocardial contractility with a fall in cardiac output, resulting in decreased renal blood flow and decreased GFR.[169]

Both nitrous oxide and halothane were used extensively in the large series reported by Morgan and Lumley,[156] with satisfactory results. Deutsch et al.[36] administered halothane 1.5% and oxygen to hydrated, nonpremedicated healthy subjects and reported a 19% mean reduction in GFR and a 38% reduction in effective renal plasma flow. Berry[170] reported a 30% reduction in RBF with deep halothane anesthesia.

Methoxyflurane is regarded as nephrotoxic in chronic renal failure because of the adverse effects of the high serum levels of fluoride ions produced as a result of metabolism.[171] Enflurane is metabolized to a lesser extent than methoxyflurane, with serum fluoride levels considerably below the nephrotoxic threshold.[172] However, the threshold for fluoride-induced nephrotoxicity may be lower in diseased or transplanted kidneys, and enflurane should be used with great caution.[173] Isoflurane is metabolized with very low levels of inorganic fluoride.[174] This fact, along with its low arrhythmogenic potential, makes it an ideal agent for patients with chronic renal failure.[151]

Surgical Considerations

Intraoperative

Patients with chronic renal failure may develop superimposed acute renal failure; ischemia or nephrotoxins are the major mechanisms causing the renal insult.[78] Careful attention to fluid balance and an effort to maintain cardiac output and renal perfusion are essential. Severe hypertension occurring during or immediately after surgery is usually related to the infusion of excessive amounts of fluid.[153] Drugs such as the aminoglycosides, cisplatin, and radiographic contrast media are well-known nephrotoxins and should be avoided, especially in the patient with chronic renal failure.[61] Careful intraoperative monitoring of direct arterial pressure is preferable in patients with severe hypertension or coronary artery disease. Patients whose volume status is unclear before or during surgery should have a central venous line placed or a Swan-Ganz catheter placed for measurement of pulmonary capillary wedge pressure.[66]

Strict antiseptic technique should be employed in all surgical procedures. Infection is a significant cause of postoperative morbidity; 26% of the patients with chronic renal failure reported by Brenowitz et al.[175] developed infections after major surgery.

The use of indwelling catheters should be limited to the intraoperative and immediate postoperative period. Patients in renal failure are particularly prone to develop urinary tract infections due to *Proteus, Pseudomonas,* or other coliform organisms in the presence of an indwelling catheter.[176] Occasionally these infections result in gram-negative septicemia, hypotension, and death.

Intraoperative blood loss should be carefully estimated and replaced only if excessive. Overtransfusion of patients in chronic renal failure may lead to volume overload, thrombosis of arteriovenous shunts, and decreased erythropoietin production.

Postoperative

Several authors[153,175,177] in large series report that patients in renal failure who are on chronic hemodialysis can undergo major surgical procedures with a mortality of 2% to 4%. However, the incidence of nonfatal complications is high; 60% of the patients in one series had at least one postoperative complication.[175]

After surgery, the normal patient becomes antidiuretic because of increased production of renin, angiotensin, and aldosterone, which limits sodium excretion; water excretion is also limited by ADH. The patient with chronic renal failure has a decreased response to these hormones and may continue to be polyuric. Salt and water losses in the postoperative period should be quantified rather than estimated from normal physiology.

Hyperkalemia resulting from tissue breakdown and blood administration will often occur if renal potassium excretion is limited. The routine addition of potassium to postoperative fluids can be harmful. Frequent laboratory determinations of serum electrolytes in the postoperative period are wise. In the series by Hampers et al.,[153] hyperkalemia was the major indication for postoperative dialysis. Hemodialysis is preferable to conservative measures and ion exchange resins in the face of rapidly progressive hyperkalemia and hypercatabolism.

Thrombosis of arteriovenous fistulas occurred in 22% of the surgical series reported by Brenowitz et al.[175] and in 6 of 33 patients reported by Hampers et al.[153] The reasons for the increased clotting of the arteriovenous fistulas are unknown but may have been related to a hypercoagulable state present after operation.[178] Wound healing is impaired in chronic renal failure, and dehiscence may occur. Delayed healing of wounds in uremia has been noted by Balch et al.[179] and Stein and Wiersum.[180] Wound healing is best aided by control of uremia with dialysis and by adequate nutritional support in the postoperative period.[181] Postoperative infections, especially pneumonia and wound infections, are prevalent.[175] Bilateral pneumonia was identified at autopsy in over 50% of 201 patients who died in chronic renal failure.[176]

Uremic patients have a tendency to bleed postoperatively, but this tendency is reduced in well-dialyzed patients. A delay following dialysis will allow the effect of the heparin to dissipate and will help prevent the bleeding complications of heparinization during and after surgery. To lessen postoperative morbidity, the following recommendations are applicable for patients with chronic renal failure who are to undergo major surgery: (1) dialysis should be performed on the day before surgery, (2) hypertension should be adequately controlled, either by dialysis or with antihypertensive medications, and (3) the serum potassium concentration should be below 5.5 mEq/L on the day of surgery.[153]

References

1. Prough DS, Foreman AS: Anesthesia and the renal system. In Barash PG, Cullen BF, Stoelting RK (eds): Clinical Anesthesia, 2nd ed, pp 1125–1155. Philadelphia: JB Lippincott, 1992.
2. Notley RG: Ureteral morphology. Urology 12:8, 1978.
3. Thompson JD: Vesicovaginal fistulas. In Te Linde's Operative Gynecology, 7th ed, pp 785–817. Philadelphia: JB Lippincott, 1992.
4. Woodburne RT: Essentials of Human Anatomy, 4th ed, pp 474–515. New York: Oxford University Press, 1969.
5. Masterson JG: An experimental study of ureteral injuries in radical pelvic surgery. Am J Obstet Gynecol 73:359, 1957.
6. DeLancey JOL: Anatomy of the female bladder and urethra. In Ostergard DR, Bent AE (eds): Urogynecology and Urodynamics: Theory and Practice, 3rd ed, pp 3–18. Baltimore: Williams & Wilkins, 1991.
7. Ricci JV, Lisa JR, Thom CH: The female urethra: A histologic study as an aid in urethral surgery. Am J Surg 79:499, 1950.
8. Woodburne RT: Anatomy of the bladder and bladder outlet. J Urol 100:474, 1968.
9. DeLancey JOL: Anatomy of the female pelvis. In Thompson JD, Rock JA (eds): Te Linde's Operative Gynecology, 7th ed, pp 33–65. Philadelphia: JB Lippincott, 1992.
10. Gosling JA: The structure of the female lower urinary tract and pelvic floor. Urol Clin North Am 12:207, 1985.
11. Krantz KE: The anatomy of the urethra and anterior vaginal wall. Am J Obstet Gynecol 62:374, 1951.
12. DeLancey JOL: Anatomy and embryology of the lower urinary tract. Obstet Gynecol Clin North Am 16:717, 1989.
13. Berkow SG: The corpus spongeosum of the urethra: Its possible role in urinary control and stress incontinence in women. Am J Obstet Gynecol 65:346, 1953.
14. Rud T, Andersson KE, Asmussen M, Hunting A, Ulmsten U: Factors maintaining the intraurethral pressure in women. Invest Urol 17:343, 1980.
15. Power RMH: An anatomical contribution to the problem of continence and incontinence in the female. Am J Obstet Gynecol 67:302, 1954.
16. McGuire EJ: Urethral sphincter mechanisms. Urol Clin North Am 6:39, 1979.
17. Rubenstein M, Meyer R, Bernstein J: Congenital abnormalities of the urinary system: I. A postmortem survey of developmental anomalies and acquired congenital lesions in a children's hospital. J Pediatr 58:356, 1961.
18. McKenna H: A significant increase in developmental malformations of the renal tract in perinatal autopsies at Royal Women's Hospital, Brisbane, 1972–1973. Med J Aust 1:108, 1974.
19. Barakat AJ, Drougas JG: Occurrence of congenital abnormalities of kidney and urinary tract in 13,775 autopsies. Urology 38:347, 1991.
20. Miller ED Jr: Anesthesia and the kidney. Welcome Trends Anesthesiol II(no 1):3–10, 1993.
21. Prough DS, Zaloga GP: Management of acute oliguria in the elderly patient. Int Anesthesiol Clin 26:112, 1988.
22. Mirenda JV, Grissom TE: Anesthetic implications of the renin-angiotensin system and angiotensin converting enzyme inhibitors. Anesth Analg 72:667–683, 1991.
23. Cohen JD, Neaton JD, Prineas RJ, Daniels KA: Diuretics, serum potassium and ventricular arrhythmias in the Multiple Risk Factor Interventional Trial. Am J Cardiol 60:548–554, 1987.
24. Schrier RW: Body fluid volume regulation in health and disease: A unifying hypothesis. Ann Intern Med 113:155–159, 1990.
25. Bevan DR: Renal Function in Anesthesia and Surgery. London: Academic Press, 1979.
26. Sladen RN: Effect of anesthesia and surgery on renal function. Crit Care Clin 3(2):373–389, 1987.
27. Mazze RI: Renal physiology. In Miller RD (ed): Anesthesia, vol 1, pp 601–617. New York: Churchill Livingstone, 1990.
28. Bastron RD, Perkins FM, Pyne JL: Autoregulation of renal blood flow during halothane anesthesia. Anesthesiology 46:142, 1977.
29. Mujais SK: Transport and renal effects of general anesthetics. Semin Nephrol 6(3):251–258, 1986.
30. Walker LA, Buscemi-Bergin M, Gellai M: Renal hemodynamics in conscious rats: Effects of anesthesia, surgery, and recovery. Am J Physiol 245:F67–F74, 1983.
31. Gelman S, Fowler KC, Smith LR: Regional blood flow during isoflurane and halothane anesthesia. Anesth Analg 63:557–565, 1984.
32. Price HL, Linde HW, Jone RE, et al: Sympathoadrenal responses to general anesthesia in man and their relation to hemodynamics. Anesthesiology 20:563, 1959.

33. Burnett CH, Bloomburg EL, Shortz G, et al: A comparison of the effects of ether and cyclopropane anesthesia on the renal function of man. J Pharmacol Exp Ther 96:380, 1949.

34. Habif DV, Papper EM, Fitzpatrick HF, et al: The renal and hepatic blood flow, glomerular filtration rate, and urinary output of electrolytes during cyclopropane, ether and thiopental anesthesia, operation, and the immediate postoperative period. Surgery 30:241, 1951.

35. Mazze RI, Schwartz FD, Slocum HC, et al: Renal function during anesthesia and surgery: I. The effects of halothane anesthesia. Anesthesiology 24:279, 1963.

36. Deutsch S, Goldberg M, Stephen GW, et al: Effects of halothane anesthesia on renal function in normal man. Anesthesiology 27:793–799, 1966.

37. Everett GB, Allen GD, Kennedy WF, et al: Renal hemodynamic effects of general anesthesia in out-patients. Anesth Analg 52:470–479, 1973.

38. Warren DJ, Ledingham JGG: Renal circulatory responses to general anesthesia in the rabbit: Studies using radioactive microspheres. Clin Sci 48:61–66, 1975.

39. Barry KG, Mazze RI, Schwartz FD: Prevention of surgical oliguria and renal hemodynamic suppression by sustained hydration. N Engl J Med 270:1371–1377, 1964.

40. Johnson MC, Malvin RL: Plasma renin activity during pentobarbital anesthesia and graded hemorrhage in dogs. Am J Physiol 22:1098–1101, 1975.

41. Yun JCH, Kelly GD, Bartter FC, et al: Mechanism for the increase in plasma renin activity by pentobarbital anesthesia. Life Sci 22:1545–1554, 1979.

42. Ishihara H, Ishida K, Oyama T, et al: Effects of general anaesthesia and surgery on renal function and plasma ADH levels. Can Anaesth Soc J 25:312–318, 1978.

43. Roizin MF, Moss J, Henry DP, et al: Effect of general anesthetics on handling- and decapitation-induced increases in sympathoadrenal discharge. J Pharmacol Exp Ther 204:11–18, 1978.

44. Crandell WB, Pappas SG, Macdonald A: Nephrotoxicity associated with methoxyflurane anesthesia. Anesthesiology 27:591, 1966.

45. Mazze RI, Shue GL, Jackson SH: Renal dysfunction associated with methoxyflurane anesthesia: A randomized prospective clinical evaluation. JAMA 216:278, 1971.

46. Mazze RI, Trudell JR, Cousins MJ: Methoxyflurane metabolism and renal dysfunction: Clinical correlation in man. Anesthesiology 35:247, 1971.

47. Goldman L, Caldera DL: Risks of general anesthesia and elective operation in the hypertensive patient. Anesthesiology 50:285–293, 1979.

48. Schwartz SI, Shires GT, Spencer FC, Storer EH (eds): Principles of Surgery, 4th ed, pp 125–129. New York: McGraw-Hill, 1983.

49. Myers BD, Moran SM: Hemodynamically mediated acute renal failure. N Engl J Med 314:97–105, 1986.

50. Pringle H, Maunsell RCB, Pringle S: Clinical effects of ether anaesthesia on renal activity. Br Med J 2:542, 1905.

51. Kennedy WF, Sawyer TK, Gerbershagen HU, et al: Systematic cardiovascular and renal hemodynamic alterations during peridural anesthesia in normal man. Anesthesiology 31:414, 1969.

52. Hayes MA, Goldenberg IS: Renal effects of anesthesia and operation mediated by endocrines. Anesthesiology 24:487, 1963.

53. Silvarian M, Amory DW, Lindbloom LE, et al: Systemic and regional blood flow changes during spinal anesthesia in the rhesus monkey. Anesthesiology 43:78–88, 1975.

54. Mazze RI, Barry KG: Prevention of functional renal failure during anesthesia and surgery by sustained hydration and mannitol infusion. Anesth Analg 46:61, 1967.

55. Miller ED Jr: The renin-angiotensin system in anesthesia. In Brown BR Jr (ed): Anesthesia and the Patient with Endocrine Disease, pp 19–28. Philadelphia: FA Davis, 1980.

56. Grossman RA: Oliguria and acute renal failure. Med Clin North Am 65:413, 1981.

57. Hegeman TF: Oliguria: A frequent problem in the critically ill patient. Indiana Med 77:864, 1984.

58. Byrick RJ, Rose DK: Pathophysiology and prevention of acute renal failure: The role of the anesthetist. Can J Anaesth 37:457, 1990.

59. Anderson RJ, Schrier RW: Acute renal failure. In Wilson JD, Braunwald E, Isselbacher KR (eds): Harrison's Principles of Internal Medicine, 12th ed, chap 223. New York: McGraw-Hill, 1991.

60. Brenner BM, Lazarus JM: Chronic renal failure. In Wilson JD, Braunwald E, Isselbacher KJ (eds): Harrison's Principles of Internal Medicine, 12th ed, pp 1150–1157. New York: McGraw-Hill, 1991.

61. Dixon BS, Anderson RJ: Nonoliguric acute renal failure. Am J Kidney Dis 6:71, 1985.

62. Sweny P: Is postoperative oliguria avoidable? Br J Anaesth 67:137, 1991.

63. Miller TR, Anderson RJ, Linas SL, et al: Urinary indices in acute renal failure: A prospective study. Ann Intern Med 89:47, 1978.

64. Tilney NL, Lazarus JM: Acute renal failure in surgical patients. Surg Clin North Am 63:357, 1983.

65. Hagar D: Renal insufficiency after intravenous pyelography. Surg Gynecol Obstet 150:236, 1980.

66. Samii K, Conseillar C, Viasrs P: Central venous pressure and the pulmonary wedge pressure: A comparable study in anesthetized surgical patients. Arch Surg 111:1122, 1976.

67. Shah DM, Browner BD, Dutton RE, et al: Cardiac output and pulmonary wedge pressure. Arch Surg 112:1161, 1977.

68. Espinel CH, Gregory AW: Differential diagnosis of acute renal failure. Clin Nephrol 13:73, 1980.

69. Hou SH, Bushinsky DA, Wish JB, et al: Hospital acquired renal insufficiency: A prospective study. Am J Med 74:243, 1983.

70. Wilson DR: Pathophysiology of obstructive uropathy. Kidney Int 18:281, 1980.

71. Suki WN, Guthrie AG, Martinez-Maldonado M, Eknoyan G: Effects of ureteral pressure elevation on renal hemodynamics and urine concentration. Am J Physiol 228:38, 1971.

72. Hoffman LM, Suki WN: Obstructive uropathy mimicking volume depletion. JAMA 236:2096, 1976.

73. Gourdie RW, Rogers ACN: Bilateral ureteric obstruction due to endometriosis presenting with hypertension and cyclic oliguria. Br J Urol 58:224, 1986.

74. Saw KC, Bullock KN: Leaking iliac artery aneurysm causing bilateral ureteric obstruction and oliguria. Br J Urol 64:431, 1989.

75. Hedegaard CK, Wallace D: Percutaneous nephrostomy: Current indications and potential uses in obstetrics and gynecology. Literature review and report of a case. Obstet Gynecol Surv 42:671, 1987.

76. Ellison DH, Bia MJ: Acute renal failure in critically ill patients. J Intensive Care Med 2:8, 1987.

77. Abreo K, Moorthy AV, Osborne M: Changing patterns and outcome of acute renal failure requiring hemodialysis. Arch Intern Med 146:1338, 1986.

78. Mandal AK, Lightfoot BO, Treat RC: Mechanisms of protection in acute renal failure. Circ Shock 11:245, 1983.

79. Anderson RJ, Linas SL, Berns AS, et al: Nonoliguria acute renal failure. N Engl J Med 296:1134, 1977.

80. McMurray SD, Luft FC, Maxwell DR, et al: Prevailing patterns and predictor variables in patients with acute tubular necrosis. Arch Intern Med 138:950, 1978.

81. Rasmussen HH, Ibels LS: Acute renal failure: Multivariate analysis of causes and risk factors. Am J Med 73:211, 1982.

82. Frankel MC, Weinstein AM, Stenzel KH: Prognostic patterns in acute renal failure: The New York Hospital, 1981–1982. Clin Exp Dial Apheresis 7:145, 1983.

83. Madias NE, Harrington JT: Platinum nephrotoxicity. Am J Med 65:307, 1978.

84. Blachley JD, Hill JB: Renal and electrolyte disturbances associated with cisplatin. Ann Intern Med 95:628, 1981.

85. Meyers C, Roxe DM, Hano J: The clinical course of nonoliguric acute tubular necrosis. Proc Am Soc Nephrol 7:62, 1974.

86. Singh R, Leb D, Brooks D, et al: Nonoliguric acute tubular necrosis. Proc Am Soc Nephrol 7:85, 1974.

87. Diamond JR, Yoburn DC: Nonoliguric acute renal failure. Arch Intern Med 142:1882, 1982.

88. Hollenberg NK, Adams DF, Solomon HS, et al: What mediates the renal vascular response to a salt load in normal man? J Appl Physiol 33:491, 1972.

89. Kleinknecht D, Ganeval D, Gonzalez-Duque LA, Fermanian J: Furosemide in acute oliguric renal failure: A controlled trial. Nephron 17:51, 1976.

90. Parker S, Carlon GC, Isaacs M, et al: Dopamine administration in oliguria and oliguric renal failure. Crit Care Med 9:630, 1981.

91. Barry KG, Cohen A, Knochel JP, et al: Mannitol infusion: II. Prevention of acute functional renal failure during resection of aneurysms of the abdominal aorta. N Engl J Med 264:967, 1961.

92. Hoch WM, Kursh ED, Persky L: Early aggressive management of intraoperative ureteral injuries. J Urol 114:530, 1975.

93. Zinman LM, Libertino JA, Roth RA: Management of operative ureteral injury. Urology 12:290, 1978.

94. Flynn JT, Tiptaft RC, Woodhouse CRJ, Parts AMI, Blandy JP: The early and aggressive repair of iatrogenic ureteric injuries. Br J Urol 51:454, 1979.

95. Symmonds RE: Prevention and management of genitourinary fistula. J Cont Ed OB/GYN 21:13, 1979.

96. Miyazawa K: Urological injuries in gynecological surgery. Hawaii Med J 39:11, 1980.

97. Benson RC, Hinman F: Urinary tract injuries in obstetrics and gynecology. Am J Obstet Gynecol 70:467, 1955.

98. Buchsbaum HF, Schmidt JR: Gynecologic and Obstetric Urology, p 90. Philadelphia: WB Saunders, 1978.

99. Graber EA, O'Rourke JJ, McElrath T: Iatrogenic bladder injury during hysterectomy. Obstet Gynecol 23:26, 1964.

100. Thompson JD: Operative injuries to the ureter: Prevention, recognition, and management. In Thompson JD, Rock JA (eds): Te Linde's Operative Gynecology, 7th ed, pp 759–783. Philadelphia: JB Lippincott, 1992.

101. Mengert WF, discussion of paper by VC Freida. Am J Obstet Gynecol 83:408, 1962.

102. Everett HS, Mattingly RF: Urinary tract injuries resulting from pelvic surgery. Am J Obstet Gynecol 71:502, 1956.

103. Guerriero WG: Operative injury to the lower urinary tract. Urol Clin North Am 12:339, 1985.

104. Richardson EH: A simplified technique for abdominal panhysterectomy. Surg Gynecol Obstet 48:298, 1929.

105. Mattingly RF, Borkowf HI: Acute operative injury to the lower urinary tract. Clin Obstet Gynecol 5:123, 1978.

106. Burch JC: Cooper's ligament urethroversion suspension for stress incontinence. Am J Obstet Gynecol 100:764, 1968.

107. Marshall VF, Manchetti AA, Krontz KL: The correction of stress incontinence by simple vesico-urethral suspension. Surg Gynecol Obstet 88:509, 1949.

107a Peyreyra AJ, Lebherz TB: Combined urethrovesical suspension and vaginourethroplasty for correction of stress incontinence. Obstet Gynecol 30:537, 1967.

108. Tancer ML: Observations on prevention and management of vesicovaginal fistula after total hysterectomy. Surg Gynecol Obstet 175:501, 1992.

109. Lee RA, Symmonds RE, Williams TJ: Current status of genitourinary fistula. Obstet Gynecol 72:313, 1988.

110. St. Martin EC, Trichel BE, Campbell JH, Locke CM: Ureteral injuries in gynecologic surgery. J Urol 70:51, 1953.

111. Bresette JF, Patterson JA: Strategy for repairing vesicovaginal fistulas. In: Update on General Surgery. Contemp Ob/Gyn [special issue] 68, 1983.

112. Moir JC: Vesicovaginal fistula. Proc R Soc Med 59:1019, 1966.

113. Robertson JR: Vesicovaginal fistulae. Obstet Gynecol 42:611, 1973.

114. Kelly J: Vesicovaginal fistulae. Br J Urol 51:208, 1979.

115. Wang Y, Hadley JR: Non-delayed transvaginal repair of high lying vesicovaginal fistula. J Urol 144:34, 1990.

116. Latzko W: Postoperative vesicovaginal fistulas. Am J Surg 58:211, 1942.

117. Falk HC, Kurman M: Repair of vesicovaginal fistula: Report of 140 cases. J Urol 89:226, 1963.

118. Kaser O: The Latzko operation for vesicovaginal fistulae. Acta Obstet Gynecol Scand 56:427, 1977.

119. Bright TC, Peters PC: Ureteral injuries secondary to operative procedures. Urology 9:22, 1977.

120. Schwartz WG, Hofmeister FJ, Mattingly RF: Value of intravenous urograms in pelvic surgery. Obstet Gynecol 23:584, 1964.

121. Burchell RC: Physiology of internal iliac artery ligation. J Obstet Gynaecol Br Commonw 75:642, 1968.

122. Shingleton HM: Repairing injuries to the urinary tract. In: Update on General Surgery. Contemp Ob/Gyn 23:76–90, 1984.

123. Spence HM, Boone T: Surgical injuries to the ureter. JAMA 176:1970, 1960.

124. Mushlin AI, Thornbury JR: Intravenous pyelography: The case against its routine use. Ann Intern Med 111:58, 1989.

125. Thompson JD, Benigno BB: Vaginal repair of ureteral injuries. Am J Obstet Gynecol 111:601, 1971.

126. Shingleton HM: Recognizing injuries to the urinary tract. In Sanz LE (ed): Gynecologic Surgery, chap 40. NJ: Medical Economics Books, 1988.

127. Riss P, Koelbl H, Neuntenfel W, Janisch H. Wertheim radical hysterectomy 1921–1986: Changes in urologic complications. Arch Gynecol Obstet 291:249, 1988.

128. Van Nagell JR, Roddick JW Jr: Vaginal hysterectomy, the ureter and excretory urography. Obstet Gynecol 39:784, 1972.

129. Symmonds RE: Ureteral injuries associated with gynecologic surgery: Prevention and management. Clin Obstet Gynecol 19:623, 1976.

130. Smith AM: Injuries of the pelvic ureter. Surg Gynecol Obstet 140:761, 1975.

131. Fry DE, Milholen L, Harbrecht P: Iatrogenic ureteral injury. Arch Surg 118:454, 1983.

132. Politano VA, Leadbetter WF: An operative technique for the correction of vesicoureteral reflux. J Urol 79:932, 1958.

133. Boari A: Contributo sperimentalle alla plastica dell' uretere. Atti Acad Sci Med Nat Ferrara 68:149, 1984.

134. Ockenblad NF: Perimplantation of the ureter into the bladder by a flap method. J Urol 57:845, 1947.

135. Bischoff PF: Boari-plasty and vesicorenal reflux. In Whitehead ED (ed): Current Operative Urology, pp 708–772. New York: Harper and Row, 1975.

136. Thompson IM, Ross G Jr: Long-term results of bladder flap repair of ureteral injuries. J Urol 111:483, 1974.

137. Harrow BR: A neglected maneuver for ureterovesical implantation following injury at gynecologic operations. J Urol 100:280, 1968.

138. Harada N, Tanimura M, Fukuyama K, et al: Surgical management of a long ureteral defect: Advancement of the ureter by descent of the kidney. J Urol 92:192, 1964.

139. Turner-Warwick R, Worth PH: The psoas bladder hitch procedure for the replacement of the lower third of the ureter. Br J Urol 41:701, 1969.

140. Prout GR Jr, Koontz WW Jr: Partial vesical immunobilization: An important adjunct to ureteroneocystostomy. J Urol 103:147, 1970.

141. Lee RA, Symmonds RE: Ureterovaginal fistula. Am J Obstet Gynecol 109:1032, 1971.

142. Cohen EN, Winslow-Brewer H, Smith D: The metabolism and elimination of d-tubocurarine H_3. Anesthesiology 28:309, 1967.

143. Ehrlich RM, Skinner DG: Complications of transureteroureterostomy. J Urol 113:467, 1975.

144. Sandoz IL, Paul DP, MacFarlane CA: Complications with transureteroureterostomy. J Urol 117:39, 1977.

145. Brown R, Barnes R, Wensell G, Asghan M: Ureteroureterostomy and cutaneous ureterostomy. J Urol 106:658, 1971.

146. Dowling RA, Corriere JN, Sandler CM: Iatrogenic ureteral injury. J Urol 135:912, 1986.

147. Witters S, Cornelissen M, Vereecken R: Iatrogenic ureteral injury: Aggressive or conservative treatment. Am J Obstet Gynecol 155:582, 1986.

148. Kaskarelis D, Sakkas J, Aravantines D, Michalas S, Zolotas J: Urinary tract injuries in gynecologic and obstetrical procedures. Int Surg 60:40, 1975.

149. Beland G: Early treatment of ureteral injuries found after gynecologic surgery. J Urol 118:25, 1977.

150. Shapiro SR, Bennett AH: Recovery of renal function after prolonged unilateral ureteral obstruction. J Urol 115:136, 1976.

151. Weir PHC, Chung FF: Anesthesia for patients with chronic renal disease. Can Anaesth Soc J 31:468, 1984.

152. Gilbert PL, Stein R: Preoperative evaluation of the patient with chronic renal disease. M Sinai Med J 58:69, 1991.

153. Hampers CL, Bailey GL, Hager EB, Vandam LD, Merrill JP: Major surgery in patients on maintenance hemodialysis. Am J Surg 115:747, 1968.

154. Stewart JH, Castaldi PA: Uraemic bleeding: A reversible platelet defect corrected by dialysis. Q J Med 143:409, 1967.

155. Lofstrom B: Anaesthetic problems in renal transplantation. Scand J Urol Nephrol 1:161, 1967.

156. Morgan M, Lumley J: Anesthetic considerations in chronic renal failure. Anaesth Intens Care 3:218, 1975.

157. Rabiner SF, Drake RF: Platelet function as an indication of adequate dialysis. Kidney Int 7:S144, 1975.

158. Ghoneim PH: Plasma protein binding of thiopental in patients with impaired renal or hepatic function. Anesthesiology 42:545, 1975.

159. Spector S, Vesell ES: Disposition of morphine in man. Science 174:421, 1971.

160. Don HF, Dieppa RA, Taylor P: Narcotic analgesics in anuric patients. Anesthesiology 42:745, 1975.

161. Gillies IDS: Anaemia and anaesthesia. Br J Anaesth 46:589, 1974.

162. Katz J, Kountz SL, Cohn R: Anesthetic considerations for renal transplant. Anesth Analg 46:609, 1967.

163. Jacobsen E, Christiansen AH, Lunding M: The role of the anaesthetist in the management of acute renal failure. Br J Anaesth 40:442, 1968.

164. Miller RD, Way WL, Hamilton WK, Layzer RB: Succinlycholine-induced hyperkalemia in patients with renal failure? Anesthesiology 36:138, 1972.

165. List WF: Serum potassium changes during induction of anaesthesia. Br J Anaesth 39:480, 1967.

166. Deutsch S: Anesthetic management of patients with chronic renal disease. South Med J 68:65, 1975.

167. Katz RL, Wolf CE: Neuromuscular and electromyographic studies in man: Effects of hyperventilation, carbon dioxide inhalation and d-tubocurarine. Anesthesiology 25:781, 1964.

168. Walts LF, Lebowitz M, Dillon JB: The effect of ventilation on the action of tubocurarine and gallamine. Br J Anaesth 39:845, 1967.

169. Deutsch S, Bastron RD, Pierce EC Jr, Vandam LD: The effects of anaesthesia with thiopentone, nitrous oxide, narcotics and neuromuscular blocking drugs on renal function in normal man. Br J Anaesth 41:807, 1969.

170. Berry AJ: Respiratory support and renal function. Anesthesiology 55:655, 1991.

171. Cousins MJ, Mazze RJ: Methoxyflurane nephrotoxicity: A study of dose response in man. JAMA 225:1611, 1973.

172. Cousins MJ, Greenstein CR, Hitt BA: Metabolism and renal effects of enflurane in man. Anesthesiology 44:44, 1976.

173. Lochning R, Mazze RI: Possible nephrotoxicity from enflurane in patients with severe renal disease. Anesthesiology 40:203, 1974.

174. Mazze RI, Cousins MJ, Barr GA: Renal effects and metabolism of isoflurane in man. Anesthesiology 40:536, 1974.

175. Brenowitz JB, Williams CD, Edwards WS: Major surgery in patients with chronic renal failure. Am J Surg 134:765, 1977.

176. Schreiner GE, Maher JF: The patient with chronic renal failure and surgery. Am J Cardiol 12:317, 1963.

177. Lissos I, Goldberg B, Van Blerk PJP, Meijers AM: Surgical procedures on patients in end-stage renal failure. Br J Urol 45:359, 1973.

178. Warren R: Medical progress: Postoperative thombophilia. N Engl J Med 249:99, 1953.

179. Balch HH, Meroney WH, Sako Y: Observations on the surgical care of patients with post-traumatic renal insufficiency. Surg Gynecol Obstet 100:439, 1955.

180. Stein AA, Wiersum J: The role of renal dysfunction in abdominal wound dehiscence. J Urol 82:271, 1959.

181. Burke JF Jr, Francos GC: Surgery in the patient with acute or chronic renal failure. Med Clin North Am 71:489, 1987.

Complications in Gynecologic Surgery: Prevention, Recognition, and Management,
edited by James W. Orr, Jr., and Hugh M. Shingleton.
J. B. Lippincott Company, Philadelphia, © 1994.

Chapter 6

Wound Healing

James W. Orr, Jr.
Peyton T. Taylor, Jr.

Biologic Basis for Wound Repair

*The creation and successful repair of a surgical wound is of fundamental interest to all surgical specialists. We wish to create a wound with the **least trauma** and to have it heal, without complications, resulting in a strong, inapparent yet functional scar.*

While individual subspecialties must acquire different surgical techniques, the general aspects of wound repair should be an integral aspect of every surgeon's training. These important principles of wound management are based on decades of clinical studies combined with a continually evolving understanding of the physiologic basis of the healing process. Unfortunately, clinical observations, opinion, and even dogma vary greatly between surgeons and institutions. Thus, many aspects of wound care have been passed anecdotally from one generation of surgeons to the next, frequently without scientific scrutiny. These clinical biases often exist with little emphasis on the physiologic basis of wound healing that has been developed from laboratory studies of cellular and subcellular events, animal models, and clinical studies involving patients with specific surgical diseases.

Wound repair is the result of a complex but orderly, integrated cascade of molecular and chemical events (Fig. 6–1). Although only specific components are well understood, the important aspects of wound healing, while varying in duration, are remarkably similar in various tissues throughout the body.[1]

Once initiated, the healing cascade can be easily impeded by any number of variables (Fig. 6–2). In general, the negative effects of technical factors predominate, but clinical factors such as vitamin deficiency, malnutrition, obesity, corticosteroid use, poorly controlled diabetes, uremia, radiation therapy, and chemotherapy may also be important. Despite the recent emphasis on specific growth factors, currently there are few clinical methods to accelerate the healing process after routine incisions. However, attempts to "revascularize" or minimize tissue trauma may be of specific benefit in some clinical situations.

The importance of attention to technical factors to facilitate optimal wound healing cannot be overemphasized. The earliest medical writings from the Smith Papyrus (1700 B.C.) describe wounds and their management.[2] The methods of gentle tissue handling and other aspects of wound management taught by surgeons in ancient times were lost in European surgery during the Dark Ages and did not reappear until after the Renaissance, when Ambrose Paré in the 16th century rediscovered and emphasized gentle surgical technique. This reemphasis on the technical aspects of wound healing and wound care has largely occurred since the turn of the century, endorsed by such surgical figures as Alexis Carrel and William Halsted.

The tendency will always be in the direction of exercising greater care and refinement in operating, and that the surgeon will develop an increasing respect for tissues, a sense which recoils from inflicting unnecessarily, insult to structures concerned in the process of repair.[2]

167

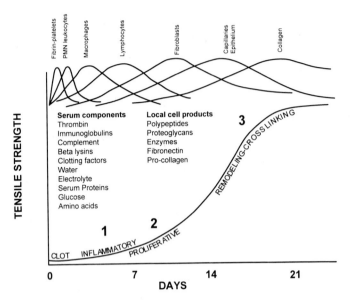

FIGURE 6–1. A wound healing curve indicating important cellular components, serum components, and local cell products. (Modified with permission from Schilling J: Wound healing. Surg Rounds, July 1983.)

It is well recognized that technical factors, *almost entirely under the surgeon's control,* are the most common potential impediments to the optimal healing of surgical wounds. Tissue contusion, thermal injury, excessive or poorly chosen suture material, foreign bodies, bacterial contamination, incomplete hemostasis, improper drainage, and excessive tension on coapted edges are but a few of the important aspects of surgical care. Unfortunately, attention to technical detail may be lost as a result of the intensity and pace of surgical training programs. In fact, aspects of wound healing and wound care are more often recited as important by medical students than by surgeons in training or in practice. In many institutions, a 10-minute lecture on the principles of wound healing involves 9 minutes of silence, 45 seconds of testimonials, and 15 seconds of science.

The guiding principle for the management of a surgical wound involves the creation of an optimal healing environment. This occurs only when tissues are viable, free of excessive bacterial contamina-

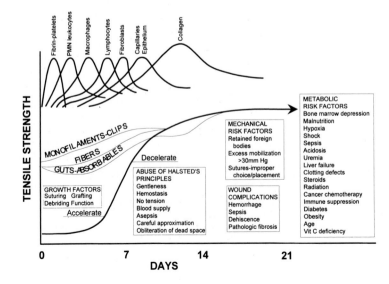

FIGURE 6–2. Wound healing curve demonstrating the aspects of accelerating factors and the broad array of technical, mechanical, and metabolic factors that may interfere with wound healing. (Modified with permission from Schilling J: Wound healing. Surg Rounds, July 1983.)

tion, and contain minimal amounts of foreign body. This environment can only be created when routine clinical techniques incorporate sound physiologic principles gleaned from laboratory and clinical investigations that have been subjected to scientific scrutiny. In fact, "failure of a wound to heal is in the great majority of cases a consequence of failure of decision making and technique."[3] Acute wound failure (disruption, infection) or delayed wound failure (hernia) may relate to local or systemic factors, including metabolic disturbances, drug administration (steroids, cytotoxic agents), or other immunosuppressive states that require the surgeon to modify routine techniques.

Unfortunately, even under optimal circumstances the normal response to tissue injury does not always produce an excellent functional result. The same healing process that results in abdominal wall incision strength can also produce strictures, keloids, or adhesions. The practicing pelvic surgeon should have a basic understanding of all aspects of the healing process and modify specific variables in an attempt to create an optimal wound environment.

Biologic Phases of Wound Repair

> *The biologic phases of wound repair involve an integrated continuum of events that are dynamic, continuous, and interrelated but which, for conceptual purposes, are often divided into three arbitrary phases (Table 6–1).*

The Inflammatory Phase

> *The inflammatory phase of wound healing describes those events occurring during the first few hours after unintentional or intentional wounding. The migration of large numbers of neutrophils into an uncontaminated wound is the microscopic hallmark of the inflammatory phase.*

Tissue injury is followed by inflammation characterized by both vascular and cellular components designed to protect the body against alien substances and to dispose of dying tissue preparatory to the repair process.[4] Acute tissue incision is accompanied by transient (5–10 minutes) local capillary vasoconstriction (intended to minimize blood loss), followed by vasodilation, reduced flow, and increased vascular permeability. The last is mediated by prostaglandins ($PGE_{1,2}$), prostacyclin (PGI_2), various kinins, histamines (released by mast cells and platelets), and serotonin (released from mast

TABLE 6–1. **Stages in Wound Healing**

First Stage (Inflammation)
Vascular changes
- Vasodilation
- Slow flow
- Increased permeability
Cellular changes
- PMN and monocyte migration
- Platelet release of chemotactics
- Endothelial cell production
- Fibroblasts appear

Second Stage (Proliferative Phase)
- Macrophage predominance
- Increased fibroblasts, ground substance
- Collagenolysis
- New capillary formation

Third Stage (Collagen Maturation and Remodeling)
- Decreased cellularity
- Decreased vascularity
- Collagen remodeling and cross-linking

cells). At the injury site, neutrophils initially adhere to capillary walls and, with increased capillary permeability, diapedese into the extravascular space of the wounded area. Serum and other blood components accumulate between tissue surfaces. Platelets agglutinate and release a phospholipid that stimulates the intrinsic coagulation cascade. The extrinsic coagulation cascade is concurrently initiated by thromboplastins released from traumatized tissues. This process culminates in a wound filled with a fibrin-rich clot, composed of neutrophils, erythrocytes, platelets, and plasma proteins. The amount of this wound coagulum is directly related to the duration of exposure. Prolonged exposure (i.e., an open wound) can result in an excessive coagulum secondary to an exaggerated inflammatory response. In this situation, the excessive wound fibrin can actually engulf bacteria and provide an anatomic sanctuary that protects them from the bactericidal effects of prophylactic antibiotics.[5]

This inflammatory process, which continues for approximately 72 hours,[2] has been termed the lag phase, as the wound has essentially no collagen deposition or strength.

In parallel to early fascial healing, epithelialization, the process by which cells from the basal layer of the epidermis migrate across a denuded percutaneous wound, also occurs. Epithelialization begins within hours of wounding, and there is general acceptance that cell migration, not cell division, is the mechanism of epithelial cover. Epithelialization is controlled in part by epidermal growth factor (EGF), and epithelial migration is thought to be initiated by the loss of contact inhibition. Epithelial proliferation continues from the basal layer of the opposing wound edges until epithelial cells come in contact with cells of *similar* origin—the process of contact inhibition. When cells of unlike origin come in contact, the process of contact inhibition is not as precise and results in a chronic inflammatory reaction or the piling up of tissue in ridges. The basal cells of the epidermis and exposed epidermal appendages enlarge, extend out, flatten, and migrate out from the opposing skin edges. In wounds closed primarily, this watertight seal is apparent within 48 hours.[6,7]

Proliferative Phase

The proliferative phase is characterized by the production by the cellular components of their specialized products. The hallmark of the proliferative phase is the production and orderly deposition of collagen and the gain of wound tensile strength.

As the transient phase of white cell migration ends and the short-lived neutrophils die, the population of longer-lived monocytes predominates in the wound and continues its "debriding" activity for weeks.[2] It is clear that neutrophil phagocytosis plays a dominant role in the earliest phase of wound repair by reducing the number of contaminating bacteria and decreasing the amount of cellular debris. However, neutrophils do not appear necessary for normal repair of sterile or minimally contaminated wounds. In contrast, monocytes must be present to create normal fibroblast production and wound space invasion.[2] Importantly, macrophages are considered an obligate cellular component of normal wound healing and can promote collagen synthesis and angiogenesis. The absence of macrophages results in suboptimal wound healing.

Activated macrophages synthesize a wide variety of substances collectively referred to as either essential regulatory peptides or cytokines. These cytokines fundamentally affect both the surrounding cells (paracrine effect) and the cells that produce them (autocrine effect). It is during this early phase of cell commitment that exposure to cytotoxic drugs or radiation therapy has the biggest impact in terms of impeding wound healing. Other factors, including hypoxia (which increases angiogenesis promotion), may explain the wide variation in the wound healing process observed clinically.

This proliferative phase begins about 3 days after wounding and continues for approximately 21 days.[1] Following specific cellular signals, collagen and long chain mucopolysaccharides are synthesized and secreted by fibroblasts. Although small amounts of collagen are produced in the first 2 days after wounding, the rate of collagen synthesis greatly increases 5 days after wounding and continually increases for a period of 3 weeks.

Fibroblasts (factory cells) are attracted to or develop in the wound in numbers by both fibronectin and platelet-derived growth factor (PDGF).[8,9] Although still debated, most of the fibroblasts observed in healing wounds are thought to have been derived from local mesenchymal cells.[2] Angiogenesis factors, related both to PDGF and to macrophage-derived growth factors,[10,11] induce the influx of vascular smooth muscle cells and the growth of capillaries from existing blood vessels. Once established, fibroblasts produce collagen from the third day after injury for weeks or months. By the fourth or fifth week, however, the absolute number of fibroblasts has decreased dramatically, and the capillary network has shrunk to a few well-defined capillary systems.[2] Lymphatic channels begin to appear within 4 to 5 days of wounding, and lymphatic canalization is nearly normal within 3 weeks. Although the first collagen fibers appear 4 to 5 days after wounding, they appear as thin, randomly oriented fiber bundles. However, as the fibroblast population decreases, collagen fibers become the dominant anatomic component of wounds and produce a dense collagenous structure that firmly binds the injured tissues. PDGF, a glycoprotein, can promote the migration and proliferation of fibroblasts and endothelial cells as well as stimulate collagen synthesis in vitro.[3,12] Recombinant DNA technology and biochemical purification have permitted the identification of a number of other cytokines, including transforming growth factor, acidic fibroblast growth factor, and basic fibroblast growth factor/heparin-binding growth factors, EGF, transforming growth factor-*a*, epidermal cell–derived growth factor, insulin-like growth factor-1/somatomedin C, interleukin 1, and interleukin 2, which modulate healing.[13,14] Tumor necrosis factor administered locally in collagen may potentiate hematopoiesis and angiogenesis and increases wound strength in an Adriamycin-treated animal model.[15]

Myofibroblasts, thought to be derived from fibroblasts, also appear in large numbers during this phase.[7] These cells contain bundles of microfilaments and are contractile. Proliferation of myofibroblasts contributes to wound closure by contractile effects, pulling the wound edges together. The action of the myofibroblasts and closure by contraction are most important in wounds that are not closed primarily or in wounds where tissue mass has been lost.[16]

Early collagen synthesized during wound repair is loosely cross-linked and contributes little to wound tensile strength. Within days, however, intra- and intermolecular covalent cross-linking occurs with extracellular aggregation of collagen molecules. It is the intermolecular bonding that produces the fibrils and fibers of the quaternary helical collagen structure.[17] This orderly aggregation of collagen is associated with an increase in wound tensile strength. Variations occur in dermis, fascia, and bone, and distinct differences in collagen types and subtypes are found throughout the body. Types I and III are the most common types in soft tissues and elastic viscera. Type II appears limited to cartilage. The amino acids found only in collagen and used to identify it in analytical procedures are hydroxyproline and hydroxylysine.[7]

Oxygen is an important substrate for collagen synthesis and is required for the hydroxylation of lysine and proline, which is required for the release of collagen from cells. Adequate oxygen delivery is important and can be enhanced by ensuring adequate perfusion, administration of supplemental oxygen, using well-vascularized flaps, and smoking cessation.[18]

Ground substance, a term used to describe the coagulum of various glycosaminoglycans-mucopolysaccharides (chondroitins, chondroitin sulfate, heparin sulfate, and keratin sulfate), can be divided into two major groups: the sulfated and nonsulfated mucopolysaccharides.[19] These huge macromolecules exist as a nonfibrillar matrix within which collagen is deposited. The glycosaminoglycans are in highest concentration during the first 3 to 4 days after wounding. It is hypothesized that the ground substance plays a role in the formation of collagen fibrils, perhaps serving as a latticework for formation of a fibrin network.[20] Additionally, fibronectin, a glycoprotein present in both circulating blood and ground substance, probably has a central role in the organization of connective tissue structure.[3]

Collagen Remodeling Phase

The hallmark of the remodeling phase is the extracellular aggregation of collagen with complex intra- and intermolecular cross-linking of collagen fibrils. The process of remodeling (an equilibrium between collagen synthesis and collagen degradation) lasts for several years as scars become more pliable, stronger, and change color, size, and configuration.

Total wound collagen content does not increase after approximately 6 weeks, yet wounds slowly continue to gain tensile strength.[21,22] Secondary scar remodeling dominates wound repair after 21 days, and during the remodeling phase, wound tensile strength gradually increases, reaching a plateau *several years* after wounding. The collagen in the wound undergoes constant degradation and replacement—an equilibrium between collagen synthesis and collagen degradation. During this phase, collagenolysis results from the action of a number of tissue collagenases. Newly synthesized collagen, elaborated by specialized fibroblasts, is aligned along the lines of tissue stress and is highly cross-linked and is structurally much stronger than loosely cross-linked collagen elaborated during the initial days after wounding. The measurable increase in bursting strength and tensile strength in experimental wounds is thought to be a result of the more complexly cross-linked form of collagen,[20] and the process is thought to continue for at least 1 year.[3] This increase in tensile strength occurs without an increase in the total amount of collagen in the wound.[18,19]

Scar tissue in most incisions always remains firm and strong; however, defects in late remodeling may result in tissue thinning and actual loss of strength in some incisions. Late incisional hernias may occur after 2, 3, or even 5 years, suggesting that this remodeling phase may continue for prolonged periods of time.[2]

Tissue Strength

Tensile strength (load per cross-sectional area) and bursting strength (load to bursting regardless of dimension) are minimal the first 5 days after wounding. The strength that exists in the first 2 days is thought to be due to intercellular forces, fibrin polymerization, and epithelialization.[2] By 5 days there is enough collagen cross-linking to allow successful removal of skin sutures without disruption unless there is undue wound tension. Most wounds have developed less than 15% of their ultimate tensile strength by 3 weeks.[2] Fortunately, this 15% may be sufficient to resist normal stress.

Within any given population, different tissues heal at different rates, with five- to tenfold differences existing in measured wound strength.[1] Individual tissues also regain strength at different rates. At 10 days, skin incisions have regained 10% of their unwounded strength. By 21 days, skin wounds have significant bursting strength.[23] However, delayed removal of skin clips ($\geq$7 days) offers no benefit in late tensile strength (measured at 14–20 days) over removing clips at 5 days. Obviously, skin wounds under stress may suffer superficial separation if clips or sutures are removed early.

There is less data on the gain in bursting strength of human fascial wounds, but these wounds seem to gain tensile strength more slowly than skin wounds.[24] In comparison, fascial incisions heal slowly. Only 5% of unwounded fascial tensile strength is present at 1 week, 20% to 25% at 3 weeks, and 40% at 8 weeks.[1] This fact becomes clinically important when selecting suture material for fascia closure that is subjected to strain, especially episodic peak forces, such as abdominal closures that may be stressed during coughing or retching.

Collagen maturation occurs rapidly in intestinal anastomosis with nearly normal strength achieved by 4 months.[1] The integrity of bladder epithelium also returns rapidly.

The individual and variable return of wound strength only emphasizes the need to select sutures and closure techniques related to the specific needs and healing characteristics of the injured tissue.

Early human trials suggest the potential benefit of autologous PDGF, topical EGF, and recombinant human growth hormone to accelerate healing. In animals, ultrasound accelerates wound healing via local temperature regulation, fibroblast stimulation, or alteration of cytoplasmic factors.[25] Unfortunately, there is no clinically applicable biochemical method to consistently enhance wound healing.

When incised wounds are allowed to heal, intentionally dehisced, and immediately resutured, they develop strength significantly faster than those left with a primary closure.[2] Clinically, this suggests the need to incise the same incision when acute reoperative intervention is necessary.

Factors Complicating Wound Healing

Technical Factors

> *Wound complications add significant morbidity, lengthen the hospital stay, increase the cost of care, and often impair the patient's vocational and domestic rehabilitation.*

Technical factors under the surgeon's control can significantly contribute to altered healing and wound problems. In the great majority of cases, failure of a wound to heal is a consequence of failure of decision making and technique.[3] Additionally, a significant proportion of wound problems is associated with concurrent wound infection, and efforts to decrease the latter are important and likely to result in improved wound healing. In fact, optimal preparation of local tissues for operation requires a thoughtful surgical biologist.[2]

Preoperative Stay

The duration of the preoperative hospital stay correlates with the risk of wound infection. In an oft-quoted prospective evaluation of 23,649 wounds, Cruse and Foord[26] reported that clean wound infection rates in patients operated on after more than 24 hours in the hospital were double those in patients operated on on the day of admission (2.1% vs. 1.1%). The increased risk is likely related to hospital-acquired alterations in bacterial flora. In fact, a significant alteration in a patient's normal bacterial flora occurs by 24 hours after hospitalization. Hospital-acquired bacteria are more pathogenic than community bacteria and, if given the opportunity (i.e., by a skin incision), they are statistically more likely to be associated with infection and poor wound outcome. These findings imply the importance of outpatient evaluation and the significance of minimizing preoperative patient exposure.

Preparation

SURGICAL STAFF. Maimonides first associated the importance of hand washing in the 11th century. The French surgeons DeChaulic in the 14th century and Paré in the 16th century recognized the importance of "surgical cleanliness."[27] In 1857 Pasteur proposed the important effect of microorganisms in the genesis of infection. Semmelweis in 1861 indicated the importance of hand washing (with chlorinated lime) in decreasing the risk of puerperal fever.[28] Later, Lister utilized a 1:20 solution of carbolic acid to disinfect his skin.[28]

Glove puncture occurs in as many as 60% of all surgical procedures.[6,28] Actual needle injury occurs commonly with many gynecologic procedures (Table 6–2). Regardless of technique, this risk is increased in direct proportion to the amount of surgical needle handling. However, other factors (Table 6–3) also increase these risks.[29] Thus, the surgical team's bacterial flora is frequently exposed to the incision and the patient's disease is exposed to the surgical team. It is important to decrease the risk of

TABLE 6–2. **Percutaneous Injuries and Recontacts, by Service and Surgical Procedure**

Procedure	Risk Class*	No. of Procedures	No. (%) of Procedures with One or More Injuries
Gynecology service	—	307	31 (10)
Vaginal hysterectomy	H	47	10 (21)
Abdominal hysterectomy	M	165	17 (10)
Other gynecology	L	95	4 (4)
Ovarian cystectomy	—	15	1 (7)
Salpingo-oophorectomy	—	35	1 (3)
Miscellaneous	—	45	2 (4)

Modified with permission from Tokars JI, et al: Percutaneous injuries during surgical procedures. JAMA 267:2899–2904, 1992.
*Risk class: H, high; M, medium; L, low.

disease transmission through good skin preparation of both the surgeon and the patient.

The surgeon's hands cannot be sterilized, as 20% of the resident bacterial flora are located in nail beds or appendages beyond the reach of surgical scrubs.[27] Therefore, the purpose of the surgical scrub is to remove transient and pathogenic organisms. Although subject to debate, significant evidence exists to suggest the adequacy of a 2-minute scrub if a brush is used to scrub the skin folds around the nails.[30] Friction appears necessary to remove resistant microorganisms.[30] Although preoperative preparation is paramount, a 10- to 15-second scrub with an alcohol-containing agent should be undertaken after every surgical procedure to decrease transient bacteria and inactivate the HIV virus.[30] A large variety of surgical preparation solutions are available (Table 6–4) with differing activity, onset, and duration of action.

Aqueous iodine alone is highly concentrated and irritating.[31] However, iodophors (Betadine) combine iodine with a polymer to promote slow release to overcome these effects.[31] The most commonly used solution is 10% (1% free iodine) and may be combined with a detergent to form a scrub solution. Betadine scrub should only be used on intact skin, as it is cytotoxic to fibroblasts and impedes healing of soft tissues.[31]

Chlorhexidine gluconate has broad-spectrum

TABLE 6–3. **Increasing the Risk of Glove Perforation**

Emergency procedure
Longer operative time
Inadequate muscle relaxation
Number of sutures
Wound depth
Needle handling

bactericidal activity. Solutions containing chlorhexidine gluconate, which binds to the stratum corneum (activity for 5–6 hours),[27] or an iodophor are the most effective surgical scrubs with the least stability, contamination, or toxicity problems. Chlorhexidine gluconate, a quaternary amine, is superior in decreasing the bacterial count and is a more persistent agent (i.e., in preventing regrowth in a gloved hand) than povidone-iodine.[30,31] Although alcohol produces the most rapid and quantitative reduction of bacterial counts, it does have significant drying effects on the skin and is extremely volatile.[30]

PATIENT. The skin, with an average area of approximately 1.8 m^2, is the largest body organ, accounting for 16% of body weight and 20% of body water.[4,30] Three relatively distinct microenvironments exist. Oily regions (head, trunk, upper back), moist regions (axillae, groins), and dry regions (extremities) differ in the type and quantity of bacterial flora.[30] The microflora differs dramatically between regions or organs (Table 6–5).

Currently, skin preparation involves two aspects: physical cleansing and antisepsis. Cruse and Foord suggested the benefit of a preoperative phisoHex shower.[26] Despite conflicting information, it is our opinion that the simple prophylactic technique of a shower with an antiseptic soap has great potential benefits, minimal risks, and minimal cost and should be considered before any high-risk procedure.

The initial preoperative skin preparation involves decisions regarding the necessity of benefit of hair removal. Surgical tradition suggests the need for a clean operative field, and many surgeons still experience a compulsive desire to remove hair from the surgical field. Cruse and Foord first indicated the increased infectious risks associated with shaving hair in the operative field.[26] Theoretically,

TABLE 6–4. **Antisepsis for Surgical Disinfection**

Agent	Mean Reduction in Release of Skin Bacteria (%)	
	Immediate	*>3 hr*
Liquid soap	40	0
Povidone-iodine liquid soap	90	20
Chlorhexidine detergent	75	70
Povidone-iodine aqueous solution	97	75
Isopropyl alcohol 60%	96	90
Hexachlorophene detergent	40	91
Isopropyl alcohol 70%	99.3	99.1
Isopropyl alcohol 70% plus chlorhexidine 0.5%	99.4	99.7

Modified with permission from Masterson BJ: Skin preparation. In American College of Surgeons: Care of the Surgical Patient, chap 22. New York: Scientific American, 1991.
Note: The application time for chlorhexidine detergent is 3 minutes; for all other preparations it is 5 minutes.

preoperative shaving results in significant cutaneous microinjury, which increases the risk of infection. Their original data suggested a risk reduction with "clipper" removal. A more recent prospective, randomized trial involving over 1,000 patients demonstrated the benefit of hair removal by clipping on the morning of surgery. When compared to a razor shave or clipping on the night before surgery, the morning clipping resulted in the lowest risk of infection (Table 6–6). We doubt that floor nurses or other associated floor personnel will know the planned placement of a surgical incision. We prefer to clip hair in the operating room just be-

fore starting the surgical procedure. Depilatories can be used for hair removal but are associated with a significant risk of skin irritation.[27]

The importance of surgical site preparation, including cleaning and antisepsis, became apparent during World War II, when a 1% to 10% iodine and 7% alcohol preparation was accepted methodology. A skin "cleaner" is a nonantiseptic. An antiseptic is a germicide applied to an animate object and a disinfectant is a germicide applied to an inanimate object. In 1938, Walter introduced the quaternary amines. In general, alcoholic preparations of povidone-iodine and chlorhexidine are preferable,

TABLE 6–5. **Normal Microflora**

Organ System	Total Bacterial Concentrations*	Ratio of Anaerobes to Aerobes
Skin		
Moister areas (axillae, perineum, etc.)	10^4–10^6	1:10
Drier areas (trunk, upper arms and legs)	10^1–10^3	1:5–10
Exposed areas (head, face, feet)[†]	10^4–10^6	1:5–10
Digestive System		
Stomach	0–10^5	1:1
Proximal small bowel	10^2–10^4	1:1
Ileum	10^5–10^8	1:1
Colon	10^9–10^{11}	100–1000:1
Urogenital System		
Female urethra	10^2–10^3	Aerobes
Endocervix	10^8–10^9	5–10:1
Vagina	10^8–10^9	5–10:1

*Per cm^2 of tissue.
[†]Anaerobes may outnumber aerobes in the skin of the cheeks, upper back, and presternum.

TABLE 6–6. **Wound Infections: One vs. Two Knives**

Procedure	No. of Infections/ No. of Patients (%)	
	One Knife	*Two Knives*
Clean	5/160 (3.1)	10/171 (5.8)
Clean-contaminated	5/117 (4.3)	7/138 (5.1)
Overall	10/277 (3.6)	17/309 (5.5)

Modified with permission from Hasselgren PO, et al: One instead of two knives for surgical incision. Arch Surg 119:917–920, 1984.

because alcohol itself is a disinfectant. Chlorhexidine gluconate is the agent of choice.[30] Vaginal preparation dilutes bacterial flora, and there is no distinct advantage to using an antiseptic over using normal saline.

Incision

Wound healing and outcome may be related to incision placement. The selection of the abdominal incision and its placement are related to a number of factors. The actual incision placement and incision type relate to the diagnosis, the urgency of the operation, patient habitus, the presence of a previous incision, cosmetic preferences, and the possible need for a stoma. A transverse incision has fewer adverse effects on postoperative respiratory function. In planning incisions for elective surgery, the surgeon's primary responsibility is to identify a site that allows sufficient access for successful completion of the planned operation but also allows extension of the operative field exposure if necessary. Finally, the site must allow safe closure.

The most aesthetically pleasing scar results when the long axis of the scar is in the direction of maximal skin tension.[4] A transverse incision, although not the strongest, heals with an almost invisible scar and clinically performs very well. Clinically, transverse fascial incisions rarely suffer from acute wound failure. This benefit is not related to incision strength but is likely related to less stress placed on the incision itself.[1] In most situations, the Pfannenstiel incision is adequate for benign gynecologic procedures. If necessary, exposure can be increased by incising the rectus muscle at its insertion. The converted Cherney incision then allows increased lateral pelvic exposure as well as improved upper abdominal access. If a transverse incision is used with the preoperative anticipation of the need of additional exposure, a rectus muscle-

splitting incision (Maylard) may be appropriate.[32] If this incision is chosen, care to ligate the epigastric artery is essential.

The strongest incision is a midline incision closed with widely placed sutures incorporating nearly 1.5 cm of fascial tissue and placed at intervals of 1.5 to 2.0 cm. Sutures placed close to the fascial edge result in a decrease in tensile strength.[33] There appears to be no difference in the incision strength of extended vertical incisions through or around the umbilicus.[34] Supraumbilical incisions may be appropriate to allow adequate pelvic exposure in the morbidly obese.[35]

While incision site selection is important during primary procedures, the correct decision during repeat procedures may be more critical. Although previous scars are associated with less vascularity and an increased rate of infection,[36] second or repeat incisions should be made at the same site if possible. If not, new parallel incisions or new incisions that transect previous scars at an acute angle should be avoided, as they compromise blood supply and predispose the site to poor healing. If the previous incision is used for reoperation, the pelvic surgeon must be cognizant of the increased risk of intraperitoneal adhesions and intestinal injury. Sharp dissection of the subcutaneous and fascial tissue above or below the incision may facilitate peritoneal entry into the peritoneum.

Once incision placement has been decided, the incision should be made with a single, bold stroke to decrease subcutaneous dead space. The clinical dictum, Create a bold incision with a sharp knife!, has withstood the test of time and is supported by data from clinical studies and from studies of animal models.[21,37] A series of knife sweeps through the subcutaneous tissue and fascia produces a series of stair steps, increases the amount of devitalized tissue in the wound, increases dead space, and makes coaptation of perpendicular edges suboptimal. Although dead space may occur in any incision, its presence increases the risk of wound infection and poor outcome. Unfortunately, using suture material to "close" the dead space may further increase the risk (4×) of infection and poor wound healing.[21]

Recent attention has re-focused on the role and benefit of subcutaneous suture placement. DelValle et al.[22] suggested that sutures placed to encompass the superficial fascia decreased the risk of superficial wound disruption from 16.1% to 2.5% following cesarean section. Unfortunately, this study did not evaluate wound incision type or control of other important factors such as the use of electrocautery.

Interestingly, the authors reported this benefit when plain catgut was used (loss of tensile strength in 5–7 days). Importantly, they indicated that superficial disruption was more likely to occur with longer surgery and increased weight.[22] In the laboratory, subcutaneous sutures decreased the activity of antibiotics and increased the risk of infection, although the effect is least with polyglycolic acid (PGA) and Prolene.[38]

There is no need for two surgical knives in the operative field to create a skin incision.[37] In a prospective study of 609 patients, Hasselgren et al. evaluated infection rates in incisions created with one or two different blades.[39] There was no difference in wound infection rates in clean (3.1%) or clean-contaminated wounds or in the overall infection rate whether one knife or two were used. Eliminating the second blade may in itself contribute to significant health care savings.

Both experimental and clinical evidence suggests[26] that the use of electrocautery to create a surgical incision increases the amount of necrotic tissue and the rate of wound infection. Incisions created with the surgical diathermy unit cause tissue damage and create a zone of thermal injury of several hundred microns on either side of the incision.[26] The actual amount of tissue injury increases in direct proportion to current density.[28] When compared to incisions made with a knife, wounds created with the electrosurgical unit in experimental models have a threefold increased risk of infection and decreased tensile and bursting strength.[28,37] Evaluating different methods to create a midline fascial incision, Kumagai et al. used a scalpel, electrocautery in the cutting mode, and electrocautery in the coagulation mode in an animal model.[40] The wound strength of the scalpel incision was nearly twice that of those made with electrocautery in the cutting mode (187 vs. 223) and almost three times (187 vs. 402) that of incisions made with electrocautery in the coagulation mode.

It is evident that the unselective use of electrocautery increases the risk of infection, and there is no evidence to suggest that cautery incisions sustain less blood loss clinically. Incisions created with the CO_2 laser are associated with a smaller zone of thermal injury than electrosurgical incisions but a greater zone of thermal injury than knife incisions. Experimental wounds created with the CO_2 laser have been reported to have reduced tensile strength.[28] Comparative studies of steel, electrosurgical, and laser incisions suggest little advantage of the latter two in terms of time, blood loss, and pain.[41]

Wound Hemostasis

Serum and tissue fluid collect in the incision as a requisite first step in wound repair. However, excessive blood and fluid is not desirable. Blood is an excellent culture medium, and reports relate the incidence of experimental wound infections to the hemoglobin concentration of wound fluid.[21] The necessary inoculum is decreased by a factor of 4 when the wound hemoglobin level increases from 8% to 20%.[42]

The electrosurgical cautery is a useful adjunct for achieving wound hemostasis and may be safely employed with a bipolar unit or with fine-tipped forceps to minimize thermal injury to adjacent tissue. When used in this manner, there is no reported increase in the risk of wound complications, even when compared to suture ligature.[43] As important, electrosurgical control of vessels larger than 2 mm in diameter is inconsistent,[28] and other methods of control may be necessary.

Suture Material

Decisions regarding suture selection for wound edge reapproximation or vessel ligature are of vital importance to wound outcome. Lister introduced the first monofilament absorbable suture material. His use of catgut dramatically changed many techniques.[3] In fact, today there is little role for natural suture material.

The choice of appropriate surgical suture material is primarily related to the need for suture tensile strength and the duration of activity. The ideal suture loses its tensile strength over a time interval in which the injured tissue regains tensile strength. A large number of suture materials and configurations are currently available (Table 6–7). The suture's chemical composition is more important than the physical configuration in determining wound outcome.[44]

Prospective studies evaluating permanent suture materials for fascial closure suggest a 10% risk of chronic wound problems. Long-acting absorbable sutures were developed in an attempt to bypass these problems. Although previous data suggested little difference, one recent report[45] that evaluated polyglyconate and polydioxanone sulfate suture suggested that these two presumably long-acting, absorbable materials were similar in suture reactivity but markedly different in early (14 days) and late (35 days) tensile strength.[45] Fortunately, both sutures performed well clinically.[46] Although long-acting absorbable or nonabsorbable sutures are

TABLE 6–7. **Suture Materials**

Material	Tensile Strength	Knot Security	Reactivity	Days to 10% of Tensile Strength
Permanent				
Manufactured				
Steel	4	4	1	
Polyamide (nylon)	3	3	1	
Polyesters (Dacron)	3	3	1	
Polyolefins (Prolene)	3	1	1	
Natural				
Silk	2	3	3	
Cotton	2	2	2	
Linen	2	2	2	
Absorbable				
Catgut	1	2	3	5
Chromic catgut	1	3	3	28
Polyglycolic acid	2	2	1	28
Polydioxonone sulfate	3	2	1	56
Polyglyconate	3	2	1	55

Modified with permission from Orr JW Jr: Introduction to Pelvic Surgery: Pre and Postoperative Care. In Gusberg S (ed): Female Genital Cancer. New York: Churchill Livingstone, 1988.

ideal for fascial repair, the surgeon must choose appropriate sutures for other portions of the operation.

In an elegant study, McGeehan et al.[47] evaluated the effect of suture material in the presence of synergistic wound sepsis in an animal model. When contaminated with a significant inoculum (6×10^5) of E. coli and B. fragilis, PGA suture material was associated with less risk of infection than catgut, nylon, silk, Prolene, or controls. This "antibacterial" effect may be related to specific suture breakdown products.[44] As important, PGA sutures are associated with less pain.[48] We believe that using anything other than PGA sutures during the abdominal, inguinal, or vulvar portion of the procedure increases the potential risk of infection and contributes to poor wound healing and poor surgical outcome.

Absorbable sutures are acceptable for vessel ligation. In an animal model, Hay indicated that vessel control (1.5-mm vessels) was nearly complete when sutures maintained their tensile strength for 96 hours. There appears to be little role for permanent sutures even in this clinical situation.[48a]

The choice of suture size is also important. Edlich et al. indicated that the recoverability of viable bacteria, both gram-positive (S. aureus) and gram-negative (E. coli), increased as suture size increased.[37] Currently, excluding fascial closure, the tensile strength of synthetic 2-0 and 3-0 materials is satisfactory for nearly all aspects of benign or malignant pelvic procedures.

The decision to use a suture (other than fascial) should be carefully evaluated, as it is important to minimize the amount of suture material in any surgical situation. For instance, suture approximation of ovarian surfaces does not decrease the risk of pelvic adhesions. Mirana et al.[49] evaluated 30 ovaries, half of which were sutured, the other half left unapproximated, in an animal model and reported no difference in terms of absence of adhesions, presence of avascular adhesions, presence of vascular adhesions, number of corpora lutea, or number of embryos. It is apparent that the use of specific sutures as well as suture placement should be defensible prior to use. Recent studies suggest that single-layer uterine closure with PGA sutures can save 10% of the operative time[50] without increasing the risk of acute (bleeding) or late (separation) complications.

The amount of foreign body in a wound correlates with infectious risks, and even suture length is important. In animal models, both wound infection rates and recoverability of viable bacteria are markedly increased when longer lengths of suture material are used. In the clinical situation, this information suggests that the presence of suture material should be minimized and attention should be focused on all surgical moves, even the cutting of residual suture from knots.

Adequate knot tying is vital to impart optimal tensile strengths of specific sutures. The number of knots as well as the complexity (simple vs.

surgeon's knots) may influence suture security and suture volume in the wound.[1] Von Rijessel et al.[51] evaluated suture size and knot volume resulting from three- or five-throw knot configurations with 2-0 and 4-0 suture. Knot volume increased by a factor of 1.4 with five throws, regardless of suture size, and increased by a factor of 6.2 when the same knot configuration was made with 4-0 rather than 2-0 suture. These results emphasize the need to minimize both suture size and the number of knots placed in any suture material. Additional throws or larger suture size only contribute to foreign body presence, potential infection, and poor healing.

Although PGA is a superior suture material, many physicians are uncomfortable tying PGA sutures and continue to use less optimal materials. Terra and Aberg[52] compared the strength of knots made in monofilament, steel, chromic, Prolene, and Dexon sutures. (Dexon is a proprietary form of PGA.) In relating knot configuration to maximum tensile strength, they found that two sequential surgeon's knots in Dexon brought the material to 75% of the maximum unknotted strength of PGA. Additional knots had minimal effect on suture strength but did increase the volume of suture material, with the potential problems already discussed. Prolene, commonly used for fascial closure, reached its maximum strength (98%) with three consecutive surgeon's knots.

The principle of wound stapling dates to the turn of the century. Although criticized for introducing a rigidity that makes the tissue conform to the suture rather than the other way around, staples create a reproducible repair and may actually increase blood flow in specific anastomotic sites. Their use decreases operative time,[53] and currently the majority of gastrointestinal procedures are performed using B-shaped staples. A wide variety of staplers are available. It is imperative that the surgeon understand the role and place of specific stapling devices before using them. The role of staplers in laparoscopic gynecologic surgery has been expanded but not yet critically reviewed. In specific instances they may contribute significant costs,[54] and current information has not shown their benefit when compared to other, less expensive methods such as electrocautery or sutures.[55]

Absorbable staples have been used for vaginal cuff closure and for uterine closure following cesarian section[19] but have not gained popularity. Although individual reports have suggested a decrease in operative time, a lowered risk of infection and reduced hospital stay have not been consistently demonstrated.[56] The use of vaginal staples may require more extensive vaginal dissection, which may contribute to bleeding and inadequate cuff support.

The use of staples for skin approximation is an accepted norm and allows excellent tissue approximation with minimal time. "Clipped" skin wounds are more resistant to infection than sutured incisions.[28] Interestingly, subcuticular closures do not necessarily lessen scar formation.[57]

The popularity of taped skin closure is limited despite the potential benefits. Difficulty in achieving accurate skin edge approximation and the need for a dry field contribute to the limited use.

Other methods of tissue approximation, including glues, absorbable clips, or even laser welding, require further evaluation.

Vasoconstrictors

Any condition that decreases delivery of white cells to an area of bacterial contamination increases infectious risks and contributes to poor healing.[58] There is little role for the use of vasoconstrictors in the management of any abdominal or vaginal wound. England et al.[59] evaluated the effect of epinephrine (1:200,000) in women undergoing vaginal surgery. The frequency of cuff cellulitis and cuff abscess was significantly higher in patients given epinephrine than in controls. There was no objective evidence of decreased blood loss (310 mL vs. 280 mL) or alteration in postoperative hematocrit. It makes little sense to decrease wound vascularity, potentially decrease the concentration of prophylactic antibiotics, or increase the risk of tissue hypoxia by using vasoconstrictors. Additionally, these agents significantly increase heart rate, ventricular irritability (50% of women have premature ventricular contractions), and systolic pressure (to a mean of 190 mm Hg).[60] Although many surgeons use vasoconstrictors to improve tissue dissection, we find little benefit to their use. If necessary, normal saline may be injected to assist in dissection.

Drains

There is little historical or current information to validate the role of routine pelvic or abdominal wall drainage.[61] In Cruse and Foord's initial study,[26] drain placement increased the risk of infection in clean wounds, although closed suction drainage decreased risks when compared to passive drainage. The infection rate in clean, undrained wounds, 1.5%, rose to 1.8% in those with closed suction drainage, increased again to 2.4% when Penrose drains were brought out through a stab wound, and dramatically increased to 4% when Penrose drains were placed in the wound. Unfortunately, the use of closed suction drainage increases patient cost, increases nursing requirements, and potentially removes valuable serum proteins.

Edlich et al.[37] indicated that the type of drain material made little difference in the risk of wound infection. When Silastic drains and latex drains were compared with no drains in an animal model, any drain (foreign body) increased the potential risk of wound infection.[62] This information, coupled with the data from Cruse and Foord, suggests that Penrose drainage or passive drainage is to be avoided.

In a prospective randomized study, Farnell et al.[63] evaluated the role of subcutaneous drainage in clean, clean-contaminated, and dirty incisions. Over 1,000 patients were randomly assigned to primary closure following irrigation with an antibiotic solution (neomycin, Polymyxin, or gentamicin), primary closure with a subcutaneous drain and antibiotic irrigation, a primary subcutaneous drain with saline irrigation, or primary closure with a subcutaneous drain alone. The infection rate did not differ for clean or clean-contaminated procedures, regardless of the use of drains. However, there was a trend toward a decreased infection rate in class IV incisions when catheters and antibiotic irrigation were used. In fact, 94% of contaminated wounds were successfully closed primarily with this technique. These findings have been reproduced by Lubowski and Hunt,[64] whose prospective evaluation failed to demonstrate a benefit of drains in 349 abdominal incisions.

As important, pelvic drainage after abdominal hysterectomy or pelvic lymphadenectomy[65,66] does not decrease febrile morbidity, the incidence of lymphocyst formation, or lymphedema. It only increases operative time and potential expense. In a recent study by Jensen et al.,[67] closed suction drains placed after radical hysterectomy increased the rate of rehospitalization or drain site infection. Pelvic drains are not helpful when wound infection occurs, as cultures from closed suction[68] drainage do not predict infection risk or response.[69]

Topical Applications

After World War I, Alexander Fleming claimed that the local instillation of antiseptics would harm the wound. Today it is common knowledge that scrubs and detergents damage tissue defenses and potentiate infection.[5]

The routine use of topical antiseptics or antibacterial solutions has no scientific basis. Although the subcutaneous tissues (with lowered antibiotic levels) may provide an anatomic sanctuary for bacteria, the use of topical antibiotics is of little benefit except in the most contaminated cases.[70,71] We urge that contamination be prevented with technique rather than treated with topical agents. In cases of gross contamination, however, such as in operations on an unprepared intestinal tract, antibiotic solutions should be considered for wound irrigation.

Although topical antibiotics may not be important, there may be a role for wound irrigation at the time of closure. Investigational data suggest little benefit of irrigation unless used under pressure.[37] In contaminated wounds, irrigation at ≥7 psi removes contaminants and decreases infectious risk. Continuous irrigation is superior to pulsatile irrigation.[72] This pressure can be attained with a 35-mL syringe and a 19-gauge needle.[37]

Wound Closure

Most abdominal wall closure techniques are based on anecdotal experience, familiarity, prejudice, and previous training. Few prospective studies in the gynecologic literature have addressed optimal methods of wound closure.

Wound closure has classically been divided into three categories: (1) *primary closure,* in which wound edges are approximated at the completion of the surgical procedure, (2) *secondary closure,* in which the wounds are allowed to heal without reapproximation ("granulate in"), and (3) *tertiary* or *delayed primary closure,* in which wound reapproximation is delayed for 4 or more days.

After incision and closure, the abdominal wall fascia regains little strength for 2 to 3 weeks.[1] Therefore, closure with a suture that loses the majority of its tensile strength before that time could place the wound at risk. Additionally, collagen maturation or remodeling (and wound strength accumulation) continues for a prolonged period. An optimal closure would incorporate suture that loses its tensile strength in a mirror image to the fascia regaining its tensile strength. Both laboratory[73] and clinical[46] evidence suggest the potential benefit of using long-acting absorbable sutures for fascia closure.

The concept of mass abdominal wall closure was introduced by Jenkins (in Eckersley[3]) and significant clinical evidence suggests a benefit.[46,74] The strongest fascia closure incorporates a Smead-Jones internal retention mass closure. However, this closure is not necessary in all patients. We conducted a randomized prospective study of 402 women undergoing gynecologic procedures to evaluate and compare the Smead-Jones mass closure and continuous mass closure with a long-acting absorbable suture (polyglyconate). We found no difference in the rate of seroma formation, infection, or hernia formation (at 6 months). No patient had fascial dehiscence. Importantly, the use of a continuous closure decreased fascial closure time from 12.10 minutes to 4.75 minutes, potentially resulting in significant cost savings.

There is no apparent benefit to parietal peritoneal closure, as these defects exhibit mesothelial integrity at 48 hours and are indistinguishable at 5 days. Tulandi et al.[75] used second-look laparoscopy to evaluate the effects of peritoneal closure. There was no difference in the wound infection rate between open and closed methods (2.4% vs. 3.6%). The incidence of infection in those patients undergoing second-look laparoscopy (15.8% vs. 22.2%) and the incidence of bowel obstruction were not significantly different. Peritoneal closure at cesarean section only increases operative time, with no effect on analgesic requirements, infection risk, or return of bowel function.[76] Peritoneal approximation may increase the risk of adhesions by creating local tissue ischemia.

Skin closure can be successfully accomplished using nonreactive sutures, clips, or tape. Taped wounds are extremely resistant to infection.[77] The timing of skin suture removal relates to the desired cosmetic effect, the amount of tension on the wound edges, regional blood supply, nutritional status, concurrent steroid use, concurrent chemotherapy or radiation therapy, and infection. Of the various factors under surgical control, the length of time the skin suture remains in place is the most important determinant.[4] The size of either the suture or needle is not as important as the inherent skin tension in the predisposition to the development of sutural scars.[4] Early suture removal may result in less scarring in wounds with minimal tension[25]; however, wound evaluation is a better index than counting days.[7] In most situations, removing several sutures and evaluating the extent of wound adhesion allows safe removal of skin sutures.[7]

Specific tactics used for contaminated wound closure include delayed primary closure. This method was first described by Guy DeChaulic in 1363[78] but was not developed or used clinically until World War II, when military wounds necessitated a different management scheme. Importantly, experimental evidence suggests that the early tensile strength of primary and delayed closures is comparable, but at 60 days the delayed closure is significantly stronger.[3]

Open wound management involves the placement of sterile fine mesh gauze covered by a sterile dressing. There is little need for changing or disturbing this gauze pack during the first 4 postoperative days unless there is postoperative fever. Management is often associated with a reduction in bacterial flora to critical levels ($<10^5$/g tissue). Unnecessary inspection during this interval only increases the risk of contamination and subsequent infection. Although wound healing following clean or clean-contaminated procedures usually occurs by primary intention, delayed primary closure might be considered in contaminated wounds. Primary closure in this situation has a high ($\geq$50%) infection risk. Although quantitative bacterial wound cultures might be used, existing evidence from clinical and animal studies suggests that the wound should not be closed prior to the fourth day, and that a longer delay (in the absence of macroscopic infection) is of little benefit.[5] Wound margins can be approximated after the fourth day with minimal risk of infection.[4] At that time, the sutures placed but left untied intraoperatively can be used to reapproximate the incision as a delayed primary closure (Table 6–8).

Dressings

Following closure, the wound should be covered. Unfortunately, much of the information available on postoperative wound management and dressings has little scientific merit. Surgical dressings should protect the wound from contamination during epithelialization; however, their use can alter pH, cellular infiltration, moisture, or oxygen concentration.[79] Increased moisture under occlusion facilitates epithelial migration and epithelialization. Therefore, an occlusive dressing, if not contaminated by blood or serum, should be left in place for 48 hours. Clear, semipermeable dressings allow easy wound inspection; however, collections of serum or blood should be avoided, as they may accentuate poor wound healing or result in maceration.[25] The semipermeable dressings clearly have different characteristics that can affect bacterial growth (Table 6–9).[80] One recent prospective study in human volunteers suggested no clinical difference in the healing of superficial wounds. While providing a physical barrier, no dressing had the ability to stave off infection once bacteria were present.[80]

TABLE 6–8. Infection Rates in Clean-Contaminated (Type II), Contaminated (Type III), and Dirty (Type IV) Wounds, by Closure Technique

	Type II Infections		Type III Infections		Type IV Infections	
Closure Technique	*No.*	*%*	*No.*	*%*	*No.*	*%*
Primary closure and DAB*	27/659	(4.1)	6/99	(7.1)	7/45	(15.5)
Catheter and saline	26/678	(3.8)	5/105	(4.8)	5/53	(9.4)
Catheter and DAB	29/678	(4.3)	7/97	(7.2)	3/53	(5.7)
Catheter alone	29/659	(4.4)	4/103	(3.9)	12/53	(22.6)
$p = \chi^2$ test	0.959		0.667		0.055	

Modified with permission from Farnell MB, et al: Closure of abdominal incisions with subcutaneous catheters. Arch Surg 121:641–648, 1986.

*DAB indicates solution of 0.5 g of neomycin sulfate, 0.1 g of polymyxin B sulfate, and 80 mg of gentamicin sulfate per liter of normal saline.

> *Surgical dressings in wounds closed secondarily are of vital import. The presence of necrotic tissue leads to contamination and infection and inhibits epithelial cell migration.[18] Following physical debridement, optimal humidity must be maintained. Absorbent dressings remove serum, and normal saline-soaked wet-to-dry dressings are satisfactory. The addition of other substances may significantly impair healing. The use of hydrogen peroxide as a chemical debridement, Dakin's solution, and acetic acid should be discouraged.[31]*

Antibiotic Prophylaxis

Surgical site infections are the cause, directly or indirectly, of a majority of postoperative wound complications. As with most phenomena, infections and other wound complications are both multifactorial and interrelated and prolong hospital stay, increase the risk of wound separation and dehiscence, and may increase the risk of potentially lethal thromboembolic disease. They directly increase patient suffering as well as the cost of care.

Perioperative antibiotics effectively decrease the number of patients who develop postoperative wound infections. This is true for a wide range of surgical procedures, including vaginal hysterectomy, abdominal hysterectomy, radical abdominal hysterectomy with lymphadenectomy, and for an increasing number and variety of class I wounds. Although important, perioperative antibiotic therapy only complements a well-conceived, well-executed procedure with hemodynamic, respiratory, and nutritional support.[81]

SELECTION OF ANTIBIOTIC AGENTS. For gynecologic procedures the principles of prophylaxis include the use of agents with activity against potential aerobic and anaerobic pathogens. Single-agent cephalosporins are the most widely used drugs (Table 6–10). For patients who have cephalosporin

TABLE 6–9. Recovery of Bacterial Pathogens

Organism/ Treatment	Time (hr)		
	24	*48*	*72*
Staphylococcus aureus			
Air exposed	7.0 ± 0.2	6.5 ± 0.6	6.8 ± 0.5
DuoDERM	7.0 ± 0.2	7.3 ± 0.2	7.0 ± 0.5
Opsite	6.4 ± 0.1	6.7 ± 0.5	6.0 ± 0.1
Vigilon	7.9 ± 0.3	7.8 ± 0.2	7.7 ± 0.1
Clostridium perfringens			
Air exposed	2.8 ± 1.0	3.0 ± 0.8	2.7 ± 0.7
DuoDERM	6.2 ± 0.7	6.7 ± 0.2	6.1 ± 0.7
Opsite	3.7 ± 0.4	3.9 ± 0.9	5.7 ± 1.6
Vigilon	5.8 ± 0.5	6.5 ± 0.4	6.2 ± 0.4
Pseudomonas aeruginosa			
Air exposed	4.3 ± 1.1	4.9 ± 0.3	5.0 ± 0.3
DuoDERM	5.9 ± 0.7	6.4 ± 0.6	6.1 ± 0.4
Opsite	6.5 ± 0.1	7.4 ± 0.3	6.9 ± 0.4
Vigilon	7.0 ± 0.4	7.3 ± 0.2	6.9 ± 0.3
Bacteroides fragilis			
Air exposed	1.3 ± 1.8	0.0 ± 0.0	0.0 ± 0.0
DuoDERM	6.4 ± 0.3	8.0 ± 0.1	8.2 ± 0.2
Opsite	1.9 ± 2.7	2.7 ± 3.8	5.0 ± 3.2
Vigilon	6.1 ± 0.7	7.6 ± 0.2	7.0 ± 0.8

Modified with permission from Katz S, et al: Semipermeable occlusive dressings. Arch Dermatol 122:58–62, 1986.

Note: Values are given as geometric mean log colony-forming units per milliliter, ± SD.

TABLE 6–10. **Antibiotic Prophylaxis Regimens for Gynecologic Cancer Surgery**

Cancer	Antibiotic Regimen
Cervical Cancer	
Conization	Rarely indicated
Total hysterectomy	First- or second-generation cephalosporin* (<3 doses)
Radical hysterectomy	First- or second-generation cephalosporin (<3 doses)
Pelvic exenteration	Bowel preparation (mechanical and antibiotic)
	Intraoperative antibiotic irrigation
	Second-generation cephalosporin (<5 days)
	TMP-SMX[†] with stent removal (<3 days)
Endometrial Cancer	
Hysterectomy with lymphadenectomy	First- or second-generation cephalosporin (<3 doses)
Ovarian Cancer	
Primary resection	Bowel preparation (mechanical and antibiotic)
	Intraoperative antibiotic irrigation
	First- or second-generation cephalosporin (<3 doses)
Second-look procedure	Prophylaxis rarely indicated
Palliative (or secondary) resection	Second-generation cephalosporin
	Intraoperative antibiotic irrigation
Vulvar Cancer	
Vulvectomy (± node dissection)	Cephalosporin with good gram-positive coverage (<3 doses)
Trophoblastic Disease	
Suction evacuation	Doxycycline (1 wk)

Modified with permission from Orr JW Jr, Taylor PT: Reducing postoperative infection in the patient with gynecologic cancer. Infec Surg 6: 666, 1987.
*Metronidazole may be used in those with penicillin allergy.
[†]Trimethoprim-sulfamethoxazole (Bactrim, Septra).

allergy or who have profound penicillin allergy, either aminoglycosides or metronidazole are effective for prophylaxis for gynecologic or general abdominal procedures.[70]

TIMING OF ANTIBIOTIC ADMINISTRATION. There is experimental and clinical evidence that the timing of antibiotic administration is of critical importance. Antibiotics administered *before or with* the creation of the incision are much more effective than antibiotics administered for several days before surgery or begun postoperatively.[82] Attention should also be paid to the half-life of the antibiotics selected. For procedures lasting longer than the half-life of the antibiotics, specific drugs may need to be readministered every half-life to achieve uniform therapeutic levels. It seems reasonable that the same principles regarding redosing should apply when procedures are associated with large blood loss and large-volume crystalloid replacement or blood transfusion. Recent information suggests the importance of enterococcal coverage when significant contamination occurs.

DURATION OF ANTIBIOTIC ADMINISTRATION. Long-term antibiotic "prophylaxis" was shown to

be ineffective and inadvisable almost two decades ago.[70] Current recommendations for most class II and III procedures are for prophylaxis of short duration; three-dose regimens are as effective as, or more effective than, multiple-day regimens.[70] For many procedures, single-agent/single-dose therapy is as effective as multiple-dose therapy.[70]

Patient-Related Factors

In addition to technical factors, a variety of important patient-related factors exist. Some may be recognized and corrected preoperatively.

Vitamin Deficiency

Scurvy, a deficiency in vitamin C, is the classic example of a clinical vitamin deficiency adversely affecting wound healing. Ascorbic acid is an essential element for a variety of important oxidation-reduction systems as well as both collagen synthesis and collagen cross-linking. Collagen synthesis, fibroblast formation, and neutrophil bacterial killing require vitamin C. Clinically, wound dehiscence is eight times more likely to occur in patients deficient in vitamin C.[18] Fortunately, patients with profound vitamin C deficiency are rare in industrialized nations except for people who are also suffering from alcoholism. When encountered, vitamin C deficiency can be effectively treated with replacement using supplementation doses of 100 to 2,000 mg/day.

Administration of vitamin A can counteract the local effects of corticosteroids. A topical dose of 200,000 IU is locally effective with minimal systemic effect if given within 3 to 4 days of wounding.[18] Supplemental vitamin E may increase the breaking strength of irradiated wounds and may increase wound fibroblast content. However, to date there is little apparent benefit to routine supplementation with these or other vitamins in the absence of a documented deficiency.

Serum zinc levels of less than 100 mg/dL are also associated with poor healing.[18] Although zinc plays an important role in cell mitosis and proliferation, zinc supplements (zinc sulfate, 220 mg b.i.d.) are of no benefit unless measured serum levels are low.

Malnutrition

Specific nutritional deficiencies can interfere with the wound healing process. Malnutrition alters tissue regeneration, the inflammatory reaction, and immune function. Carbohydrate provides the substrate for cell proliferation and phagocytic activity. Fat is a vital component of cell membranes, and protein-derived amino acids are essential for tissue synthesis and repair. When compared to wounds in well-nourished control patients, wounds in malnourished patients contain less hydroxyproline.[18]

Chronic and profound malnutrition, common in patients with advanced malignancy, has long been associated with impaired wound healing. In animal models, malnutrition is associated with a decrease in wound bursting strength and colonic anastomotic bursting pressures.

Clinical studies have shown that the adverse effect of malnutrition on wound healing can be significantly improved by a short period of preoperative feeding and does not require absolute correction of the protein-calorie deficit.[25] In addition, randomized prospective trials have suggested a substantial reduction in both surgical morbidity and mortality in patients (with and without cancer) who receive perioperative parenteral nutritional support.[25]

Corticosteroid Use

Corticosteroids inhibit the influx of inflammatory cells, the migration and proliferation of macrophages, and the proliferation of wound fibroblasts; stunt angiogenesis and capillary budding; and decrease the rate of epithelialization.[2] High-dose corticosteroid therapy used before or immediately after wounding significantly delayed wound healing in experimental systems.

Although few clinical evaluations document this problem, the use of long-acting absorbable or permanent sutures should be considered for fascial closure in an attempt to minimize acute wound failure.

Diabetes

Poorly controlled insulin-dependent diabetes adversely affects wound healing. The rate of wound infection is increased, as is the rate of wound separation and dehiscence. A component in some diabetic patients is related to impaired blood supply related to microangiopathy.[25] In addition, hyperglycemia results in an impaired inflammatory response, multifactorial leukocyte dysfunction, and alterations in cellular and humoral immunity. In experimental systems, decreased wound collagen content, decreased wound granulation, and decreased wound breaking strength have been reported. Although several reports suggest that patients with diabetes have an increased risk of wound infection and wound separation, other reports suggest that with strict perioperative control of blood glucose levels, most of these impediments can be reversed.[25] Although many methods exist, it behooves the pelvic surgeon to monitor and maintain control during the perioperative period.

Renal Failure/Uremia

Patients with acute and chronic renal failure have been reported to have an increased incidence of wound infections as well as delayed or impaired wound healing. In experimental animals this seems to be related to the toxic effects of elevated levels of urea on the formation of granulation tissue without alteration in wound collagen content or composition. Dialysis and nutritional support have been reported to reverse the grossly measurable clinical defects, and near normal wound healing has been reported in carefully managed patients.

Radiation Therapy

Therapeutic dosages of radiation therapy create a unique set of surgical problems. The most profound effects of therapeutic irradiation on wound repair are observed when operations are performed *within* a treatment field many months or years after completion of therapy. After sufficient time has elapsed, the treatment volume is characterized by a loss of elastic fibers, the development of often extensive regional fibrosis, and the development of obliterative endarteritis.[83] This abnormality poses a significant problem if a later operation is performed in the irradiated field.[83]

Therapeutic radiation given 2 to 4 weeks *prior to* wounding is associated with increased capillary dilation within the treatment field ("wound hyperemia") with attendant increase in wound vascularity and operative blood loss. There is a therapeutic window: if surgery is delayed until the hyperemic phase has resolved (4–6 weeks after completion of radiation), there is little if any disruption of acute wound healing. Therapeutic radiation delivered at the time of wounding (or up to 6 days after wounding) results in an impaired inflammatory response, delayed myofibroblast transformation, and a decrease in collagen synthesis and cross-linking within the wound.[84]

Because radiation wounds present a unique problem related to inadequate vascularity and poor oxygenation as a result of progressive obliterative endarteritis,[18] management of these wounds often requires revascularization procedures with a well-vascularized flap. There appears to be little difference in the healing capacity of flaps between irradiated and nonirradiated recipient areas.[84]

Chemotherapy

Almost every cytotoxic agent available for clinical chemotherapy has been demonstrated to interfere with the early phases of wound healing in laboratory and animal models, including impairment of the initial inflammatory response, recruitment of fibroblasts, and neovascularization.[18] Clinical correlation of these observations is, however, lacking. Indeed, several studies have reported no increase in wound complication rates in patients treated with postoperative chemotherapy, even when efforts were made to administer chemotherapy as soon as possible after surgery.[85] One recent study found that clinical wound repair in patients treated with chemotherapy who developed postoperative wound complications was at least as good as wound repair in "normal" general obstetric and gynecologic patients reported in the literature.[85] Additionally, the early use of chemotherapy (before the 11th postoperative day) did not increase wound complication rates when compared with later treatment. Although laboratory studies suggest a detrimental effect on wound healing, chemotherapy should not be delayed in those who may potentially benefit from immediate cytotoxic therapy.[86]

Hypoxemia

Prolonged low tissue oxygen tension (PO_2) impairs healing.[2,87] However, wounds with a high PO_2 are resistant to infection. Molecular oxygen, an essential factor in wound healing, is required for energy-dependent processes, including cell replication, protein synthesis, protein export, and the hydroxylation of proline and lysine prior to their incorporation into collagen. Oxygen is essential to produce toxic superoxide radicals used by granulocytes to kill phagocytized bacteria. Neutrophil phagocytosis triggers a series of metabolic events that results in a 15- to 20-fold increase in oxygen consumption.[88]

Methods to measure tissue PO_2 are not clinically available, and therefore tissue PO_2 can only be estimated by measuring arterial PO_2 and assessing peripheral perfusion. It must be remembered that changes in FiO_2 produce small changes in actual arterial oxygen content but can produce large changes in tissue PO_2. In fact, inspiring an FiO_2 of 45% may alter tissue PO_2 from 10 mm Hg to 40 mm Hg.[88]

Wound perfusion is paramount to maintaining tissue oxygenation.[89] Dehydration or hypovolemia (which further increases sympathetic tone) should be avoided to maximize the wound environment. In women with normal cardiopulmonary reserve, tissue PO_2 does not fall until hemoglobin levels fall below 6 g/dL.[18] Supplemental oxygen decreases infection risk as much as prophylactic antibiotics and is most effective when combined with antibiotics.[54] Oxygen supplementation should be considered in all patients, as they may suffer from hypoxemia, and advocated in patients with specific vascular disease.

Special Circumstances

Wound Infection

The risk of abdominal wound infection is significant following gynecologic surgery. The frequency of infection is at least 5.0%[90] after abdominal hysterectomy for benign indications and increases after more radical procedures.

The presence of erythema, induration, or late unexplained postoperative fever necessitates careful evaluation of the surgical incision. Simple removal of several sutures or clips with wound probing will often release an undrained seroma or purulence, with minimal cosmetic sequelae. If purulence is discovered, immediate drainage alters pH and decreases the adverse effect of specific binding proteins or inactivating enzymes.[91] The placement of normal saline–soaked wet-to-dry dressing (three times daily) and secondary closure is an alternative. In most situations, drainage suffices; however, staphylococcal or streptococcal infections (suggested by a wide zone of diffuse erythema) may require appropriate antibiotic administration. Cultures should be considered if clinical problems persist.[91] Anaerobic cultures may be important, as these organisms are present in approximately 30% of wound abscesses.[9]

Recent attention has focused on the role of "early" reclosure of disrupted incisions.[92] In one prospective study of wounds reclosed after 4 days, the success rate was 85.7% (30/35) with a mean healing time of 15.8 days. These findings compared favorably to those wounds not successfully reclosed (67.2 days) and those allowed to heal by secondary intention (71.8 days to healing).[92] There may be a role for broad-spectrum antibiotics in the treatment of severe abscesses that are successfully reclosed.[93] "Early closure" can also be successfully performed following the diagnosis of an infected dehiscence of an episiotomy. One recent report suggested a 94% success rate with early (3–13 days) closure.[94]

Wound Disruption

The published rates of complete wound disruption vary from 0% to 3%. The risk of dehiscence is greater for vertical (1% to 3%) than transverse incisions (0.37%–0.69%).[34] In most gynecologic procedures, this risk should be less than 1%.

The potential causes include suture knot problems (breaking or untying), suture rupture, or fascial tear secondary to improper suture placement or weakened tissue in patients with coexisting disease or malnutrition. Clinically, improper suture placement (<1.5 cm from the fascial edge) is the most common correctable problem. In the laboratory, sutures tied with tension lead to increased neutrophil accumulation and decreased wound strength.[95]

Wound disruption most frequently occurs in the elderly (>60 years) and is often associated with increased intra-abdominal pressure. The problem is seen clinically on the seventh to tenth postoperative day and is often preceded by leakage of peritoneal fluids from the abdominal incision.

Fascial evisceration should be considered a surgical emergency, as it carries a mortality of 10% to 30%. In this situation, the intestinal tract should be managed with moistened, sterile laparotomy pads (or towels) with immediate mass closure using permanent suture after incision debridement.

In cases associated with infection and late fascial disruption, conservative management may be appropriate; however, these patients will develop late wound complications in the form of hernias.

Incisional Hernia

Late wound failure (hernia) is a common problem following abdominal closure. Although the reported incidence varies, it may approach 7% to 15% with sufficient follow-up.[96] Long-term follow-up is important, as 5.6% of patients may develop wound hernias at 2½ to 5½ years.[96]

In one study of more than 1,000 laparotomies, herniation was more likely to occur in the elderly, those who underwent colonic surgery, and those with incisions larger than 18 cm.[96] Others suggest the role of increased abdominal pressure and obesity.[24] Late risks of wound failure could not be correlated with surgical experience, but 48% of patients with a wound infection following surgery developed a hernia.[96] Although this study could not document a difference between transverse and vertical incisions, the risk was significantly higher in incisions closed with absorbable suture.[96]

Repair must minimize wound tension and may necessitate a mesh graft.[36] Herniorrhaphy of a previously infected wound is associated with a higher risk (3.5×) of infection, even with complete skin healing and the absence of current infection.[97] For this reason, this operative procedure should not be strictly considered a clean operation, and patients may benefit from antibiotic prophylaxis.

Despite method of repair, recurrent incisional hernias are common, with a recent reported rate of 41% at 5 years.[98] The re-recurrence rate was greater than 50%. The only important risk factor was hernia size, with the risk almost doubled for hernias larger than 4 cm.

Stoma

The formation of an intestinal stoma is an important aspect of a number of operative procedures.[99] If possible, the site should be marked preoperatively to ensure that it is away from bony prominences, skin folds, or existing scars. In general, lower abdominal placement is preferable; however, upper abdominal placement may be superior in the obese. If so, the site should be at least 2 cm below the costal margin and lateral to the umbilicus.[99]

In contrast to ileostomy, the sigmoid colon can be matured with little rosebud as the semisolid fecal matter is evacuated twice daily. Some believe that a flush end colostomy is preferable, as it facilitates irrigation.[99] It would appear that the entire fecal stream is diverted with a loop colostomy.

Immediate postoperative stoma care is important. A normal stoma invariably has a moderate amount of venous engorgement and edema and usually appears dusky.[100] If necrosis occurs, a test tube can be placed into the stoma to allow illumination to determine the depth. If necrosis is below the fascia, immediate revision may be necessary.[99,101]

Late complications such as retraction (usually related to inadequate mobilization or stoma necrosis), stricture (stomal necrosis), prolapse, or parastomal hernia are not common.

References

1. Orr JW Jr: Sutures and closures. Ala J Med Sci 23:36–41, 1986.
2. Madden JW, Arem AJ: Wound healing: Biologic and clinical features. In Sabiston DC Jr (ed): Textbook of Surgery: The Biological Basis of Modern Surgical Practice, 14th ed, p 165. Philadelphia: WB Saunders, 1991.
3. Eckersley JRT, Dudley HAF: Wounds and wound healing. Br Med Bull 44:423–436, 1988.
4. Edlich RF: Biology of wound repair: Its influence on surgical decision. Facial Plast Surg 1:169–180, 1984.
5. Edlich RF: The biology of wound repair and infection: A personal odyssey. Ann Emerg Med 14:1019–1025, 1985.
6. Chan P, Lewis AAM: Influence of suture technique on surgical glove perforation. Br J Surg 76:1208–1209, 1989.
7. Peacock EE Jr: Wound healing and wound care. In Schwartz SI (ed): Principles of Surgery, 5th ed, chap 8. New York: McGraw-Hill, 1989.
8. Seppa H, Grotendorst G, Seppa S, et al: Platelet-derived growth factor is chemotactic for fibroblasts. J Cell Biol 92:584, 1982.
9. Grinnell F, Billingham RE, Burgess L: Distribution of fibronectin during wound healing in vitro. J Invest Dermatol 76:1279, 1982.
10. Knighton DR, Hunt TK, Thakral KK, et al: Role of platelets and fibrin in the healing sequence: An in vitro study of angiogenesis and collagen synthesis. Ann Surg 196:379, 1982.
11. Thakral KK, Goodson WH, Hunt TK: Stimulation of wound blood vessel growth by wound macrophages. J Surg Res 26:430, 1979.
12. Miyazawa K: Role of epidermal growth factor in obstetrics and gynecology. Obstet Gynecol 79:1032–1040, 1992.
13. Pessa ME, Bland KI, Copeland EM III: Growth factors and determinants of wound repair. J Surg Res 42:207–217, 1987.
14. Fong Y, Lowry SF: Cytokines and the cellular response to injury and infection. In: Trauma, chap 7. Chicago: American College of Surgeons, 1990.
15. Mooney DP, O'Reilly M, Gamelli RL: Tumor necrosis factor and wound healing. Ann Surg 211:124–129, 1990.
16. Christou NV: Predicting infectious morbidity in elective operations. Am J Surg 165:52S–58S, 1993.
17. Bryant CA, Rodeheaver GT, Reem EM, et al: Search for a nontoxic surgical scrub solution for periorbital lacerations. Ann Emerg Med 13:317–321, 1984.
18. Ehrlichman RJ, Seckel BR, Bryan DJ, Moschella CJ: Common complications of wound healing. Surg Clin North Am 71:1323–1350, 1991.
19. Burkett G, Jensen LP, Lai A, et al: Evaluation of surgical staples in cesarean section. Am J Obstet Gynecol 161:540–547, 1989.
20. Carucci DJ, Scott R, Pearce C, et al: Evaluation of hemostatic agents for skin graft donor sites. J Burn Care Rehabil 5:321–323, 1984.
21. Deholl D, Rodeheaver G, Edgerton T, Edlich RF: Potentiation of infection by suture closure of dead space. Am J Surg 127:716–720, 1974.
22. DelValle GO, Combs P, Qualls C, Curet LB: Does closure of camper fascia reduce the incidence of post-cesarean superficial wound disruption? Obstet Gynecol 80:1013–1016, 1992.
23. Cho JY, Cha K, Kim MI: Interrupted circular suture: Bleeding control during cesarean delivery in placenta previa accreta. Obstet Gynecol 78:876–879, 1991.
24. Lazaro da Silva A, Petroianu A: Incisional hernias: Factors influencing development. South Med J 84:1500–1504, 1991.
25. Care of the surgical wound. In: Care of the Surgical Patient, chap 7. New York: Scientific American, 1991.
26. Cruse PJE, Foord R: A five-year prospective study of 23,649 surgical wounds. Arch Surg 107:206–214, 1973.
27. Mackenzie I: Preoperative skin preparation and surgical outcome. J Hosp Infect 11(suppl B):27–32, 1988.
28. Edlich RF, Rodeheaver GT, Thacker JG: Technical factors in the prevention of wound infections. In Simmons RL, Howard RJ (eds): Surgical Infectious Diseases, chap 22. New York: Appleton-Century-Crofts, 1982.
29. Tokars JI, Bell DM, Culver DH, et al: Percutaneous injuries during surgical procedures. JAMA 267:2899–2904, 1992.
30. Masterson BJ: Skin preparation. In: Care of the Surgical Patient, chap 2. New York: Scientific American, 1991.
31. Brantley SK, St. Arnold PA, Das SK: Antiseptic use in wound management. Infect Surg:33–39, 1990.
32. Helmkamp BF, Krebs HB: The Maryland incision in gynecologic surgery. Am J Obstet Gynecol 163:1554, 1990.
33. Sanders RJ, Diclementi D, Ireland K: Principles of abdominal wound closure: I. Animal studies. Arch Surg 112:1184–1187, 1977.
34. Johnson JC, Barnes WA: How to choose the right abdominal incision. Contemp Ob/Gyn:56–73, 1993.
35. Greer BE, Cain JM, Figge DC, Shy KK, Tamimi HK: Supraumbilical upper abdominal midline incision for pelvic surgery in the morbidly obese patient. Obstet Gynecol 76:471–473, 1990.
36. Fry DE, Osler T: Abdominal wall considerations and complications in reoperative surgery. Surg Clin North Am 71:1–11, 1991.
37. Edlich RF, Rodeheaver GT, Thacker JG, Edgerton MT: Fundamentals of wound management in surgery: Technical factors in wound management. South Plainfield, NJ: Chirurgecom Inc, 1977.
38. Rodeheaver G, Edgerton MT, Smith S, et al: Antimicrobial prophylaxis of contaminated tissues containing suture implants. Am J Surg 133:609–611, 1977.
39. Hasselgren P, Hagberg E, Malmer H, et al: One instead of two knives for surgical incision: Does it increase the risk of postoperative wound infection? Arch Surg 119:917–920, 1984.
40. Kumagai SG, Rosales RF, Hunter GC, et al: Effects of electrocautery on midline laparotomy wound infection. Am J Surg 162:620, 1991.

41. Pearlman NW, Stiegmann GV, Vance V, et al: A prospective study of incisional time, blood loss, pain, and healing with carbon dioxide laser, scalpel, and electrosurgery. Arch Surg 126:1018–1020, 1991.

42. Guidelines for prevention of wound infection. In: Care of the Surgical Patient, chap 5. New York: Scientific American, 1991.

43. Ritter EF, Demas DP, Thompson DA, Devereux DF: Effects of method of hemostasis on wound infection rate. Am Surg 56:648–650, 1990.

44. Edlich RF, Panek PH, Rodeheaver GT, et al: Physical and chemical configuration of sutures in the development of surgical infection. Ann Surg 177:679–688, 1973.

45. Metz SA, Chegini N, Masterson BJ: In vivo tissue reactivity and degradation of suture materials: A comparison of Maxon and PDS. J Gynecol Surg 5:37–46, 1989.

46. Orr JW Jr, Orr PF, Barrett JM, et al: Fascial closure: Continuous or interrupted? A prospective evaluation of #1 Maxon suture in 402 gynecologic procedures. Am J Obstet Gynecol 163:1485–1489, 1990.

47. McGeehan D, Hunt D, Chaudhuri A, Rutter P: An experimental study of the relationship between synergistic wound sepsis and suture materials. Br J Surg 67:636–638, 1980.

48. Mahomed K, Grant A, Ashurst H, James D: The Southmead perineal suture study: A randomized comparison of suture materials and suturing techniques for repair of perineal trauma. Br J Obstet Gynaecol 96:1272–1280, 1989.

48a. Hay DL, von Fraunhaufer JA, Masterson BJ: Hemostasis in blood vessels after ligation. Am J Obstet Gynecol 260:737, 1989.

49. Mirana R, Luciano A, Muzzi L, et al: Reproductive outcome after ovarian surgery: Suturing vs. nonsuturing of the ovarian cortex. J Gynecol Surg 7:155, 1991.

50. Hauth JC, Owen J, Davis RO: Transverse uterine incision closure: One versus two layers. Am J Obstet Gynecol 167:1108–1111, 1992.

51. von Rijssel EJ, Brand R, Admiral C, et al: Tissue reaction and surgical knots: The effect of suture size, knot configuration, and knot volume. Obstet Gynecol 74:64–68, 1989.

52. Terra H, Aberg C: Tensile strengths of twelve types of knot employed in surgery, using different suture materials. Acta Chir Scand 142:1–7, 1976.

53. Orr JW Jr, Shingleton HM, Hatch KD, Taylor PT, et al: Urinary diversion in patients undergoing pelvic exenteration. Am J Obstet Gynecol 142:883–889, 1982.

54. Summit RL Jr, Stovall TG, Lipscomb GH, Ling FW: Randomized comparison of laparoscopy-assisted vaginal hysterectomy with standard vaginal hysterectomy in an outpatient setting. Obstet Gynecol 80:895–901, 1992.

55. Daniell JF, Kurtz BR, Lee JY: Laparoscopic oophorectomy: A comparative study of ligatures, bipolar coagulation, and automatic stapling devices. Obstet Gynecol 80:325–328, 1992.

56. Villeneuve MG, Khalife S, Marcoux S, Blanchet P: Surgical staples in cesarean section: A randomized controlled trial. Am J Obstet Gynecol 163:1641–1646, 1990.

57. Winn HR, Jane JA, Rodeheaver GT, et al: Influence of subcuticular sutures on scar formation. Am J Surg 113:257–259, 1977.

58. Barker W, Rodeheaver GT, Edgerton MT, Edlich RF: Damage to tissue defenses by a topical anesthetic agent. Ann Emerg Med 11:307–310, 1982.

59. England GT, Randall HW, Graves WL: Impairment of tissue defenses by vasoconstrictors in vaginal hysterectomies. Obstet Gynecol 61:271–274, 1983.

60. Cunningham AJ, Donnelly M, Bourke A, Murphy JF: Cardiovascular and metabolic effects of cervical epinephrine infiltration. Obstet Gynecol 66:93–98, 1985.

61. Moss JP: Historical and current perspectives on surgical drainage. Surg Gynecol Obstet 152:517–527, 1981.

62. Magee C, Rodeheaver GT, Golden GT, et al: Potentiation of wound infection by surgical drains. Am J Surg 131:547–549, 1976.

63. Farnell MB, Worthington-Self S, Mucha P, et al: Closure of abdominal incisions with subcutaneous catheters. Arch Surg 121:641–648, 1986.

64. Lubowski D, Hunt DR: Abdominal wound drainage: A prospective randomized trial. Med J Aust 146:133–135, 1987.

65. Orr JW Jr, Barter JF, Kilgore LC, et al: Closed suction pelvic drainage after radical pelvic surgical procedures. Am J Obstet Gynecol 155:867–871, 1986.

66. Clarke-Pearson D, Cliby W, Soper J, et al: Morbidity and mortality of selective lymphadenectomy in early stage endometrial cancer. Presented at the 22nd annual meeting of the Society of Gynecologic Oncologists, Orlando, Fla, Feb 17–20, 1991.

67. Jensen JK, Disaia PJ, Lucci JA III, et al: To drain or not to drain? A retrospective study of closed-suction drainage following hysterectomy with lymphadenectomy. Presented at the 24th annual meeting of the Society of Gynecologic Oncologists, Palm Desert, Calif, Feb 7–10, 1993.

68. Becker GD: Ineffectiveness of closed suction drainage cultures in the prediction of bacteriologic findings in wound infections in patients undergoing contaminated head and neck cancer surgery. Otolaryngol Head Neck Surg 93:743–747, 1985.

69. Creasman WT, Hill GB, Weed JC Jr, Gall SA: A trial of prophylactic cefamandole in extended gynecologic surgery. Obstet Gynecol 59:309–314, 1982.

70. Orr JW Jr, Taylor PT: Reducing postoperative infection in the patient with gynecologic cancer. Infect Surg 12:361–372, 1987.

71. Scher KS, Peoples JB: Combined use of topical and systemic antibiotics. Am J Surg 161:422–425, 1991.

72. Madden J, Edlich RF, Schauerhamer R, et al: Application of principles of fluid dynamics to surgical wound irrigation. Curr Topics Surg Res 3:85–93, 1971.

73. Foresman PA, Edlich RF, Rodeheaver GT: The effect of new monofilament absorbable sutures on the healing of musculoaponeurotic incisions, gastrotomies, and colonic anastomoses. Arch Surg 124:708–710, 1989.

74. Gallup DG, Nolan TE, Smith RP: Primary mass closure of midline incisions with a continuous polyglyconate monofilament absorbable suture. Obstet Gynecol 76:872–875, 1990.

75. Tulandi T, Hum HS, Gelfand MM: Closure of laparotomy incisions with or without peritoneal suturing and second look laparoscopy. Am J Obstet Gynecol 158:536–537, 1988.

76. Hull DB, Varner MW: A randomized study of closure of the peritoneum at cesarean delivery. Obstet Gynecol 77:818–821, 1991.

77. Edlich RF, Rodeheaver G, Kuphal J, et al: Technique of closure: Contaminated wounds. J Am Coll Emerg Phys 3:375–381, 1974.

78. Dougherty SH, Fiegel VD, Nelson RD, et al: Effects of soil infection potentiating factors on neutrophils in vitro. Am J Surg 150:306–311, 1985.

79. Marshall DA, Mertz PM, Eaglstein WH: Occlusive dressings. Arch Surg 125:1136–1139, 1990.

80. Katz S, McGinley K, Leyden JJ: Semipermeable occlusive dressings. Arch Dermatol 122:58–62, 1986.

81. Bohnen JMA, Solomkin JS, Patchen E, et al: Guidelines for clinical care: Anti-infective agents for intra-abdominal infection. Arch Surg 127:83–89, 1992.

82. Wenzel RP: Preoperative antibiotic prophylaxis (editorial). N Engl J Med 326:337–338, 1992.

83. Miller SH, Rudolph R: Healing in the irradiated wound. Clin Plast Surg 17:503–508, 1990.

84. Aitasalo K, Aro HT, Virolainen P, Virolainen E: Healing of microvascular free skin flaps in irradiated recipient tissue beds. Am J Surg 164:662–666, 1992.

85. Kolb BA, Buller RE, Connor JP, et al: Effects of early postoperative chemotherapy on wound healing. Obstet Gynecol 79:988–992, 1992.

86. Omura GA, Bundy BN, Berek JS, et al: Randomized trial of cyclophosphamide plus cisplatin with or without doxorubicin in ovarian carcinoma: A Gynecologic Oncology Group study. J Clin Oncol 7:457–465, 1989.

87. Jonsson K, Jensen JA, Goodson WH, et al: Tissue oxygenation, anemia, and perfusion in relation to wound healing in surgical patients. Ann Surg 214:605–613, 1991.

88. Knighton DR, Halliday B, Hunt TK: Oxygen as an antibiotic: A comparison of the effects of inspired oxygen concentration and antibiotic administration on in vivo bacterial clearance. Arch Surg 121:191–195, 1986.

89. Jensen JA, Goodson WH, Vasconez LO, Hunt TK: Wound healing in anemia. West J Med 144:465–467, 1986.

90. Dicker RC, Greenspan JR, Strauss LT, et al: Complications of abdominal and vaginal hysterectomy among women of reproductive age in the United States. Am J Obstet Gynecol 144:841–847, 1982.

91. Brook I, Frazier EH: Aerobic and anaerobic bacteriology of wounds and cutaneous abscesses. Arch Surg 125:1445–1451, 1990.

92. Walters MD, Dombroski RA, Davidson SA, et al: Reclosure of disrupted abdominal incisions. Obstet Gynecol 76:597–602, 1990.

93. Gottrup F, Gjode P, Lundhus F, et al: Management of severe incisional abscesses following laparotomy. Arch Surg 124:702–704, 1989.

94. Ramin SM, Ramus RM, Little BB, Gilstrap LC: Early repair of episiotomy dehiscence associated with infection. Am J Obstet Gynecol 167:1104–1107, 1992.

95. Hogstrom H, Haglund U, Zederfeldt B: Tension leads to increased neutrophil accumulation and decreased laparotomy wound strength. Surgery 107:215–219, 1990.

96. Ellis H, Bucknall TE, Cox PJ: Abdominal incisions and their closure. Curr Prob Surg 22:5–51, 1985.

97. Houck JP, Typins EB, Sarfeh IJ, et al: Repair of incisional hernia. Surg Gynecol Obstet 169:397–399, 1989.

98. Hesselink VJ, Luijendijk RW, Dewilt JHW, et al: An evaluation of risk factors in incisional hernia recurrence. Surg Gynecol Obstet 177:228–234, 1993.

99. Abcarian H, Pearl RK: Stomas. Surg Clin North Am 68:1295–1305, 1988.

100. Doberneck RC: Revision and closure of the colostomy. Surg Clin North Am 71:193–201, 1991.

101. Edlich RF, Kenney JG, Morgan RF, et al: Antimicrobial treatment of minor soft tissue lacerations: A critical review. Emerg Clin North Am 4:561, 1986.

Complications in Gynecologic Surgery: Prevention, Recognition, and Management,
edited by James W. Orr, Jr., and Hugh M. Shingleton.
J. B. Lippincott Company, Philadelphia, © 1994.

Chapter 7

Vascular Access

Victoria L. Seewaldt
Benjamin E. Greer

The development of central venous catheters has had an enormous impact on the practice of medicine. Their use has revolutionized critical care, facilitated the development of total parenteral nutrition (TPN), and permitted many advancements in the care of cancer patients. Central venous catheters and access have become such an integral part of medicine that it is difficult for a physician currently in training to conceive of a time when the ability to achieve safe, central access at the bedside was not possible.

History

Central venous catheterization was first reported in 1952, when Aubaniac[1] described the infraclavicular approach to subclavian vein catheterization for rapid volume replacement. Ten years later Wilson et al.[2] described infraclavicular subcutaneous venous cannulization as a method for monitoring central venous pressure. Ashbaugh and Thompson[3] attempted to popularize this technique in the early 1960s but met with much criticism, owing to the high rate of complications in catheter placement and maintenance, including pneumothorax and thrombosis.[4] In 1965 Yoffa[5] described the supraclavicular approach to subclavian cannulization, claiming it to be both safer and simpler than the infraclavicular approach. Internal jugular vein cannulization was first described in 1966 by Hermosura et al.,[6] and a detailed description of this technique was reported by English et al. in 1969.[7] To date, three different approaches to catheterizing the internal jugular vein have been described.

The development of permanent venous access began with the advent of chronic hemodialysis. In 1960 Quinton et al. (Scribner)[8] devised the external arteriovenous shunt, the first device that allowed long-term access to venous circulation. The silicone rubber elastomer proved to be an excellent biocompatible material, producing minimal thrombosis and trauma to the vessel intima. In 1966 the Bresica-Cimino fistula, a surgically created internal fistula between the radial artery and vein, was introduced. The fistula decreased the risks of clotting and infection that occurred frequently with the external shunt.[9]

The introduction of TPN in 1968 provided the stimulation for further refinements in permanent venous access techniques and catheters. Dudrick et al.[10] demonstrated that growth, development, and a positive nitrogen balance could be achieved with parenteral feeding alone. This was a major breakthrough in surgical care, because for the first time it became possible to overcome the hypercatabolic state in patients whose postoperative courses were complicated by prolonged ileus, sepsis, or poor wound healing. TPN allowed nonoperative as well as operative intervention to be successful in patients with fistulas and chronically infected wounds directly related to nutritional defects.[11] It made survival possible for patients who might otherwise have died of postoperative complications directly related to nutritional defects. The nutrient solution, however, was too irritating and sclerosing to be administered long term by peripheral vein and required infusion into a temporary catheter threaded into the superior vena cava. This method of administration allowed rapid dilution and peripheral distribution of the nutrients at isotonic concentrations. The major obstacle to long-term TPN was maintaining safe, permanent access to the central venous circulation.

To overcome the obstacles of long-term venous access, Scribner et al. in 1970 devised the "artificial gut" system.[12] Nutrient solution was introduced through an external arteriovenous shunt, allowing patients to receive TPN at home. However, unlike patients with chronic renal failure, patients with chronic intestinal disease did not have uremic platelet dysfunction, and clots tended to accumulate in these shunts. For this reason attention again focused on developing other methods of permanent central access.

Broviac et al. in 1973[13] developed a soft silicone rubber elastomer catheter that was inserted into the subclavian vein by a venous cutdown or through a skin incision. An extravascular segment of the catheter ran through a subcutaneous tunnel within the anterior chest wall, exiting near the sternal border below the level of the nipple. A Dacron cuff placed 2 to 3 cm from the exit site was incorporated along the extravascular segment, providing for a strong anchoring point for the surrounding tissue as fibroelastic scar tissue grew into the Dacron material. This tissue barrier also discouraged the migration of skin flora into the central circulation along the catheter tract.

In the late 1970s right atrial catheters were routinely employed for the delivery of TPN to bone marrow transplant patients; however, these small-diameter catheters could not be used to deliver blood products. Patients undergoing transplantation needed to receive multiple solutions including chemotherapy, blood products, and antibiotics, and to have blood drawn frequently. Unfortunately, these patients typically had been extensively treated before transplantation and had few usable veins for access. Robert Hickman[14] in collaboration with oncologists at the Fred Hutchinson Cancer Research Center developed a modified right atrial catheter that helped solve some of the venous access problems in bone marrow transplant patients. The Hickman catheter was similar to the one developed by Broviac but had a slightly thicker wall and an internal diameter of 0.32 mm rather than the commonly used 0.22 mm. The larger lumen allowed infusion of blood products and the drawing of blood (Fig. 7–1).

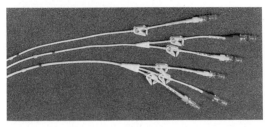

FIGURE 7–1. Three sizes of permanent venous catheters. *Top,* single lumen; *middle,* double lumen; *bottom,* triple lumen. Reprinted by permission of Chapman & Hall, from Hickman RO, et al: Central venous access. In Greer B, Berek J (eds): Gynecologic Oncology: Treatment Rationale and Techniques, p 286. © 1991 Elsevier Science Publishing Co, Inc.

The single-lumen Hickman catheter rapidly gained acceptance. However, it became apparent that more than one port or access line was needed to meet the antibiotic, hyperalimentation, and blood product requirements of transplant recipients. A double-lumen Hickman catheter was developed in 1981.[15] Initial nutritional studies demonstrated that patients with double-lumen Hickman catheters received a greater percentage of their TPN calorie requirements than did control patients with a single-lumen catheter, with a similar frequency of septicemia in both groups.[15] Today the Hickman catheter has become an integral part of the care of cancer patients and others with long-term antibiotic and TPN requirements. However, this line requires regular attention. Patients or their caregivers must use sterile technique, frequently flush the ports, and be able to recognize signs of infection. Moreover, the ports are visible externally and may be cosmetically undesirable for some patients.

In 1982 Niederhuber's group[16] developed a totally implantable subcutaneous port system for long-term venous access, called the Port-a-Cath. The device, made of stainless steel, titanium, or plastic, consists of a subcutaneous injection port attached to a catheter that enters into the central venous circulation. It is accessed by a noncoring needle through a self-sealing septum made of silicone rubber. If properly managed, the septum will allow 2,000 punctures. Between injections the system is "locked" with heparin and requires no maintenance except a heparin flush every 6 weeks. The port is palpable but not visible at the skin surface, and requires no dressing changes (Fig. 7–2).

The Groshong catheter,[17] a thin-walled silicone catheter with a subcutaneous extravascular segment with or without a Dacron cuff, is a further refinement of the right atrial catheter that also attempts to minimize maintenance requirements. It employs a

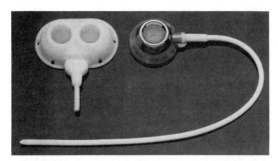

FIGURE 7–2. Subcutaneous port system. The right port is a single port made of stainless steel. The left port is made of plastic and is a dual-port version. Reprinted by permission of Chapman & Hall, from Hickman RO, et al: Central venous access. In Greer B, Berek J (eds): Gynecologic Oncology: Treatment Rationale and Techniques, p 286. © 1991 Elsevier Science Publishing Co, Inc.

two-way slit valve that allows infusion and blood return but remains closed when not in use. This decreases the need for frequent flushing and theoretically reduces the rate of associated thrombosis.[18]

The most recent developments in central venous access have come about in response to the need for cost containment and a tendency toward decreased hospital stays. In the 1990s home intravenous (IV) therapy has become a mainstay of medical management in many clinical situations. This out-of-hospital care places a greater burden on home care nurses to maintain vascular access. A new peripheral central venous catheter, the peripherally inserted central catheter, or PICC,[19] provides reliable central access and can be inserted at the bedside by specially trained nurses. The risk of mechanical catheter insertion complications such as pneumothorax or hemothorax is eliminated by the peripheral insertion site. The catheter tip can be placed in either the superior vena cava or the subclavian vein, depending on the type of solution to be infused. Tip placement is estimated by external measurement and the catheter is trimmed accordingly. Placement is confirmed with a postinsertion chest radiograph. The PICC line can be used to deliver chemotherapy, TPN, and sclerosing solutions, as well as IV fluid and antibiotics.

Temporary Venous Access

Central Venous Catheterization

Central venous catheters, Swan-Ganz catheters, and arterial lines are frequently needed perioperatively as well as in the care of critically ill nonsurgical patients. Central venous catheters are also useful in the care of chronically ill but medically stable patients and patients with poor venous access. The decision to use a particular method of venous or arterial access is situation dependent; there is no list of absolute indications for line placement. However, there are many situations in which central venous and Swan-Ganz lines are helpful.

Common indications for central venous catheterization include poor or inadequate peripheral venous access, rapid large-volume or transfusion requirements, administration of sclerosing agents such as TPN or chemotherapy, emergency access, and the measurement of central venous pressures (Table 7–1). With the exception of extensive thrombosis of the superior vena cava, there are few absolute contraindications to central venous catheterization. Relative contraindications include uncorrected coagulopathies, superior vena cava syndrome, previous neck surgery, an uncooperative patient, severe orthopnea, and the presence of a contralateral hematoma, hemothorax, or pneumothorax.

Preoperative indications for Swan-Ganz catheterization and radial artery catheterization are controversial and are based on risk assessment data. In 1977 Goldman[24] reported attempts to risk stratify patients to predict cardiac risks and complications of noncardiac surgery. He developed a scoring system (Table 7–2) to assess perioperative cardiac risk based on the severity of the underlying heart failure, the occurrence of a recent myocardial infarction or arrhythmias, the presence of aortic stenosis, the patient's age and medical condition, and the type of surgery to be performed. Goldman recommended perioperative hemodynamic monitoring

TABLE 7–1. **Indications for Central Venous Access**

Poor venous access

Emergency venous access

Rapid volume replacement

Large-volume blood product administration

Central venous pressure measurements

Pulmonary artery catheter placement

Transvenous pacing

Administration of sclerosing agents

Chemotherapy

Total parenteral nutrition

Hemodialysis

Plasmapheresis

TABLE 7–2. Goldman Criteria: Multifactorial Index Score to Estimate Cardiac Risk in Noncardiac Surgery

Factor	Points
S_3 gallop or jugular venous distention on preoperative physical examination	11
Transmural or subendocardial myocardial infarction in the previous 6 months	10
Premature ventricular beats, more than 5/min	7
Rhythm other than sinus, or presence of premature atrial contraction	7
Age >70 years	5
Emergency operation	4
Intrathoracic, intraperitoneal, or aortic valve surgery	3
Evidence for important valvular aortic stenosis	3

Poor general medical condition
    Potassium < 3.0 mEq/L
    Bicarbonate < 20 mEq/L
    Blood urea nitrogen > 50 mg/dL
    Creatinine > 3.0 mg/dL
    Pao_2 < 60 mm Hg
    $Paco_2$ > 50 mm Hg
    Abnormal liver status
    Chronically bedridden
	3

Scoring System

Class I: (0–5 points)   0.7% nonfatal but life-threatening complications, 0.2% fatal complications

Class II: (6–12 points)   5% nonfatal but life-threatening complications, 2% fatal complications

Class III: (13–25 points)   11% nonfatal but life-threatening complications, 2% fatal complications

Class IV: (26 or more points)   22% nonfatal but life-threatening complications, 56% fatal complications

Reproduced with permission from Goldman L: Cardiac risks and complications of noncardiac surgery. Ann Intern Med 98:504, 1983.

for patients in class IV of his multifactorial risk assessment or those in class III who had evidence of moderate to severe congestive heart failure, aortic stenosis, or a recent myocardial infarction. Detsky et al. refined Goldman's scoring system by including variables that reflected the severity of coronary artery disease such as angina pectoris.[25] A comprehensive discussion of preoperative assessment may be found in Chapter 1.

Peripheral Venous Catheterization

Two types of needles are used for peripheral vein cannulization: hollow needles, including butterfly catheters, and indwelling plastic catheters that are inserted over a hollow needle. The most frequent sites used for peripheral IV line insertion include the dorsum of the hands, the wrists, and the antecubital fossae. Peripheral venous catheters should be routinely monitored for evidence of infection, and access sites should be changed every 48 to 72 hours. If infection is suspected, the IV catheter should be immediately removed. The largest possible catheter should be inserted in patients who need or may need large-volume fluid replacement. The flow rate of a 14-gauge catheter averages 125 mL/min and accommodates respectively two and three times the flow rate of 16- and 20-gauge catheters.[26] In emergency situations only antecubital veins should be used, as hypotension results in peripheral vasoconstriction and more peripheral placement will limit fluid delivery to the central circulation. Central lines are preferable to peripheral venous access for patients who are unstable or who require rapid fluid resuscitation. However, in emergency situations it is important not to delay therapy while obtaining central venous access.

Temporary Venous Access: Approach and General Consideration

Internal Jugular Vein Catheterization

Anatomy of the Internal Jugular Vein

The internal jugular vein collects blood from the skull, brain, superficial parts of the face, and much of the neck. It emerges from the base of the skull via the posterior compartment of the jugular foramen and descends posterior to the internal carotid artery in the carotid sheath, running posterolateral to the internal and common carotid artery. It unites with the subclavian vein to form the brachiocephalic vein. At its termination, the internal jugular vein is lateral and anterior to the common carotid artery. The right internal jugular vein, the brachiocephalic vein, and the superior vena cava form a short, almost direct line to the right atrium. The left internal jugular vein is a relatively less desirable site for cannulation, as the left brachiocephalic vein is longer and enters the subclavian vein at an angle.

The superior segment of the internal jugular vein is overlapped by the posterior belly of the digastric muscle and is medial to the sternocleidomastoid muscle. The vein may be cannulated in its midportion, which is located in the depression between the sternal and clavicular heads of the sternocleidomastoid, in the lesser supraclavicular fossa. The inferior portion lies behind the anterior portion of the clavicular head, terminating just above the medial end of the clavicle.

The internal jugular vein is in close proximity to many vital structures. It shares the carotid sheath with the internal carotid artery and cranial nerves IX, X, and XII. The thoracic duct opens near the union of the left subclavian and internal jugular veins and the smaller right lymphatic duct enters at the same juncture on the right. Both right and, especially, left internal jugular veins pass close to the apex of the lung at their confluence with the subclavian veins.[20]

Approach

A central approach to the internal jugular vein is described below (Fig. 7–3).[27,28]

1. The patient is placed supine in the Trendelenburg position (approximately 15 to 20 degrees) to distend the vein, facilitate its identification, and prevent air embolism. The patient's head is turned opposite from the side chosen for cannulization. This positioning stretches the vein, thereby fixing it, and also accentuates muscular landmarks.

2. The triangle formed by the sternal and clavicular heads of the sternocleidomastoid muscle and the clavicle is identified. If the patient is awake, lifting her head slightly facilitates identification of the triangle. The carotid artery lies within the carotid sheath just medial to the internal jugular vein. The carotid artery is a valuable landmark, but its proximity increases the likelihood of inadvertent arterial puncture.

3. The operator palpates the medial aspect of the triangle along the sternal head of the muscle to locate the pulsation of the carotid pulse. Once the pulse has been identified, the operator places two fingers along the artery to retract it medially and to serve as a guide for localizing the internal jugular vein.

4. The patient is prepared and draped in sterile fashion.

5. A finder needle is attached to a 5 to 10 cc syringe filled with 3 to 5 mL of sterile saline or heparin flush. Standing at the patient's head the operator inserts the needle at the apex of the triangle formed by the two heads of the sternocleidomastoid muscle.

6. Maintaining slight negative pressure on the syringe, the operator directs the needle caudally toward the ipsilateral nipple and parallel to the medial border of the clavicular head at a 45-degree angle to the frontal plane. If the vein is not cannulated after the needle has been advanced a few centimeters, the

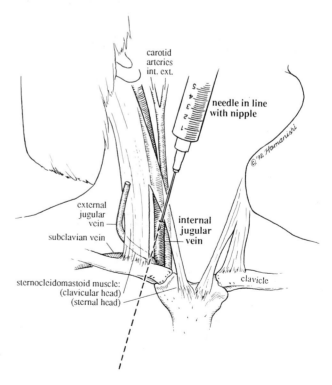

FIGURE 7–3. Central approach to internal jugular venipuncture.

needle is slowly withdrawn with the operator maintaining slight negative pressure. If this approach is not successful, the needle is withdrawn completely and redirected 5 to 10 degrees more laterally. If this does not result in successful cannulation, the needle is redirected along the sagittal plane. The operator should not direct the needle medial to the sagittal plane, as this will likely result in carotid artery cannulization.

7. Once the position of the internal jugular vein has been ascertained, the finder needle can be removed. The intracath needle is then inserted in the same position and angle. When the vein is cannulated the syringe is removed. A gloved finger should be quickly placed over the opening of the intracath to prevent air embolism.

8. A guidewire is then inserted and the needle is withdrawn over the wire. The catheter is then carefully advanced over the stabilized guidewire.

9. After patency of the catheter is established, the catheter is flushed with heparin and sutured into position. A chest radiograph is obtained to ensure proper positioning and to rule out pneumothorax.

Advantages of Internal Jugular Vein Catheterization

There are several advantages of internal jugular vein catheterization. Compared to a subclavian vein approach, this approach is associated with a significantly lower risk of pleural puncture and subsequent pneumothorax. The internal jugular vein is more accessible to the anesthesiologist during surgery, and cannulation is more easily performed during cardiopulmonary resuscitation. If a hematoma forms during internal jugular catheterization, it is visible and easily compressed. Last, it may be easier to insert a Swan-Ganz catheter via the (right) internal jugular than the subclavian vein because of its direct anatomic alignment with the right atrium.

Disadvantages of Internal Jugular Vein Catheterization

The internal jugular approach carries all the usual nonspecific risks of catheter insertion, including infection, sepsis, thrombophlebitis, and malpositioning. In addition, the anatomic position of the internal jugular vein gives rise to specific difficulties and complications. The surface landmarks needed to cannulate the internal jugular vein successfully are more difficult to identify in the obese patient or in patients with a thick neck. Therefore, in these patient subsets a subclavian approach may be preferable. Although the risk of pneumothorax and air embolism is lower with internal jugular cannulization than with the subclavian approach, these complications do occur. The apical pleura lies close to the inferior segment of the internal jugular vein, and a pneumothorax may occur if the needle is advanced too far in the caudal direction.

Subclavian Vein Catheterization

Anatomy of the Subclavian Vein

The subclavian vein, a continuation of the axillary vein, joins the internal jugular vein to form the brachiocephalic vein. In the adult, the subclavian vein is 3 to 4 cm long and 1 to 2 cm in diameter.

The axillary vein runs inferior to the clavicle through the axillary space, between the pectoral humeral grove and the lateral margin of the first rib. It becomes the subclavian vein at this juncture and crosses over the first rib, passing in front of the anterior scalene muscle. The vein then runs below the medial portion of the clavicle, where it is anchored by attachments to the rib and the clavicle. The subclavian vein meets the internal jugular vein behind the sternocostoclavicular joint to form the brachiocephalic vein.[21,22]

Despite its short course, the subclavian vein passes close to several vital structures. Posterosuperiorly, the subclavian vein is separated from the subclavian artery and the brachial plexus by the anterior scalene muscle, which is only 10 to 15 mm thick in the adult. Medial to the attachment of the anterior scalene muscle to the first rib, the apical pleura is in contact with the inferior portion of the subclavian vein. The thoracic duct on the left and the lymphatic duct on the right both lie superior to the subclavian vein near its junction with the internal jugular vein. Thus, from anatomic considerations alone, subclavian vein cannulation carries the risk of damage to the pleura, lung, thoracic duct, and subclavian artery.

Approach

The subclavian vein can be cannulated using the direct infraclavicular approach (Fig. 7–4).[27,28,29]

1. The supine patient is placed in about 15 degrees of Trendelenburg position. The shoulder of the side desired for cannulation should be abducted by placing a towel behind the back. The skin is prepared and draped in sterile fashion.

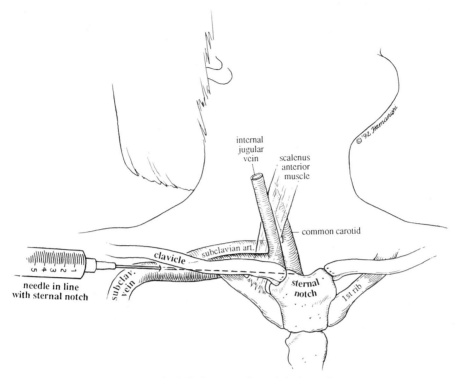

FIGURE 7-4. Infraclavicular approach to subclavian venipuncture.

2. The junction of the middle and medial thirds of the clavicle is located. The skin approximately 1 cm caudal to this position and the periosteum surrounding the clavicle is infiltrated with lidocaine.

3. A 5 to 10 cc syringe attached to an intracath is filled with 3 to 5 mL of heparin flush or sterile saline. The syringe and the needle are then held parallel to the plane of the patient's chest wall.

4. The sternal notch is identified to provide a reference point for directing the needle. Maintaining a slight negative pressure on the syringe, the operator advances the needle through the skin with its tip directed medially and slightly cephalad, toward the sternal notch and posterior to the clavicle. The needle must be kept parallel to the chest wall to avoid puncturing the pleura and causing a pneumothorax. By maintaining negative pressure in the syringe the operator can determine when the venous lumen has been entered. It is important to ensure that the return flow is not pulsating, which would indicate arterial cannulization. Once the vein is entered, the bevel of the needle is rotated caudally to facilitate the downward turn of the guidewire into the brachiocephalic vein.

5. As the syringe is separated from the intracath, the lumen should be occluded to prevent air embolism. Again, the catheter return should be checked for pulsatile flow. If entry into an artery is a possibility, blood gas values can be determined at this point to ascertain the location of the catheter.

6. A guidewire is inserted through the intracath and stabilized while the needle is withdrawn over the wire. Loss of the guidewire can result in wire embolization.

7. The catheter is inserted over the wire and the wire is removed. Once patency of the line is established the catheter is flushed with heparin and sutured in place. A chest radiograph is obtained to confirm correct placement and to rule out pneumothorax.

Advantages of Subclavian Vein Catheterization

The subclavian vein approach allows rapid access to the central circulation. It allows more freedom of neck movement than does the internal jugular approach. In obese patients or patients with a history of neck surgery, the anatomy may be easier to identify, making it a simpler approach.

Disadvantages of Subclavian Vein Catheterization

Complications of subclavian venipuncture and catheterization occur in 3% to 6% of all patients and include infection, pneumothorax, hemothorax, air embolism, thrombosis, and perforation of the subclavian artery.

Complications that are relatively specific to a subclavian approach are pneumothorax and hemothorax. The subclavian vein lies close to the pleura; therefore, a needle directed under the first rib, beneath or through both walls of the vein, can penetrate the pleural space and lung and produce a pneumothorax. Vessel injury during this process results in a hemothorax.

Hematoma and bleeding complications are also potential problems in patients with an underlying coagulopathy or who are receiving thrombolytic agents. The subclavian vein, unlike the femoral or internal jugular veins, is noncompressible. Thus, vessel laceration may be difficult to identify immediately, and the formation of a hematoma, even if identified, cannot be tamponaded by direct pressure.

Femoral Vein Catheterization

Anatomy of the Femoral Vein

The femoral vein occupies the middle compartment of the femoral sheath medial to the femoral artery and lateral to a fat pad containing lymphatics. It begins as a continuation of the popliteal vein at the adductor canal and becomes the external iliac posterior to the inguinal ligament. The femoral vein has many tributaries, including the vena profunda femoris, the great saphenous vein, and the lateral and medial femoral veins.[23]

Approach

The femoral vein may be cannulated as follows.

1. The skin overlying the femoral vein is prepared. In nonemergency situations the pubic hair may be shaved as needed. This is an important step and should be performed carefully to reduce the risk of contamination from bacterial flora from the groin. The site is covered with a sterile drape. The operator locates the femoral artery by palpating its pulse. If there is no pulse (as may occur in a code situation), the operator finds the midpoint between the symphysis pubis and the anterior superior iliac spine. The skin overlying this point is infiltrated with lidocaine.

2. A 5 to 10 cc syringe is filled with 3 to 5 mL of sterile saline or heparin flush and the finder needle is attached. The operator identifies the location of the femoral vein, medial to the pulsation of the femoral artery and two fingerbreadths below the inguinal ligament. Maintaining a slight negative pressure, the operator advances the needle slowly at a 45-degree angle to the skin until blood appears in the syringe. The finder needle can then be withdrawn and the femoral vein cannulated with the larger intracath using the same approach. Once blood return is obtained the syringe can be detached.

3. A guidewire can be inserted through the intracath and the intracath removed over the wire. The catheter is inserted over the guidewire and the guidewire is removed. Care is taken to establish return from each port. Once this is accomplished the ports are flushed with heparin. The catheter is then sutured in place.

Advantages of Femoral Vein Catheterization

The chief advantages of femoral vein catheterization are accessibility and safety for cannulation. If basic life support is being carried out there is no need for interruption during insertion. The femoral vein does not lie near major critical structures and is easily compressed with external pressure. Cannulation of the femoral vein can be of benefit in an agitated patient or one who cannot tolerate the Trendelenburg position. Femoral vein catheterization is probably the safest way to obtain central access in patients with bleeding disorders or who are receiving thrombolytic therapy. Once the vein is cannulated it provides access to the central circulation for Swan-Ganz catheterization or balloon angioplasty.

Disadvantages of Femoral Vein Catheterization

Complications arising from femoral vein catheterization include hematoma, infection, thrombosis, and femoral artery cannulization. Femoral vein catheterization has been associated with a higher rate of infection and thrombosis than catheterization at other sites.[30,31] Much of the data supporting higher rates, however, were collected when femoral vein catheterization was first developed. Recent reports of long-term femoral catheterization in pediatric patients[32] and short-term catheterization in adults[33] suggest that the complication rates of this approach are comparable to those of catheterization by other routes.

Cannulization of the Radial Artery

Radial arterial lines can provide important perioperative information about the patient's arterial pH, oxygenation, and ventilatory status. This procedure is generally without serious complications if specific guidelines are followed.[34]

Radial artery thrombosis occurs in more than 50% of radial artery cannulizations. It is important to determine the existence of collateral flow from the ulnar artery via the superficial arch. If absent, there is a high risk of ischemic injury to the hand in the event of radial artery thrombosis. The modified Allen test was developed to assess collateral flow and is performed as follows.

1. The operator instructs the patient to open and close the hand several times and then clench the fist.

2. The operator occludes both the radial and ulnar artery, then asks the patient to open the hand.

3. As pressure over the ulnar artery is released, the operator observes the patient's palm for return of normal color. Return within 6 seconds indicates adequate collateral flow. A delay of 7 to 15 seconds indicates marginal flow. Persistent blanching for more than 15 seconds is a contraindication to radial artery cannulization.

The radial artery can be cannulated as follows.

1. A towel roll is placed behind the patient's wrist and the hand is dorsiflexed 60 degrees. The wrist and forearm are then secured to a flat support with tape.

2. The wrist is prepared and draped in sterile fashion and the skin overlying the radial artery is infiltrated with 1% lidocaine.

3. The radial artery is identified by palpation.

4. The catheter is inserted at a 45-degree angle to the skin and advanced, while the operator gently palpates the radial artery to assist with directing the needle. When there is a flash of blood in the catheter hub, the needle should be held stationary and the catheter advanced over the needle. Care should be taken to thread the catheter gently to avoid causing shear damage to the artery. Once the catheter is positioned the needle is removed.

5. The operator briefly observes the blood return for arterial pulsations and then connects the hub of the catheter to the arterial tubing.

6. The catheter is secured in place with a 3-0 or 4-0 silk suture, and the tape and towels employed to fix the hand in a dorsiflexed position are removed. The catheter should then be covered with a non-occlusive surgical dressing.

Complications of Temporary Central Venous Access

The complications associated with central venous access are summarized in Table 7–3. The more clinically significant and life-threatening complications are discussed here.

Infection

Infection is a potentially fatal complication of central venous catheterization. Although the risk of sepsis is only 1%, sepsis carries a 10% to 20% mortality.[35] The frequent use of central lines in an intensive care setting makes sepsis an important diagnosis to consider in any patient who has fever and an indwelling central line.

The pathogenesis of catheter-related infections is multifactorial. The use of broad-spectrum antibiotics in the intensive care unit fosters the emergence of multiresistant and atypical organisms. In addition, the presence of a foreign body alters natural defense mechanisms, and thus nonpathogenic organisms such as coagulase-negative staphylococci can become significant pathogens. Most catheter-related infections occur as a result of migration of skin flora along the external surface of the catheter toward its tip.[36] Organisms may adhere to the catheter surface as a result of electrostatic forces.[37,38] Coagulase-negative staphylococci may produce a polysaccharide substance that helps the organisms

TABLE 7–3. **Complications of Central Venous Catheterization**

Pneumothorax
Air embolism
Hemothorax
Hematoma
Thoracic duct injury
Vocal cord nerve injury
Thrombosis
Pulmonary embolism
Infection
Sepsis
Arrhythmias
Pericardial tamponade

bond to the catheter and inhibits localized immune responses.[39] The most common organisms causing catheter infections are coagulase-negative staphylococci, *Staphylococcus aureus,* and yeast. Other organisms include enterococci, *E. coli,* and *Klebsiella,* which can infect catheters by hematologic seeding.[35]

The diagnosis of a catheter-related infection is established by clinical observation and semiquantitative culture. The isolation of an organism in broth culture alone is not typically diagnostic, owing to the high frequency of false positive results. The presence of more than 15 colony-forming units (CFUs) from catheter tip cultures has been associated with a 16% to 34% incidence of bacteremia.[40] Fewer than 15 CFUs is not felt to be clinically significant. Gram stain of the catheter tip is also useful in immediate identification of the colonizing organisms. The diagnosis of bacteremia is made on isolation of organisms that are not common contaminants, such as *S. aureus, E. coli,* or *Pseudomonas aeruginosa.* Alternatively, bacteremia may be diagnosed when two or more blood cultures are positive for organisms commonly considered contaminants, such as coagulase-negative staphylococci, diphtheroids, or *Propionibacterium.* Bacteremia is also diagnosed when a single blood culture is positive for any organism that has also been isolated from the catheter tip. During the evaluation of fever, simultaneous peripheral and central line cultures should be obtained, as line cultures have a higher rate of false positives. The diagnosis of yeast infections, especially in immunocompromised patients, is problematic because systemic invasion may occur without resulting in positive blood cultures.

The most important factor for central venous catheter infections is the duration of catheterization.[41] Norwood reported that the number of catheter infections rose markedly after 4 days; therefore, the general recommendation is to change the catheter every 3 to 4 days. Changing the catheter over a guidewire remains a controversial alternative to selecting a new site for insertion. Corona et al.[35] and other authors[42,43] believe that it is a viable alternative as long as there is no evidence of ongoing bacteremia.

Multilumen catheters may confer a higher risk of infection over single-lumen catheters. Hilton et al.[44] reported a catheter tip colonization rate of 8% for single-lumen catheters and 32% for triple-lumen catheters. These figures are controversial, for multilumen catheters may be used in the care of sicker patients with longer hospital stays and in those who require additional procedures.

Other measures, including dressings, may affect the overall infection rate. The use of plastic transparent dressings is associated with a higher degree of moisture retention than occurs with gauze dressings and results in a significantly increased rate of catheter infections. For this reason, occlusive nonpermeable dressings are discouraged.[45] Topical antibiotics (polymyxin/neomycin, bacitracin ointment) applied at the entry site may decrease the rate of infection.[46]

If a catheter infection is suspected, the insertion site should be carefully inspected for erythema and purulent drainage. Blood for culture should be obtained peripherally and through the catheter. The catheter should be removed and the tip cultured. If there is high clinical suspicion of infection, if bacteremia is present, or if culture of the tip yields more than 15 CFUs, then the line should be removed immediately and the site of insertion changed. Septic thrombophlebitis and endocarditis should always be considered in a patient with recurrent infections. Antibiotic therapy should be directed toward any known or suspected pathogen. Empirical treatment should always provide coverage for gram-positive cocci.[35]

Pneumothorax

Pneumothorax is the most common major complication following central venous catheterization. It is a rare complication of catheterization by the internal jugular route but occurs in 1% to 5% of catheterization by a subclavian route.[29] Factors that increase the risk of pneumothorax include morbid obesity, emergency catheter placement, high positive end-expiratory pressure, and cachexia.[29] A pneumothorax may be suspected when air is aspirated through the syringe during insertion or if the patient experiences respiratory distress during or after insertion. For this reason, a chest radiograph should be obtained after all attempted or successful central venous catheterizations. Patients with asymptomatic or small (<10%) pneumothoraces may be clinically observed and followed with serial chest radiographs. In all other circumstances a chest tube should be promptly inserted.

Hemothorax

Perforation of venous or arterial structures during catheter insertion may result in a hemothorax. This complication can be suspected when the catheter aspiration fails to provide a good blood return. Immediate diagnosis is important. A suspected hemothorax may be confirmed with a chest radiograph. Treatment includes removing the catheter and inserting a chest tube. Coagulation deficiencies, if present, should be corrected before line insertion to minimize the risk of hemothorax. If this is not possible, a noncompressible vein such as the subclavian vein should be avoided.

Air Embolism

Air embolism is a rare complication of central venous catheterization, occurring in 0.4% of placements.[28,47] It is, however, an important complication both to recognize and to prevent because it carries a 29% to 43% mortality.[48,49] Air embolism must be suspected if a patient develops severe respiratory distress associated with cardiovascular compromise or neurologic defects. The differential diagnosis in the clinical situation includes arrhythmias, massive pulmonary embolism, cardiac tamponade, acute myocardial infarction, and aortic dissection.

The most common cause of air embolism, accounting for 71% to 93% of all cases,[48,49] relates to disconnection of the IV line between the catheter hub and the administration apparatus. Other sites for air entry include stress fractures in the lines or hub. Air embolism can also occur during insertion when the needle hub is opened to allow guidewire insertion. Prevention, vastly preferable to management of this deadly complication, involves placing the patient in a 30-degree Trendelenburg position during catheter placement and not allowing air to enter through the needle as the guidewire is inserted. The acute management of an air embolism includes immediate aspiration through the catheter and placing the patient in a steep left lateral Trendelenburg position. As a last resort, aspiration of the right ventricle can be attempted.[29]

Permanent Venous Access

Indications

Permanent central venous access should be considered for any patient who requires long-term IV therapy, including patients receiving chronic TPN, chemotherapy, or long-term antibiotics. Permanent lines provide secure access for the administration of chemotherapy, blood transfusions, fluids, and TPN. They reduce the risk of extravasation and decrease patient discomfort and anxiety from frequent venipuncture. Permanent access can also be useful for home hospice care in that it can provide reliable access for pain medications with minimal requirements for skilled nursing care.

Many factors must be considered in deciding if long-term access is indicated for a particular patient. Medical indications include the duration of the treatment, the toxicity of the substances to be infused, and the anticipated side effects of the therapy. Certain situations mandate a central line. For example, most oncology patients will have a permanent central venous catheter emplaced at the onset of treatment, as the need for repeated venipunctures and IV access makes the need for a permanent line inevitable. Permanent venous lines in patients managed in an outpatient setting require additional considerations before placement, including the ability of the patient to care for the line, the potential for the line to be used for nonmedical purposes (e.g., illicit drug use), and the reliability of the patient in seeking medical attention should complications occur.

Line Selection

Selection of a permanent central line depends on many factors such as treatment regimen, patient preference and body habitus, and the experience of the individual institution. There are two general categories of permanent lines. The first type is the external catheter, examples of which include the Hickman, Broviac, and Groshong lines. The second type is the subcutaneous port system. Examples are the Mediport, Infus-a-Port, and Port-a-Cath. Each type of catheter has its advantages and disadvantages.

External catheters are easy to access and can accommodate complicated infusion regimens. Once placed, the external catheters have a 4- to 8-inch catheter segment visible at the chest wall and terminating in the catheter ports. These ports do not require special access equipment and are immediately available for use. External catheters such as the Hickman line allow greater regimen flexibility because they are made with single, double, and triple lumens, allowing the simultaneous infusion of blood products, TPN, and antibiotics. The large bore of the external catheter allows rapid volume infusion, which is particularly useful in an inpatient setting. The disadvantages of the external catheters are that they require frequent maintenance, may prohibit certain activities, and are visible when not in use. The external catheter requires flushing with a heparin solution three times a week, and the catheter cap must be changed weekly. In an outpatient setting the patient or a family member learns to perform catheter maintenance. If no one is available to maintain the line, frequent home nursing visits are necessary, even when the ports are not being actively used for therapy. Patients may shower or bathe with an external line, but swimming and the use of a hot tub are restricted. Precautions must be taken by the patient not to cut, tear, or pull the external segment of the catheter. Another disadvantage of the external line is that many patients do not like having a line visible at their chest surface. This can be especially important to cancer patients, who are struggling with an altered body appearance from recent surgery or chronic illness.

The subcutaneous port system has been used in both in-patient and outpatient settings. It is ideal for patients receiving infrequent infusions in an outpatient setting. The port is placed in the subcutaneous tissue with only a small protrusion visible at the site. To access the port system, a special noncoring needle called a Huber needle is inserted through the skin until it punctures the septum and accesses the port. The septum permits 2,000 punctures. The gauge of the Huber needle limits the rate at which fluids can be infused, making the port inappropriate for large-volume emergency resuscitations. The major advantages of the port system include ease of care, improved body image, and a decreased risk of infection.[51] The port system requires minimal maintenance. It is flushed once a month, and there are no caps or dressings to change. All activities, including swimming, can be pursued without restriction. There is no danger of dislodging the catheter because there is no external segment.

The disadvantages of the subcutaneous port include its limited adaptability for multi-drug induction regimens, infusion rate limitations, and difficulty accessing the port. Many clinics do not have the equipment or personnel to access a subcutaneous port. The discomfort of venipuncture is not eliminated because each time the port is accessed the patient experiences a needle poke. There is also a risk of the needle dislodging during infusion, thus causing drug extravasation. Obese patients pose a special challenge because the subcutaneous port system can be difficult to place and, once placed, can migrate. Cachectic patients also pose a problem because they have minimal subcutaneous tissue in which to implant the port system, and therefore the catheter can erode through the skin with time.

Certain clinical settings are ideal for one or another type of catheter. For example, patients undergoing bone marrow transplantation receive a double- or triple-lumen external catheter for rapid simultaneous infusions of blood products, TPN, and antibiotics and for frequent blood sampling. A subcutaneous port system is ideal in elderly, debilitated patients who need infrequent infusions in a home setting.

Placement of Permanent Central Lines

A detailed description of the placement of permanent venous catheters is beyond the scope of this discussion but is available in a report from Hickman's group.[50] Figure 7–5 shows the central venous catheter in position.

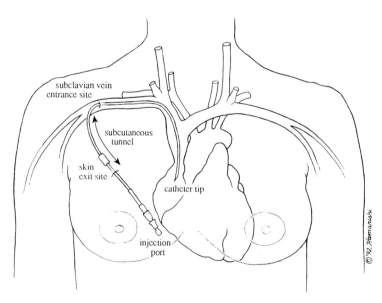

FIGURE 7–5. Anatomy of a central venous catheter.

External catheters and subcutaneous ports can be placed by using either a percutaneous approach or by a surgical cutdown technique. The percutaneous approach may be used with the subclavian vein, internal and external jugular veins, or the femoral vein. The catheter is tunneled subcutaneously for a variable length (typically 10–25 cm)[50] to stabilize the catheter and prevent infection.[51] The procedure is usually performed in an operating room or in a sterile procedures room. Sterile technique must be used during catheter placement. A "seeking" needle is used to locate the vessel. Doppler imaging can be helpful in identifying the course of the target vessel, particularly in obese or emaciated patients, whose anatomic landmarks are difficult to locate. Once the vein has been entered, a guidewire can be introduced and directed into the superior vena cava. Fluoroscopy may be helpful in confirming proper guidewire placement. Once the guidewire is in position the catheter may be brought through the subcutaneous tunnel with the Dacron cuff positioned 2 to 3 cm from the exit site. The vein dilator and peelaway sheath are then passed over the guidewire. Once the peel-away sheath is in position the wire and vein dilator are removed and the catheter is passed down the peel-away sheath under fluoroscopy. When properly positioned the tip of the catheter should reside deep within the superior vena cava or at the junction of the superior vena cava and the atrium. Contrast medium is then injected into the catheter to document patency and position. The catheter is secured to the exit site with a suture, which ensures stability until the Dacron cuff scar tissue forms.[50]

The subcutaneous port system catheters are implanted in much the same manner as external catheters. The reservoir is placed in a subcutaneous pocket with at least 1 to 1.5 cm of overlying skin and subcutaneous tissue. If the port is placed too deep, it may migrate and will be difficult to access. Alternatively, if it is placed too superficially, it may erode through the skin surface. The anterior chest is the most common placement site, but other sites, including the dorsum of the arm, have been used at our institution.

The placement of a permanent central venous line is typically a safe and short procedure. There are certain clinical situations, however, that make catheter placement extremely risky. For example, subclavian or superior venous thrombosis is a contraindication to that approach, and entry through the femoral vein should be considered. In patients with a tracheostomy, an external or internal jugular vein approach should be avoided because of contamination of the skin by tracheostomy drainage. Coagulopathies should be corrected as much as possible before catheter placement. Active, uncontrolled infections are a contraindication to line placement.

Care of Permanent Central Venous Lines

Catheter care guidelines vary from institution to institution. General guidelines are as follows. All persons taking care of a long-term catheter should employ rigorous hand washing technique. Caregivers should be trained to recognize signs of catheter infection. Patients should have access to a trained nurse or physician to immediately report complications. The catheter should not be used unless it is functioning properly. Only sterile solutions should be utilized. The care of external catheters and port systems is outlined in Table 7–4.

Complications of Permanent Central Venous Lines

Complications associated with permanent central venous catheters can be divided into three categories. In the first category are acute complications related to catheter placement, in the second category is catheter obstruction, and in the third category are catheter infections (Table 7–5).

Catheter placement is a relatively safe and simple procedure. It is estimated that in 1988 2.5 million catheters were placed, with only 1,800 complications and 32 deaths.[52] The deaths were associated with pneumothorax, hemothorax, air embolism, pericardial tamponade, hydromediastinum, and ce-

TABLE 7–4. **Care of External Catheters and Port Systems**

External Catheters
- Heparin flush 3×/wk.
- Cap replacement weekly.
- The hubs and connecting joints should be properly prepared, preferably with Betadine or alcohol solution when the catheter is used.
- The ports should be prepared in sterile fashion when they are entered.

Port Systems
- Heparin flush 1×/mo.
- The overlying skin should be prepared in sterile fashion before cather is placed.
- Infusion should begin only after blood return is identified.

TABLE 7–5. Complications of Permanent Central Venous Catheterization

Acute complications
  Pneumothorax
  Air embolism
  Catheter or guidewire embolization
  Hemothorax
  Hemomediastinum
  Pericardial tamponade
  Arrhythmias
  Cerebral air embolus
  Vocal cord injury
  Phrenic nerve paralysis
  Cerebral infarction
Obstruction
  Fibrin sleeve formation
  Thrombosis
  Superior vena cava syndrome
  Pulmonary embolism
  Catheter migration
  Catheter erosion
Infection
  Exit site infection
  Tunnel infection
  Septicemia
  Septic thrombophlebitis
  Mediastinitis

rebral infarction.[50] To improve the safety of the procedures, a suite of recommendations has been formulated. The percutaneous approach utilizing the subclavian and internal jugular veins should be avoided in patients with chronic lung disease (cystic fibrosis, emphysema, pneumonectomy), gross obesity, prior surgery on the neck and upper thorax, or uncorrectable coagulopathies. Safety suggestions include using a small-bore seeking needle, using Doppler imaging to localize major veins, and using fluoroscopy to confirm correct catheter tip location.[50]

Pneumothorax, the most common acute complication of catheter placement, occurs in 1% to 3% of all procedures.[50] Most pneumothoraces remain asymptomatic, but a small percentage progress. Chest tube placement is indicated when the pneumothorax exceeds 15% or becomes symptomatic. Tension pneumothorax should be suspected in a patient who experiences respiratory distress, chest pain, or cardiovascular collapse following line placement.

Catheter obstruction is a common complication of permanent venous catheters, occurring in up to 25% of all catheter placements.[53] In many instances the only remedy is removal of the catheter. The most common indication of early catheter obstruction is inability to draw blood through the catheter.

Other indications of obstruction are inability to infuse through the catheter or pain during infusion. Fibrin sleeve formation is the most common cause of catheter malfunction. Actual clots within the catheter lumen are rare.[50]

The initial treatment of fibrin sleeves and thrombus formations consists of infusing 5,000 units of urokinase directly into the catheter. If this does not relieve the obstruction, a chest radiograph should be obtained to determine line position. A contrast dye study can also be useful to delineate the cause and extent of the obstruction. In the case of resistant thrombus, urokinase may also be administered as a continuous drip, 4,000 to 8,000 units/kg/hr over 12 to 72 hours or 125,000 units/1.73 m^2/hr for 3 days. These protocols require careful monitoring of thrombin time and fibrinogen levels.[53]

Infection is the most common long-term complication of permanent central venous catheterization, accounting for 50% of all catheter-related complications. The infection rate is 0.3 per 100 catheter-days.[54] The most important factors in determining the risk of infection are the expertise of the persons inserting the catheter and the care the catheters receive during use.[55] Other risk factors include venous thrombosis and exit site care. Uncontrolled bacteremia is a contraindication to permanent catheter insertion; however, fever, neutropenia, and controlled infection at a distant site do not increase the risk of infection.[50] Prophylactic administration of antibiotics before catheter insertion does not appear to reduce the rate of catheter infections.[50]

There are several types of catheter infections, which differ markedly in their prognosis and management. The following definitions are useful.[54] *Exit site infection* is characterized by the development of erythema, tenderness, induration, or purulence within 2 cm of the skin exit site of the catheter. *Tunnel infection* is characterized by the development of erythema, tenderness, and induration along the tunnel of the catheter at a distance of more than 2 cm from the skin exit site, with or without signs of inflammation or purulence at the exit site itself. *Septic thrombophlebitis* is characterized by the development of septic venous occlusion in proximity to the catheter, associated with bacteremia and fever.

The most frequent type of catheter infection is exit site infection, which accounts for 25% to 50% of all infections. Septicemia of unknown origin is the second most common type of infection, accounting for 20% to 24% of all infections. Septic thrombophlebitis is uncommon, occurring in less than 5% of cases.[54,56]

Staphylococcus epidermidis is the most common pathogen associated with permanent central venous catheter infection, being isolated in 31% to 54% of all line infections. Other common organisms include *Staphylococcus aureus* (14%–20%), *Corynebacterium* (5%–11%), *Pseudomonas* (6%–7%), *Candida* (5%–7%), and *Enterococcus* (2%–5%).[54,56,57]

Catheter-related infections generally have a good prognosis and many can be cured with antibiotics alone, without catheter removal. Press et al.[54] reported that 85% of exit site infections could be successfully treated without catheter removal. The prognosis for tunnel infection is considerably worse: only 31% can be cured without catheter removal. Neutropenia does not mandate catheter removal, and patients should be treated with IV antibiotics or colony-stimulating factors until they are no longer neutropenic.[50] Septic thrombophlebitis is an absolute indication for catheter removal and may necessitate surgical resection of the involved venous segment.[50]

Much of the information gathered on catheter-related infections has been obtained in *Staphylococcus epidermidis* infections of Hickman catheters. It is important to consider that while *S. epidermidis* infection carries a good prognosis, infections by other organisms such as *S. aureus* do not. Thus, management recommendations that apply to *S. epidermidis* infections do not apply to *S. aureus* infections. Dugdale and Ramsey[58] found that only 10% of all *S. aureus* exit site infections and no tunnel infections could be cured without catheter removal. For this reason, early catheter removal should be considered in most cases of *S. aureus* catheter infections.

If catheter salvage is attempted, clinical improvement should occur in 48 to 72 hours. If fever, inflammation, or bacteremia persists, the line should be removed. After line removal the patient should be treated with peripherally administered IV antibiotics for 48 to 72 hours before a new catheter is placed. Blood cultures should be done before the new catheter is placed to confirm the absence of bacteremia. Uncontrolled bacteremia is a contraindication to early catheter replacement.

References

1. Aubaniac R: L'injection intraveineuse sous-claviculaire: Advantages et techniques. Presse Med 60:1456, 1952.
2. Wilson NJ, Grow JB, Demong CV, Prevedel AE, Owens JC: Central venous pressure in optimal blood volume maintenance. Arch Surg 85:563, 1962.
3. Ashbaugh D, Thompson JWW: Subclavian-vein infusion. Lancet 2:1138, 1963.
4. Subclavian venepuncture (editorial). Lancet 2:1152, 1963.
5. Yoffa D: Supraclavicular subclavian venepuncture and catheterization. Lancet 2:614, 1965.
6. Hermosura B, Vanags L, Dickey MW: Measurement of pressure during intravenous therapy. JAMA 195:321, 1966.
7. English ICW, Frew RM, Pigott JF, Zaki M: Percutaneous catheterization of the internal jugular vein. Anesthesia 24:521, 1969.
8. Quinton W, Dillard D, Scribner B: Cannulation of blood vessels for prolonged hemodialysis. Trans Am Soc Artif Intern Organs 6:104, 1960.
9. Bresica MJ, Cimino JE, Appel K, Hurwich BJ: Chronic hemodialysis using venepuncture and a surgically created arteriovenous fistula. N Engl J Med 275:1089, 1966.
10. Dudrick SJ, Wilmore DW, Vars HM, Rhoads JE: Long-term parenteral nutrition with growth, development, and positive nitrogen balance. Surgery 64:134, 1968.
11. Dudrick SJ, Wilmore DW, Vars HM, Rhoads JE: Can intravenous feeding as the sole means of nutrition support growth in the child and restore weight loss in the adult? Ann Surg 169:974, 1969.
12. Scribner BH, Cole JJ, Christopher TG, Vizzo JE, Atkins RC, Blagg CR: Longterm total parenteral nutrition: The concept of an artificial gut. JAMA 212:457, 1970.
13. Broviac JW, Cole JJ, Scribner BH: A silicone rubber atrial catheter for prolonged parenteral alimentation. Surg Gynecol Obstet 136:602, 1973.
14. Hickman RO, Buckner CD, Clift RA, Sanders JE, Stewart P, Thomas ED: A modified right atrial catheter for access to the venous system in marrow transplant recipients. Surg Gynecol Obstet 148:873, 1979.
15. Sanders JE, Hickman RO, Aker BS, Hersman RD, Buckner CD, Thomas DE: Experience with double lumen right atrial catheters. JPEN J Parenter Enter Nutr 6:95, 1982.
16. Brothers TE, Von Molf LK, Niederhuber JE, Roberts JA, Walker-Andrews S, Ensminger WD: Experience with subcutaneous infusion ports in three hundred patients. Surg Gynecol Obstet 166:295, 1988.
17. Delmor JE, Horbelt DV, Jack BL, Roberts DK: Experience with the Groshong long term central venous catheter. Gynecol Oncol 34:216, 1989.
18. Malviya VK, Deppe G, Gove N, Malone JM: Vascular access in gynecologic cancer using the Groshong right atrial catheter. Gynecol Oncol 33:313, 1989.
19. Brown JM: Peripherally inserted central catheters: Use in home care. Intraven Nurs 12:144, 1989.
20. Williams PL, Warwick R, Dyson M, Bannister LH (eds): Gray's Anatomy, 37th ed, p 795. Edinburg: Churchill Livingstone, 1989.
21. Ibid., p 807.
22. Defalque RJ: Percutaneous catheterization of the internal jugular vein. Anesth Analg 53:116, 1974.
23. Gray's Anatomy, p 814.
24. Goldman L: Cardiac risks and complications of noncardiac surgery. Ann Intern Med 98:504, 1983.
25. Detsky A, Abrams HB, McLaughlin JR, et al: Predicting cardiac complications in patients undergoing non-cardiac surgery. J Gen Intern Med 1:211, 1986.
26. Graber D, Dailey RH: Catheter flow rates updated. JACEP 6:518, 1977.
27. Textbook of Advanced Cardiac Life Support, 2nd ed, pp 146–193. Dallas: American Heart Association, 1987.
28. Moosman DA: The anatomy of infraclavicular subclavian vein catheterization and its complications. Surg Gynecol Obstet 136:17, 1973.

29. Putterman C: Central venous catheterization. Acute Care 12:219, 1986.

30. Moncrief JA: Femoral catheters. Ann Surg 174:166, 1956.

31. Bansmer G, Keith D, Tesluk H: Complications following the use of indwelling catheters of the inferior vena cava. JAMA 167:1606, 1985.

32. Stenzel JP, Green TP, Furman BP, Carlson PE, Marchessault RP: Percutaneous femoral venous catheterization: A prospective study of complications. J Pediatr 114:411, 1989.

33. Williams JF, Seneff MG, Friedman BC, et al: Use of femoral venous catheters in critically ill adults: Prospective study. Crit Care Med 19:550, 1991.

34. Textbook of Advanced Cardiac Life Support, 2nd ed, pp 163–165. Dallas: American Heart Association, 1987.

35. Corona ML, Narr BJ, Thompson RL: Infections related to central venous catheters. Mayo Clin Proc 65:979, 1990.

36. Sitges-Serro A, Linares J, Garau J: Catheter sepsis: The clue is at the hub. Surgery 97:355, 1985.

37. Christensen GD, Simpson WA, Bisno AL, Beachey EH: Adherences of slime producing strains of *Staphylococcus epidermidis* to smooth surfaces. Infect Immunol 37:318, 1982.

38. Gray ED, Peters G, Verstegen M, Regelmann WE: Effect of extracellular slime substances from *Staphylococcus epidermidis* on the cellular immune response. Lancet 1:365, 1984.

39. Cooper GL: Infections associated with invasive hemodynamic monitoring. In Shoemaker WC, Aryes S, Grenvik A, Holbrook PR, Thompson WL (eds): Textbook of Critical Care, 2nd ed, p 854. Philadelphia: WB Saunders, 1986.

40. Maki DG, Weise CE, Sarafin HW: A semiquantitative culture method for identifying intravenous catheter related infections. N Engl J Med 296:1305, 1977.

41. Norwood SH: The prevalence and importance of nosocomial infections. In Civetta JM, Taylor RW, Kirby RR (eds): Critical Care, p 757. Philadelphia: JB Lippincott, 1988.

42. Bazzetti F, Terno G, Bonfanti G, et al: Prevention and treatment of central venous catheter sepsis by exchange via a guidewire: A prospective controlled trial. Ann Surg 198:48, 1938.

43. Snyder RH, Archer FJ, Endy T, et al: Catheter infection: A comparison of two catheter maintenance techniques. Ann Surg 208:651, 1988.

44. Hilton E, Haslett TM, Bornstein MT, Tucci V, Isenbery HD, Singer C: Central catheter infection: Single versus triple-lumen catheters. Am J Med 84:667, 1988.

45. Hoffman KK, Weber DJ, Samsa GP, Rutala WA: Transparent polyurethane film as an intravenous catheter dressing: A meta-analysis of the infection risks. JAMA 267:2072, 1992.

46. Maki DG, Band JD: A comparative study of polyantibiotic and iodophor ointments in prevention of vascular catheter related infections. Am J Med 70:739, 1981.

47. Malatinsky J, Faybik M, Griffith M, et al: Venipuncture, catheterization, and failure to position correctly during central venous cannulation. Resuscitation 10:259, 1983.

48. Cappa GF, Gaoge TF, Hofstetter SR: Air embolism: A lethal but preventable complication of subclavian vein catheterization. JPEN J Parenter Enter Nutr 5:166, 1981.

49. Peters JL, Armstrong R: Air embolism occurring as a complication of central venous catheterization. Ann Surg 187:375, 1978.

50. Hickman RO, Ramsey PG, Trapper D: Central venous access. In Greer BE, Berek JS (eds): Current Topics in Obstetrics and Gynecology. Gynecologic Oncology: Treatment Rationale and Techniques, pp 285–308. New York: Elsevier, 1991.

51. Sanders JE, Hickman RO, Aker S, et al: Experiences with double lumen right atrial catheters. JPEN J Parenter Enter Nutr 6:95, 1982.

52. Scott WL: Complications associated with central venous catheters. Chest 94:1221, 1988.

53. Haire WD, Liberman RP, Lund GB, Edney J, Wieczoreck BM: Obstructed central venous catheters: Restoring function with a twelve hour infusion of low-dose urokinase. Cancer 11:2279, 1990.

54. Press OW, Ramsey PG, Larson EB, et al: Hickman catheter infections in patients with malignancies. Medicine 63:189, 1985.

55. Raff JH: Results from use of 826 vascular access devices in cancer patients. Cancer 55:1312, 1985.

56. Clark DE, Raffin TA: Infectious complications of indwelling long-term central venous catheters. Chest 94:966, 1990.

57. Decker MD, Edwards KM: Central venous catheter infections. Pediatr Clin North Am 35:579, 1988.

58. Dugdale DC, Ramsey PG: *Staphylococcus aureus* bacteremia in patients with Hickman catheters. Am J Med 89:137, 1990.

Complications in Gynecologic Surgery: Prevention, Recognition, and Management,
edited by James W. Orr, Jr., and Hugh M. Shingleton.
J. B. Lippincott Company, Philadelphia, © 1994.

Chapter 8

Infection

David L. Hemsell

Surgical Procedures and Infection

Since Pasteur described the germ theory of disease in the mid-1800s, many important contributions have resulted in a reduction in the frequency and sequelae of infection after elective or emergency gynecologic surgical procedures. Before the mid-1940s, preventive measures primarily entailed using antiseptic solutions and practicing meticulous operative technique. Halstead is credited with introducing surgical gloves. In addition to protecting the hands of the operators, gloves limited the spread of infection from the surgeon's hands to the patient. Halstead reported an extremely low surgical infection rate in low-risk patients when surgical gloves were worn.[1]

The principles of surgical technique are not new. Atraumatic handling of tissue, using small tissue pedicles to minimize necrotic debris, limiting the amount of foreign material, achieving hemostasis, and eliminating dead space all contribute to decreasing the risk of surgical site infection. In 1966 Howe[2] reported that silk suture in a wound reduced host resistance to contaminating bacteria. In 1977 Blumstedt et al.[3] showed that braided suture facilitated bacterial spread. Modern suture materials have significantly reduced those problems.

The introduction of antibiotics into clinical medicine in the mid-1940s allowed effective and predictable therapy for bacterial infections. These "wonder drugs" were used not only to treat acute infection but also to prevent infection. The original prophylactic antibiotic regimen began when the pa-

tient was admitted to the hospital, and administration was often continued throughout the duration of hospitalization. It was felt that "if a little bit is good, a lot must be much better." Long-term prophylactic schemes led in some cases to superinfection, and it soon became evident that the continuous use of antibiotics may not have been the most appropriate regimen for preventing perioperative infection. In fact, prospective trials established that not all surgical procedures required antimicrobial prophylaxis. Large numbers of patients and a variety of surgical procedures were evaluated, and surgical wounds were classified as to infectious risk.[4]

Surgical Wound Classification

Clean surgical procedures include those operations in which there was no break in technique, no evidence of inflammation, and the gastrointestinal and genitourinary tracts were not entered. The incidence of infection without antibiotic administration in prospective trials was 1% to 2%, rendering the prophylactic administration of antibiotics inappropriate.

Clean-contaminated surgical procedures are comprised of those in which there was neither a break in surgical technique nor evidence of inflammation in the operative site, but either the gastrointestinal or genitourinary tracts were entered. Infection rates in these procedures ranged from 10% to 20%. When prophylactic antibiotics were administered the infection rate was reduced to a mean of about 7%. Although hysterectomy was originally considered a clean procedure, it should more appropriately be included here.

Contaminated procedures are those in which there was a break in surgical technique, gross spillage from the gastrointestinal tract, or surgery in an inflamed site. The infection rate observed in such patients ranged between 20% and 35%. This rate was significantly reduced to 10% to 15% by the administration of perioperative antibiotics.

Dirty procedures are those done in patients with a history of trauma, with a perforated viscus, or in whom it was necessary to perform a surgical procedure in the presence of purulent material. The infection rate in these patients ranged from 25% to over 50%. The use of perioperative antibiotics reduced infection by approximately 50%.

Thus, it became evident that specific procedures could be stratified for the risk of postoperative infection, and in many instances patients did not need or benefit from prophylactic antibiotic administration.

Bacterial Contamination

There is always some bacterial inoculation during any surgical procedure. As indicated by the wound classification system, the size of the inoculate is an important variable. Another important variable, although not clinically evaluable, is the virulence of the strains of inoculated bacteria. Virulence factors include β-lactamase, the single most important bacterial defense mechanism in pathogens responsible for perioperative pelvic infection; bacterial adherence; the elaboration of proteases and other enzymes; and the presence of pili or a capsule. As important to the risk of infection is the complex and poorly understood patient host defense system. Uniformly, immunocompromised patients and patients of lower socioeconomic status are at greater risk for infection, as are those exposed to a greater bacterial inoculum.

Lower Reproductive Tract Flora

Infections following gynecologic surgical procedures usually develop during the initial hospitalization, although in a small percentage of women infection develops after discharge. Most late infections develop within 2 weeks of discharge from the hospital. Bacterial pathogens causing these infections are derived from the flora of the lower reproductive tract, which includes gram-negative and gram-positive aerobic and anaerobic bacteria.[5-12]

Thadepalli et al.[13] reported an increased rate of recovery of *Escherichia coli* and *Bacteroides fragilis* from the reproductive tract during the proliferative phase of the menstrual cycle. That phenomenon was reportedly associated with a higher incidence of operative site infection, and they suggested that the risk could be lowered if hysterectomy was performed during the secretory phase. However, four other clinical investigative groups[8,11,14,15] were not able to identify significant differences in bacterial flora that could be ascribed to hormonal changes in pregnant women, premenopausal women not taking hormones, premenopausal women taking oral contraceptives, and postmenopausal women.

Preoperative cultures are not beneficial in predicting which bacteria will be isolated from the operative site when pelvic infection develops after vaginal[16,17] or abdominal hysterectomy.[18] Similar findings were reported by George et al.[6] and Grossman et al.[19] who indicated that preoperative culture results were not predictive of the risk of developing postoperative infection. Current information suggests an upper reproductive tract bacterial flora,[19,20] although the existence of upper reproductive tract flora is controversial and its role, if any, in the development of postoperative infection is speculative.

There is little question that vaginal preparation before vaginal incision reduces bacterial counts. However, this is more effective on vaginal flora than on bacterial count in the endocervix.[21,22] Amstey and Jones[23] reported that even saline preparation was effective in reducing the bacterial count in the vagina. Although the vaginal bacterial count is reduced, bacteria are not completely removed with any preparation. Four different reports indicate the recovery of potential pathogens from the operative site immediately after uterine removal.[6,16,18,24] Thus the pelvic surgeon must always be cognizant of the presence of bacterial contamination and use good surgical technique to decrease the risk of surgical site infection.

Flora Change at Hysterectomy

Bacterial flora alterations occur following hysterectomy despite the use or nonuse of antibiotics perioperatively.[10,25,26] These changes include an increase in Enterobacteriaceae, *Enterococcus faecalis,* and *Bacteroides* species. Antibiotics may play a selective role in flora alteration. In one study,[27] significantly different alterations in the lower reproductive tract flora were observed in women given either a single dose of an extended-spectrum penicillin or three doses of a second-generation cephamycin. These differences could be ascribed both to the spectrum of the antibacterial agents and to the number of doses of antibiotic administered. Three doses of cefoxitin resulted in greater alteration of bacteria than did a single dose of piperacillin.[27] Infection prevention was comparable with either regimen.

Sources of Gynecologic Infections

Infections leading to hospitalization for parenteral antimicrobial therapy have been arbitrarily classified as community acquired or nosocomial, based on where the infection develops. A more important variable involves the type of bacteria responsible for the infection. In general, patients who are hospitalized for the treatment of community-acquired infections usually require less intensive care and antimicrobial therapy than patients who develop infections while in the hospital. Many hospital-acquired infections, especially those observed in older patients, are caused by bacteria that are resistant to a variety of antimicrobial agents. Although most infections that develop after gynecologic surgery develop while the patient is hospitalized, the responsible pathogens are usually those brought into the hospital by the patient. Most gynecologic infections are not associated with multiple-antibiotic-resistant, hospital-acquired bacteria; however, this situation may occur more frequently in women treated by gynecologic oncologists.

Soft tissue infections following hysterectomy have a polymicrobial etiology, and anaerobic species play a significant role.[28–31] Similar species are recovered from the endometrium of women who develop spontaneous pelvic infections, such as septic incomplete abortion, and from those who have undergone surgical procedures such as dilation and curettage or conization. Accurately identifying the true pathogens in pelvic infections is problematic, if not impossible. Collecting material for culture from any of the pelvic infection sites is complicated by the problem that the material must be obtained through the vagina, which may result in specimen contamination by lower reproductive tract flora. Theoretically, protected culture devices should be used to obtain specimens from the endometrial cavity. Double-lumen, catheter-protected brushes were used initially by many investigators, but results obtained using a Pipelle were comparable and were attained at less expense and with less effort.[31]

Another problem with pretreatment culturing is that many laboratories do not provide physicians with sensitivity profiles of anaerobic bacteria if any are identified. To further compound the problem, a physician may receive a microbiology report listing eight different species that were recovered from the culture site of a soft tissue pelvic infection. Identifying the true pathogens from among those eight species is impossible. In clinical situations a gynecologist does not have the time to wait for culture results but must initiate therapy immediately. The patient will likely be cured and at home before the pelvic infection site culture results are returned from the laboratory. For these reasons, many gynecologists do not perform cultures before initiating treatment for a pelvic infection. However, there are those who adamantly believe that such culturing should be performed before therapy. Some physicians believe that the most appropriate cultures are those performed if and when initial therapy fails. In our experience, such cultures frequently reveal only a single organism.

In many instances, and with the delay in receiving sensitivity reports to anaerobes, therapeutic alterations in patients in whom primary therapy fails must be based on predicted weaknesses in the original therapeutic regimen. Alteration of the therapeutic regimen is also empirical and must be based on knowledge of the presumed potential pathogens as well as the coverage provided by the agent(s) selected for initial therapy. Fortunately, this is rarely a problem with the existing therapeutic drug alternatives.

Diagnosis

Temperature elevation is an important indicator of infection. Unfortunately, many patients who undergo major gynecologic surgical procedures with general anesthesia experience postoperative temperature elevation. In most women no source for the elevated temperature can be identified. Up to 40% of women who underwent abdominal hysterectomy and 17% of women who underwent vaginal hysterectomy in Parkland Memorial Hospital in Dallas had recurring temperature elevations of 38° C or greater, were asymptomatic, had a normal physical examination, and did not need antimicrobial therapy for pelvic infection or infection in other locations.

Many more women experience recurrent temperature elevations after abdominal hysterectomy, and it is presumed that the source is pulmonary, as all patients experience some degree of atelectasis (see Chap. 2). In our experience, if a woman has no symptoms and has a normal physical examination, a pelvic examination is not necessary. Additional laboratory tests such as a complete blood cell count with differential, urinalysis, and chest radiography are nonrevealing. The routine "shotgun" laboratory testing for patients experiencing temperature elevation is unnecessary and increases the cost of health care without benefit to the patient. For example, compared to the preoperative leukocyte count, a count determined in the first several postoperative days is almost uniformly elevated. Dysuria is not uncommon in women who have had a transurethral catheter in place. Fortunately, temperature elevation is infrequently associated with urethritis or cystitis. Certainly, if symptoms and physical examination of findings indicate infection of the lungs, urinary tract, operative site, or other site, specific laboratory testing should be performed and therapy begun.

Operative Site Infections

Wound Infection

A wound infection is the easiest of all postoperative infections to diagnose because of the accessibility of infection site to examination. Universal criteria for the diagnosis of a wound infection include pain and erythema of the surgical margins. The incision may be more tender than previously, and purulent exudate and induration may be present. Some investigators classify wound infections based on findings at the time of diagnosis. The infections are classified as grade I when there is a purulent discharge, grade II when grade I wounds are associated with systemic features of infection such as fever and/or leukocytosis, or grade III if surgical intervention is necessary.

It is common for infected wounds to exude serous drainage. When opened, purulent material is frequently identified in the subcutaneous space. This material should be cultured whether or not it is obviously purulent, as it is not uncommon to isolate bacterial species in what appears to be uninfected serous fluid.

The bacteria recovered from wound infections developing after abdominal hysterectomy are frequently multiple, as are those recovered from pelvic sites in women who also develop a pelvic infection. Infections that develop after procedures in which the operative site was not exposed to lower reproductive tract flora are usually caused by gram-positive aerobic cocci.

Although some patients with a wound infection (e.g., immunocompromised patients) may need antimicrobial therapy, the foundation of treatment of a superficial abdominal incision wound infection is local wound care. This consists of wet to dry dressing changes, usually four times a day, with debridement of incision margins with hydrogen peroxide or dilute acetic acid followed by removal of those caustic agents with sterile saline. Fine mesh gauze applied evenly to the wound margins appears to provide the best stimulation to granulation tissue growth. Gauze 4 × 4 inch strips or similar material can be used to fill the space between the layers of fine mesh gauze applied to the incision margins. With a good granulation base, these wounds can be closed secondarily or allowed to heal by secondary intention. Secondary closure decreases wound healing time and the amount of wound care necessary.

Cuff Cellulitis

Cellulitis is part of normal wound healing. In my opinion, every woman who undergoes hysterectomy, irrespective of the surgical approach, experiences some degree of cellulitis in the vaginal surgical margins. Cellulitis likely contributes to the asymptomatic temperature elevation that occurs after hysterectomy, but if it were a major contributor it should occur more commonly after vaginal hysterectomy, which is not the case. The potential for bacterial inoculation is certainly greater in women undergoing vaginal hysterectomy, because inoculation begins with the initial incision and continues throughout the procedure. In women undergoing abdominal hysterectomy, on the other hand, contamination occurs only at the vaginal incision at the end of the procedure.

Host defense mechanisms, with or without the aid of antimicrobial administration, are able to contain the inflammatory response to the vaginal surgical margins in most patients. In a small number of patients, lower abdominal, pelvic, and perhaps back pain develops in association with recurring temperature elevation. On examination, greater than expected tenderness, erythema, and edema are confined to the vaginal cuff. Cuff infection develops on the third postoperative day in a few patients but is more commonly diagnosed 6 to 14 days after hospital discharge. Review of the hospital stay finds it to be uneventful, with no temperature elevations. Antibiotic therapy is necessary and will be discussed subsequently.

Pelvic Cellulitis

Pelvic cellulitis develops when the inflammatory response is not confined to the vagina and extends into contiguous pelvic soft tissues. Lower abdominal, pelvic, and perhaps back pain is the clinical hallmark of this infection and is associated with recurrent temperature elevation and tenderness in the parametrial areas on bimanual examination. There is usually abdominal tenderness that is maximal over the area of cellulitis and is elicited by gentle and deep palpation of the abdominal wall. A Pfannenstiel incision often limits one's ability to elicit this tenderness.

Phlegmon

Webster's dictionary defines phlegmon as a diffuse inflammation of soft or connective tissue due to infection.[32] It is synonymous with a maximal degree of cellulitis. *The Encyclopedia and Dictionary of Medicine, Nursing, and Allied Health* refers to a phlegmon as "a diffuse inflammation of the soft or connective tissue due to infection with microaerophilic streptococci."[33] The definition in *Stedman's Medical Dictionary* is "an obsolete term for an acute suppurative inflammation of the subcutaneous connective tissue."[34] There are often microabscesses in these infected tissues; whether these coalesce to form a true abscess or whether an abscess forms de novo is unknown. A phlegmon is usually observed in the parametrial areas.

Adnexal Infection

Although infection in an adnexa is most frequently observed after hysterectomy, it can occur after other pelvic surgical procedures. The principal symptom is lower abdominal and pelvic pain that is usually more intense on the side of involved adnexa. The infection may be cellulitis, a phlegmon, or an abscess. Tenderness elicited on pelvic examination is usually cephalad and lateral to the normal parametrial areas. Tenderness may be such that one cannot appreciate the presence of an abscess; in such instances, ultrasonography is quite helpful.

Abscess

An abscess may occur in the pelvis, or in any abdominal or vaginal incision, or in either or both adnexae. The symptoms of an abscess are similar to those of cellulitis. It may be possible to palpate a mass in a patient with an abscess, but a pelvic abscess may be difficult to palpate. Neither patient symptoms, temperature elevation, nor leukocyte count can predictively differentiate between cellulitis and abscess in an infected patient.

Treatment for an abscess includes drainage. If the abscess is easily accessible, as is true in either vaginal or abdominal incisions, drainage by opening the incision is indicated. If the abscess occupies the extraperitoneal space just above the vaginal cuff following hysterectomy, drainage can be effected in a treatment room by opening the vaginal cuff under local anesthesia. At our institution, adnexal abscesses are rare and infrequently require drainage. Computed tomography–guided drainage with local anesthesia will almost uniformly prevent the necessity for another surgical procedure.

Infected Hematoma

A hematoma may develop in any surgical site. The hematomas most frequently complicated by infection in our patient population are extraperitoneal, occur in the pelvis, and may be either lateral or just above the vaginal cuff. A noninfected hematoma rarely causes symptoms, is too soft to be palpated, and is nontender. Clinically, a hematoma should be suspected from an unexplained drop in hemoglobin concentration between pre- and postoperative measurements. The typical scenario for infection of the hematoma is the development of recurring temperature elevation on the third to fifth postoperative day in an asymptomatic woman with a normal general physical and pelvic examination. If observed and untreated, the infected hematoma will become palpable and tender.

Mechanical drainage of a hematoma facilitates treatment response. However, if the hematoma is not easily accessible, parenteral antimicrobial therapy usually results in resolution of temperature elevation.

Febrile Morbidity

An asymptomatic temperature elevation is not synonymous with infection. The temperature readings required to define febrile morbidity differ widely. There are at least 32 different definitions for this diagnosis, varying from 37.5° C on two or more consecutive days more than 24 hours after surgery[35] to 38.3° C on two occasions at least 6 hours apart and more than 48 hours after surgery.[36] Temperature elevation in the absence of symptoms and physical findings is observed in many of our patients following hysterectomy. No treatment is required, and the temperature usually returns to normal without prolongation of the hospital stay. However, Shapiro and co-workers[37] reported that febrile morbidity increases the cost of health care in their patients. Obviously, individual determination is very important, and careful selection of febrile patients who may need therapy is essential in any clinical situation.

Infection Prevention

Most gynecologic surgical procedures are elective and can be scheduled for a time when the woman is free of urinary tract, pelvic, or respiratory infection. Administration of antibiotics to a clinically uninfected patient is the definition of prophylaxis. Original prophylactic regimens began at hospital admission and continued during the entire hospital stay. It was not uncommon for patients to be discharged on oral antibiotics for an additional week. Many prospective, randomized, blinded clinical trials have evaluated the need for preventive antibiotics and the ability of such a regimen to prevent infection after a variety of gynecologic surgical procedures. These will be addressed individually.

Timing of antibiotic administration is paramount. Classen and co-workers[38] reported that the most effective time to administer antibiotic was during the 2 hours before incision. Infection rates were significantly higher ($p < 0.0001$) if antibiotic was administered more than 2 hours but less than 24 hours before surgery and more than 3 hours but less than 24 hours after surgery. The following recommendations are generalized. Specific centers may have investigated the role and effects of prophylaxis in their patient population. Individual centers may use a specific antibiotic or a specific dosing regimen for certain patients.

Intrauterine Contraceptive Device Insertion

In 1990 Sinei and co-workers,[39] in a randomized clinical trial of 1,813 women, reported that 200 mg of doxycycline given orally at the time of insertion of an intrauterine contraceptive device (IUD) reduced the incidence of pelvic inflammatory disease by 31% and decreased the rate of unplanned device-related visits to the clinic by 31%. Whereas only the latter was statistically significant ($p = 0.0004$), both are believed to be clinically significant. Contrarily, Ladipo et al. found that neither the

incidence of pelvic inflammatory disease nor the frequency of unscheduled clinic visits was reduced in 1,485 women randomly given placebo or 200 mg of doxycycline. The prevalence of pelvic inflammatory disease in their entire population was only 0.01%.[40] Jovanovic et al. reported no cases of pelvic inflammatory disease after *midcycle* insertion of an IUD in 288 women given 100 mg of doxycycline twice a day for 5 days.[41]

Recommendation. Based on data from these three prospective studies, a single 200-mg dose of doxycycline given before IUD placement is recommended. Peak serum concentrations of doxycycline are observed approximately 2 hours after oral ingestion, so the medication should be prescribed and taken at home before the woman presents for IUD placement. The majority of women with uncomplicated acute salpingitis seek treatment very soon after onset of a menstrual period, especially when *Neisseria gonorrhoeae* is recovered. Therefore, insertion should be scheduled away from menstruation to further decrease the incidence of associated pelvic infection. Specific testing for sexually transmitted diseases should be performed and known negative results should be available before the device is inserted. The cervix and vagina should be prepared prior to insertion.

Hysterosalpingography

Pelvic infection following hysterosalpingography is infrequent. However, a tubal infection is undesirable in this patient population. Most commonly, women who undergo this diagnostic procedure do so as part of an evaluation for infertility. In 1980, Stumpf and March[42] devised a severity scoring system and recommended cancellation of the hysterosalpingogram if the risk factor score was high. This was a logical recommendation, since many women could have tubal patency evaluated during laparoscopy as a part of their infertility workup. Unfortunately, the scoring system did not accurately predict the risk of postprocedure infection.

However, Pyper and associates[43] reported that bacteria were carried into the peritoneal cavity with dye in 90% of women who underwent laparoscopy with dye injection. Pittaway et al.[44] reviewed the development of acute pelvic inflammatory disease after hysterosalpingography and reported that all women who developed postprocedural infection had diagnosed tubal dilation. They then prospectively evaluated the effect of three 100-mg doses of doxycycline given to women with a previous history of hydrosalpinx. For women with a dilated tube demonstrated at hysterosalpingography, 200 mg was administered after the procedure, followed by 100 mg every 12 hours for at least 5 days. No woman given doxycycline developed acute infection.

Recommendation. Although an optimal dosing regimen has not been determined, 200 mg of doxycycline should be given orally approximately 2 hours before the scheduled radiologic procedure. If there is evidence of tubal dilation, additional doses may be beneficial. The presence of sexually transmitted disease species should be evaluated and absent before this test is performed. Again, local cervical preparation is necessary.

Abortion

Since 1985 three reports have demonstrated the benefit of perioperative antibiotic administration in reducing the incidence of pelvic infection after suction curettage. Whereas no significant reduction in infection was observed in several previous smaller studies, these large studies demonstrated statistically significant reduction ($p = 0.025$ to 0.001) associated with the administration of either metronidazole or doxycycline.[45–57]

No data on the benefit of prophylactic administration of antibiotics in women undergoing suction curettage for incomplete spontaneous abortion are available. In women undergoing elective pregnancy termination, testing for sexually transmitted diseases can be carried out, with therapy given to women with positive results before the procedure. This luxury is not available in women having a spontaneous miscarriage; however, the presence of sexually transmitted disease species should be evaluated before elective termination or at spontaneous miscarriage. Recently developed tests allow "positive" patients to be identified within hours. Only these patients may benefit from prophylaxis.

Recommendation. An oral dose of 200 mg of doxycycline should be given approximately 2 hours before the procedure. It is possible that an additional 100-mg dose given 12 hours later may further reduce the infection rate.

Ectopic Pregnancy

It is intriguing that the incidence of ectopic pregnancy is increasing despite the decrease in incidence of pelvic inflammatory disease. In 1990,

Layman and Sanfilippo[48] reported that 12% of women undergoing surgical therapy for ectopic pregnancy developed operative site infection. Berenson et al.[49] reported positive intraoperative cultures of the fallopian tube in 37% of patients undergoing surgery for ectopic pregnancy. As is true for hysterectomy, culture results did not correlate with the development of postoperative infection. There is currently a prospective, randomized, blinded study in progress at Parkland Memorial Hospital, Dallas, to establish a requirement for and identification of potential benefits from a single-dose preoperative antibiotic regimen given to women undergoing laparoscopic or open surgery for ectopic pregnancy. Although recommendations are not currently available, the presence of *Chlamydia trachomatis* and *Neisseria gonorrhoeae* should be evaluated. The patient should be treated if either organism is present.

Infertility Surgery

Cartwright et al.[50] discouraged the use of intraperitoneal antibiotic irrigation during infertility-related surgery because of the potential for enhanced adhesion formation secondary to antibiotic crystallization. As previously noted,[43] bacteria are introduced into the upper reproductive tract by transcervical and intrauterine irrigation. Therefore, it is assumed that bacterial inoculation occurs with any such procedure, placing them in a clean-contaminated category. There are no data to confirm a benefit from prophylactic administration of antibiotic to these patients. The same is true for women undergoing operative procedures involving the same pelvic organs but unrelated to infertility, such as ovarian cystectomy or adhesiolysis for pain.

Recommendation. It is possible that a 200-mg dose of doxycycline given orally with a small amount of water 2 hours before a procedure would be effective. If reproductive gynecologists or anesthesiologists are uncomfortable with such a regimen, a preoperative parenteral dose of antibiotic comparable to that given before a hysterectomy should suffice. There are currently no data indicating that any regimen is better than a single preoperative 1- or 2-gm dose of cefazolin.

Retropubic Urethropexy

Bhatia and co-workers[51] reported that three 1-gm cefazolin doses given perioperatively to women undergoing a modified Burch retropubic urethropexy with placement of a Stamey suprapubic catheter was associated with significantly less febrile morbidity ($p < 0.01$) and a significantly shorter hospital stay ($p < 0.05$) than in women not given antibiotic. Hysterectomy and other procedures were not performed. Although small, this study suggests that there may be other surgical procedures for which antimicrobial prophylaxis may be beneficial.

Vaginal Hysterectomy

There are very few reports in which the administration of prophylactic antibiotic did not significantly reduce the requirement for parenteral antibiotic treatment of operative site infection after vaginal hysterectomy. Risk factors, when sought, were not uniform. If there is a relatively uniform requirement for prophylaxis, the important decisions become which agent to select and how many doses to administer. When compared with an antibiotic having a confined bacterial spectrum, an antibiotic with a broad antibacterial spectrum should provide enhanced protection against postoperative infection. However, no clinical trials have substantiated that premise. Unfortunately, the small sample sizes evaluated in clinical trials render the power of data insufficient to detect a significant difference. Similarly, there is no uniform evidence supporting the superiority of multiple doses over a single preoperative dose.

Stiver et al.[52] recently compared a single dose of a third-generation cephalosporin and three doses of cefazolin. They reported that the costs of acquisition, preparation, and administration were greater for the single-dose agent than for three doses of cefazolin. There was no difference in patient protection. With that finding, it was their opinion that cefazolin would be the drug of choice for prophylaxis in patients undergoing uncomplicated vaginal hysterectomy in their hospital. Unfortunately, they have not reported results with single-dose cefazolin. The three-dose regimen is more expensive in our hospital.

There is information to indicate that local application of antibiotic is effective in preventing infection after hysterectomy. In 1950 Turner[53] reported a reduction in the incidence of febrile morbidity from 38% to 7% with preoperative insertion of a vaginal penicillin G suppository. Wright et al.[54] reported a significant reduction in postoperative infection using a topical antibiotic combination spray in the vagina. In one study comparing oral doxycycline with three parenteral doses of cefazolin, Smith et al.[55] reported comparable protection in a small number of patients.

Two reports published in the mid-1970s indicated that suction drainage was a successful alternative to the use of prophylactic antibiotics for women undergoing vaginal hysterectomy.[56,57] Two subsequent studies[58,59] were unable to confirm efficacy of the drain. Galle et al.[58] in 1981 reported an association of pelvic abscess with drain utilization that was not observed in women given comparative antimicrobial prophylaxis. There appears to be little benefit to the routine use of suction drainage after vaginal hysterectomy.

As previously noted, vaginal preparation has little effect on endocervical bacteria, the most likely origin of bacteria inoculated into the operative site. Osborne et al.[60] reported in 1979 that hot conization of the cervix immediately before vaginal hysterectomy was as effective in preventing postoperative pelvic infection as was the administration of perioperative antibiotics.

Recommendation. Cefazolin, 1 or 2 gm administered IV in the operating room prior to anesthesia, will allow the patient to report an allergic reaction before complete infusion.

Abdominal Hysterectomy

Perhaps the first report in the gynecologic literature regarding prophylaxis appeared in 1944.[61] As for vaginal hysterectomy, many retrospective, prospective placebo-controlled and blinded, and prospective comparative studies, with or without investigator blinding, have evaluated prophylaxis for women undergoing abdominal hysterectomy.

Some investigators sought risk factors for infection. Some of these include patient age, menopausal status, diabetes, obesity, lower socioeconomic status, anemia, history of prior salpingitis, history of immediate preceding surgery such as dilation and curettage or conization, experience or lack thereof of the surgeon, performance of additional surgical procedures with hysterectomy, long duration of surgery, and excessive blood loss. Either the results were controversial, or the variables were found not to be risk factors for infection. The implication is that individual determination is necessary.

Soper et al.[62] reported bacterial vaginosis or *Trichomonas vaginalis* vaginitis to be a risk factor for cuff cellulitis after abdominal hysterectomy. Prophylaxis was not used in their patients, and the infection rate was 35%. In another report by Larsson et al.[63] that also evaluated risks without prophylaxis, the discovery of bacterial vaginosis in a preoperative slide was associated with a 35% infection rate following hysterectomy. One hopes the effect of prophylaxis will be evaluated by these authors, because soon, with the new Clinical Laboratory Improvement Amendments (CLIA) 1988 regulations, it may be impossible to obtain this information immediately before surgery, when it will be most important.

Most of the prospective data evaluating prophylaxis for abdominal hysterectomy involved small numbers of patients in each arm. For that reason, the statistical power to identify a significant difference was limited. If one combines data from prospective and blinded placebo-controlled studies evaluating various antibiotics, a statistically significant reduction in infection rate can be identified in women given antibiotic when compared with women given placebo. While that does not mean that all women undergoing abdominal hysterectomy should be given antibiotic prophylaxis indiscriminately, it does indicate that high-risk groups may be identified that would benefit from prophylaxis. Certainly, if the incidence of major infection requiring parenteral antimicrobial therapy following abdominal hysterectomy is 10% or less, prophylaxis is not indicated for the entire patient population. Neither multiple dosing of parenteral antibiotic nor using an agent with an expanded spectrum of antibacterial activity appears to enhance efficacy at infection prevention.

In the 1970s Swartz and Tanaree[56,57] reported that suction drainage as an alternative to prophylactic antibiotics was effective in reducing the incidence of infection following abdominal hysterectomy. Two subsequent studies[59,64] indicated that suction drainage was not effective, as has been our experience. Nelson et al.[65] reported that intraoperative antibiotic irrigation resulted in a significant reduction in the incidence of major postoperative infection after abdominal hysterectomy in a nonrandomized clinical trial.

Beresford and MacKenzie[66] recently reported results of a pilot study designed to compare bacterial contamination occurring when the vaginal vault was closed with automatic stapling technique or with the regular suture method. In that small study, less bacterial contamination occurred at the operative site when the stapling device was used. Although this study is of potential benefit, a larger prospective evaluation is necessary prior to the uniform adoption of this more expensive technique. Zakut and colleagues[67] found that women treated with a povidone-iodine–soaked pack left in the va-

gina until its transection at hysterectomy had significantly ($p < 0.001$) fewer bacteria recovered at intraoperative cultures but an incidence of pelvic and wound infection comparable to that observed in women given perioperative antibiotic. Febrile morbidity and the urinary tract infection rate were, however, significantly lower in women treated with the povidone-iodine pack.

Morbidity was reported to be greater after abdominal hysterectomy than after vaginal hysterectomy.[68–70] In the initial report, this was believed to be secondary to the fact that only women undergoing vaginal hysterectomy were given prophylaxis. In the latter two prospective studies, all women received perioperative antibiotic. Abdominal wall infection after abdominal hysterectomy and patient immobility, combined with the preoperative diagnosis, are a plausible explanation.

Recommendation. Cefazolin, 1 or 2 gm, may be administered IV in the operating room before anesthesia induction. Administration in this fashion will allow the patient to detect an allergic reaction before complete infusion.

Radical Gynecologic Surgery

The incidence of pelvic infection requiring parenteral antimicrobial therapy following radical hysterectomy varies from 1.5% to 23.4%, with the wound infection rate ranging from 2.8% to 18.8%. Prospective data on the need for and the efficacy of antimicrobial prophylaxis at radical abdominal hysterectomy are controversial. In most prospective studies, the number of patients in comparative terms is small. When efficacy data from many prospective studies are combined, it appears that the overall incidence of major operative site infection is significantly reduced with prophylaxis, although the hospital stay is not necessarily shortened.[71] Orr et al.[72] in a retrospective study and van Lindert et al.[73] reported that single-dose prophylaxis was effective. Van Lindert and co-workers also measured antibiotic concentrations in serum, fat, and pelvic tissues, and reported antibiotic concentrations up to 3 hours after the beginning of surgery that were above the minimal inhibitory concentration of most pathogens found preoperatively in surveillance cultures. A blood loss of more than 1,500 mL resulted in a significant decrease in antibiotic concentration in both serum and fat when measured 1 to 2 hours after administration, when compared with women whose blood loss was less than 1,500 mL. Numbers were too small to identify a correlation between blood loss and postoperative infection. Sevin et al.[74] confirmed that a three-dose regimen of perioperative antibiotic was as effective as a 12-dose regimen.

Recommendation. Same as for vaginal hysterectomy. The work of van Lindert et al. provides at least theoretical justification for administration of a second dose of antibiotic for women who lose more than 1,500 mL of blood during a surgical procedure. This should apply to hysterectomy for benign diagnoses as well. We continually evaluate risk factors for infection in women undergoing hysterectomy for benign diagnoses and have identified decreased hemoglobin as a risk factor. Duration of surgery was not found to be a risk factor, nor was it mentioned to be by van Lindert et al.

Agent Selection

A short discussion regarding prophylactic agents for administration to patients with antibiotic allergies is warranted. Approximately 12% of our patients report an allergy to penicillin. If a woman describes other than a type I allergy to penicillin, we have routinely administered prophylactic or therapeutic cephalosporin without allergic reaction over the last 13 years. If a woman has a history of a type I reaction to penicillin or describes an allergy to cephalosporins and requires prophylaxis, there are alternatives. The broadest spectrum single agent is clindamycin. It has rarely been used in our patient population, but when given it was successful. We previously reported[75] the efficacy of administering 200 mg of doxycycline IV over 2 hours, starting 2 hours before vaginal hysterectomy. Although the infection rate with that regimen was unacceptably high, an alteration in the mode of administration has been successful. The modified regimen has not been evaluated prospectively except in women who were not able to enroll in ongoing studies because of penicillin anaphylaxis. The regimen consists of 100 mg of doxycycline given orally at bedtime the night before surgery, with another oral dose given about 3 hours preoperatively. It has been effective in preventing infection following hysterectomy for benign diagnoses.

Treatment

Since the advent of antimicrobial prophylaxis, the requirement for the therapeutic application of antibiotics has significantly decreased. A multiplicity

of antibiotics and new families of antibiotics have been developed in the past two decades. These agents are semisynthetic products, most with an expanded spectrum of antibacterial activity. This has allowed single-agent therapy to achieve cure rates comparable or superior to the cure rates associated with administration of multiple antibiotics. In addition to spectrum expansion and activity enhancement, semisynthetic substitution has also resulted in prolongation of the half-life of several antibiotics, which allows less frequent dosing.

Few studies have confirmed the efficacy of a therapeutic antimicrobial regimen in a purely gynecologic population of women with postoperative pelvic infection. However, it was recognized early that therapeutic regimens should cover gram-positive and gram-negative aerobic organisms. The agents most frequently administered were a penicillin or a first-generation cephalosporin with an aminoglycoside. It was believed that if therapy for these bacteria was adequate, then the anaerobic component of the normal lower reproductive tract flora that was inoculated at surgery would not become pathogenic. The two antianaerobic compounds available at the time were chloramphenicol and clindamycin. Since they were expensive and associated with potentially serious clinical side effects, it was recommended that they be saved for failure of initial regimens. Failure rates with initial regimens were as high as 50% in some patient populations. Anaerobic infections frequently required a surgical procedure.

In 1979, a classic article by diZerega and colleagues[76] clearly documented that the combination of clindamycin and gentamicin was superior to that of penicillin and gentamicin. This hallmark article established the requirement for and benefits from including antianaerobic activity in the initial treatment regimen for acute pelvic infection.

In fact, a principal goal of spectrum expansion during the development of newer antibiotics was the inclusion of antianaerobic activity. Single-agent regimens proven effective in the treatment of acute postoperative female pelvic infections include cefoxitin,[77-84] cefotetan,[82,83] cefotaxime,[85] cefoperazone,[86,87] and piperacillin.[84,88,89] Because one of the principal defense mechanisms of bacteria causing soft tissue pelvic infection is the production of β-lactamase enzymes, a different approach taken to enhance antibacterial activity entailed combining a β-lactamase enzyme inhibitor with an established antibiotic. Clavulanic acid was combined with ticarcillin for IV administration,[81] and with amoxicillin for oral administration. Sulbactam has been combined with ampicillin and is marketed for parenteral administration.[90,91] All provide excellent coverage for the pathogens of acute pelvic infection (Table 8–1).

A new family of antibiotics, the carbapenems, is currently undergoing expansion. The first in this family to be clinically released was imipenem. Because it is degraded by a renal dehydropeptidase enzyme, it was combined with cilastatin, a dehydropeptidase I enzyme inhibitor. This combination is available for parenteral administration as Primaxin, which has proven therapeutic efficacy.[92,93]

There are many new quinolone antibiotics that are available for clinical use, and others are being developed. Nalidixic acid, the parent compound of the quinolones, had very limited antibacterial activity. Newer representatives of this family of antibiotics are available in both parenteral and oral forms and are active against both gram-negative and gram-positive aerobic and anaerobic bacteria. Efficacy data are available on the use of ciprofloxacin as a therapeutic agent for women with acute postoperative pelvic infections.[94]

Many gynecologists still prefer to use a combination of antibiotics when treating women with a postoperative pelvic infection. These combinations include clindamycin and aminoglycoside,[87–89,94–96] with or without ampicillin, or substitution of metronidazole[90,95] for clindamycin. Clindamycin alone was effective in curing 88% of cases of acute polymicrobial pelvic infections.[97] For patients with significant renal dysfunction, in whom an aminoglycoside would be contraindicated or limited in dose, the clinically available new monobactam was successfully administered. Aztreonam[98] is very active against a wide spectrum of gram-negative aerobic pathogens, including *Pseudomonas aeruginosa,* a rare pathogen for pelvic infections. It is neither nephrotoxic nor ototoxic.[98] Like the penicillins and cephalosporins, however, it is a β-lactam antibiotic. Administration of a combination of β-lactam antibiotics has been associated with the induction of β-lactamase enzyme production by a variety of bacteria, although predominantly gram-negative aerobic bacteria.

For women truly allergic to penicillin, vancomycin is the agent of choice for gram-positive aerobic bacteria when specific coverage is required. It is not well absorbed with oral ingestion, and for that reason it can also be given for antibiotic-associated pseudomembranous enterocolitis caused by *Clostridium difficile.*

Postoperative soft tissue fungal infections and bacteremia are uncommon but may develop in the postoperative patient, especially patients who receive antimicrobial treatment for a prolonged period of time, postoperative patients, and immunocompromised patients. According to Horan et al.,[99] *Candida* spp. are more common in nosocomial septicemia than *Escherichia coli* and *Pseudomonas aeruginosa,* and up to one third of such cases occur in patients who have undergone surgery within the preceding 3 weeks.[100] Solomkin and associates[101] reported that untreated candidemia can be associated with a mortality as high as 83%. A high index of suspicion is required; Gaines and Remington[102] reported that up to 85% of *Candida*-infected patients were undiagnosed at the time of their death. In a recent report, Fraser et al.[103] discovered a 20-fold increase in the incidence of candidemic patients in the decade between the late 1970s and late 1980s. For such patients, the most recently introduced imidazole, fluconazole, can be administered orally or IV. Such infections currently are observed almost exclusively by the gynecologic oncologist.

The woman with gynecologic malignancy is at risk for infections other than those caused by lower reproductive tract bacteria. The normal flora of a

TABLE 8–1. **Antibiotics and Dosing**

Agent	Dosage
Amikacin	7.5 mg/kg IV q12h
Amphotericin B	0.4–1 mg/kg q24h
Ampicillin	2 g IV q4–6h
Ampicillin/sulbactam	3 g IV q6h
Aztreonam	1–2 g IV q8–12h
Cefoperazone	2 g IV q12h
Cefotaxime	1–2 g IV q8h
Cefotetan	2 g IV q12h
Cefoxitin	2 g IV q6h
Clindamycin	900 mg IV q8h
Fluconazole	Loading dose: 400 mg Maintenance dose: 200 mg q24h
Gentamicin	Loading dose: 2 mg/kg IV Maintenance dose: 1.5 mg/kg IV q8h
Imipenem/cilastatin	0.5–1 g IV q8h
Metronidazole	Loading dose: 15 mg/kg IV Maintenance dose: 7.5 mg/kg IV q6h
Mezlocillin	4 g IV q6h
Piperacillin	4 g IV q6h
Ticarcillin/clavulanate	3.1 g IV q6h
Vancomycin	500 mg IV q6h

woman with gynecologic malignancy may be altered by the nature of the disease and by treatment such as radiation or previous antibiotic therapy. Because many women require prolonged catheterization, numerous bacteria and fungi have access not only to the urinary tract but also to the bloodstream. Tumor may erode into adjacent soft tissues, allowing infection of these adjacent structures. Obstruction of either the gastrointestinal or urinary tract may also occur, with resulting infection. Either intraperitoneal or prolonged IV catheters are other avenues for infection, and radiation or chemotherapy may render the patient more susceptible to infection by lowering the neutrophil count. In some of the latter instances, the normal signs and symptoms of infection are lacking, making it difficult to accurately diagnose the infection. Also, a response to infection such as pyuria or purulent sputum may be absent. For this reason, frequent repeat examinations and close observation are required.

The infection risk is related to both the duration and the degree of neutropenia and becomes accelerated when the neutrophil count drops below 1,000/mm^3. Gram-positive aerobes may predominate in infection sites, but the infections are usually caused by multiple bacteria. Delay in the early and aggressive antimicrobial therapy for the febrile neutropenic patient may result in a suboptimal response. For that reason, a temperature of 38.3° C or higher for more than 2 hours that is not associated with the administration of pyogenic substances such as blood products usually indicates infection. Untreated infection rapidly disseminates. Even low-virulence bacteria can cause life-threatening infections and should not be considered to be contaminants when reported in culture results. Blood, urine, and sputum should be cultured in addition to accessible sites of potential pelvic infection.

Whereas gentamicin is sufficient for combination therapy in normopenic women, amikacin should be used in febrile neutropenic patients. Efficacy with combination therapy varies from 65% to 85%, and with single-agent therapy (ceftazidime, imipenem/cilastatin) from 68% to 92%. Therapy is usually continued for 4 days after all signs and symptoms have resolved, and usually not less than 7 days. This duration of therapy is about twice the length required for the normopenic woman who develops a postoperative infection.

For patients who fail to respond to appropriate antimicrobial therapy, granulocyte transfusion may be beneficial. Daily transfusion for 4 days appears to be optimal. Cytokines (granulocyte [G]/macrophage [M] colony-stimulating factors [CSF] and G-CSF) might reduce the need for granulocyte transfusion but are expensive. This topic was recently reviewed by Roilides and Pizzo.[104] There are also monoclonal antibodies against gram-negative aerobic bacteria that have unproved success in patients with sepsis, with or without shock.[105]

Most infections are diagnosed from clinical findings, although it may be necessary to use special studies such as sonography, computed tomography, or magnetic resonance imaging. Broad-spectrum coverage is required,[106,107] and empirical therapy is more aggressive. Abscess drainage may require a surgical procedure, but percutaneous drainage is usually successful when coupled with antimicrobial therapy.

Women with temperature elevation and pyuria and in whom a urinary tract infection is suspected should be given empirical antimicrobial therapy for such an infection pending culture results. The combination of cefazolin and gentamicin provides broad-spectrum coverage for such an infection. For women with a prolonged hospitalization or who are debilitated, and with a history of recent courses of antibiotics, substitution of a third-generation cephalosporin for cefazolin provides better coverage. The therapeutic regimen can be changed depending on culture results. Some patients with indwelling catheters may be colonized but not symptomatic. Pyuria and bacteriuria usually accompany positive urine cultures in patients with normal leukocyte counts. A positive urine culture in the absence of pyuria implies a contaminated culture. Chronic suppressive therapy is frequently given to a woman with a chronic indwelling catheter or stent.

Many patients undergoing chemotherapy who become neutropenic may develop fever without clinical symptoms or signs indicating the origin of the pyrexia. Bacteria may enter the bloodstream of such patients through the gastrointestinal tract through small intestinal mucosal ulcerations. This may be enhanced by a low platelet count. These patients may also develop obvious infections such as pneumonia, cellulitis, wound infection, meningitis, and so forth. Since these patients may not exhibit the routine signs and symptoms of infection with which physicians are familiar, early and aggressive therapy is necessary. Bacteremia in these patients may be as high as 20% and in many cases is caused by Gram-negative or Gram-positive aerobic bacteria. Enteric Gram-negative rods are the most frequent pathogens. If the patient has been in the hospital for a length of time, it is more likely that *Pseudomonas* may be the pathogen. For that reason, combining a semisynthetic penicillin with a β-lactamase inhibitor, such as ticarcillin and clavulanic acid or a third-generation cephalosporin with an aminoglycoside, should provide the broadest coverage for the patient. If a superinfection caused by bacteria resistant to the initial regimen is suspected, cultures should be repeated and therapy altered to provide coverage for the suspected pathogens. Infection profiles at the surgeon's hospital should provide information that would allow prediction of the most likely pathogens in such cases.

Central IV catheters are another source of infection. Gram-positive bacteria or yeast may cause infection in the skin, which may become locally inflamed and painful. Purulent drainage may be present around the catheter site. This diagnosis is made on clinical grounds with Gram stain; the patient with such an infection should be treated with an appropriate regimen, principally vancomycin. If the patient also has neutropenia, empirical therapy must include two agents, such as a third-generation cephalosporin and an aminoglycoside. It is possible that infused solutions may be contaminated, resulting in bacteremia with infusion. In general, bacteria causing these infections are usually gram-negative aerobic bacteria. Blood culture is required to make the diagnosis, and such a patient might have fever and chills immediately following an infusion. If blood cultures were positive before the initiation of therapy, they should be repeated and negative at the conclusion of therapy. If the patient has *Pseudomonas aeruginosa infection,* it may be necessary to treat the patient for up to 4 weeks.

Although a rarity in gynecologic patients without malignancy, fungal infections can be quite problematic. Bloodstream infection may result from IV catheter site or from gastrointestinal ulcers secondary to chemotherapy or through the urinary tract as the result of a foreign body. Pneumonia may also occur in the neutropenic patient. Most infections are caused by *Candida albicans, C. tropicalis,* or *C. parapsilos,* or *Torulopsis glabrata.* Immunosuppressive therapy, especially corticosteroids, is among the greatest of the risk factors. Blood cultures may be positive in only approximately 50% of patients with candidemia presenting as a fever of undetermined origin. It is not usually a contaminant when found in blood cultures.

Fungal pneumonia presents as does any other type of pneumonia. It is usually the result of hematogenous seeding, which may be reflected in the chest radiograph. The presence of *Candida* in a sputum culture may only indicate colonization rather than infection. Fungus balls may develop in the urinary tract and can even result in ureteral ob-

struction. Bladder irrigation with amphotericin B may be the treatment of choice. The problem for the physician is determining whether *Candida* is just colonizing a site or whether it is a truly invasive infection requiring treatment. Obviously, yeast in both pleural or peritoneal fluid or cerebrospinal fluid should be considered evidence of invasive disease and treatment should be initiated. Amphotericin B has long been the therapy of choice for patients with invasive fungal infection.

Pneumonia is also common in the postoperative gynecologic oncology patient. Pneumonia may rarely result from aspiration; more frequently it results from colonization and decreased respiratory effort. Gynecologic oncology patients may also develop pneumonia as a result of metastases to the lungs. The signs and symptoms usually associated with pneumonia are present. If chest x-ray findings are diagnostic, sputum should be examined and cultured with the expectation that the predominant organisms will be Gram-negative and anaerobic. However, it must be kept in mind that aerobes may also contribute. The patient who has been hospitalized longer or who has had courses of IV antibiotic therapy prior to the development of pneumonia is more likely to have resistant bacteria and multiple bacteria and so will benefit more from empirical therapy with combination therapy, such as an aminoglycoside added to a second- or third-generation cephalosporin or an extended-spectrum penicillin with β-lactamase inhibitor.

References

1. Halstead WS: Ligature and suture material. JAMA 15:1119, 1913.
2. Howe CW: Experimental studies on determinations of wound infection. Surg Gynecol Obstet 123:507, 1966.
3. Blumstedt B, Osterberg B, Bergstrand A: Suture material and bacteria transport. Acta Chir Scand 143:73, 1977.
4. Ad Hoc Committee of the Committee on Trauma, Division of Medical Sciences, National Academy of Sciences. National Research Council: Postoperative wound infections: The influence of ultraviolet irradiation of the operating room and of various other factors. Ann Surg 160(suppl):1, 1964.
5. Gorbach S, Menda K, Thadepalli H, Keith L: Anaerobic microflora of the cervix in healthy women. Am J Obstet Gynecol 117:1053, 1973.
6. George JW, Ansbacher R, Otterson WN, Rabey F: Prospective bacteriologic study of women undergoing hysterectomy. Obstet Gynecol 45:60, 1975.
7. Ohm MJ, Galask RP: Bacterial flora of the cervix from 100 prehysterectomy patients. Am J Obstet Gynecol 122:683, 1975.
8. Tashjian JH, Coulam CB, Washington JA II: Vaginal flora in asymptomatic women. Mayo Clin Proc 51:557, 1976.
9. Bartlett JG, Moon NE, Goldstein PR, Goren B,

Onderdonk AB, Polk BF: Cervical and vaginal bacterial flora: Ecologic niches in the female lower genital tract. Am J Obstet Gynecol 130:658, 1978.

10. Grossman JH III, Adams RL: Vaginal flora in women undergoing hysterectomy with antibiotic prophylaxis. Obstet Gynecol 53:23, 1979.

11. Mehta PV: Vaginal flora: A dynamic ecosystem. J Reprod Med 27:455, 1982.

12. Heard ML, Bawdon RE, Hemsell DL, Nobles BJ: Susceptibility profiles of potential aerobic and anaerobic pathogens isolated from hysterectomy patients. Am J Obstet Gynecol 149:133, 1984.

13. Thadepalli H, Savage EW Jr, Salem FA, Roy I, Davidson EC Jr: Cyclic changes in cervical microflora and their effect on infections following hysterectomy. Gynecol Obstet Invest 14:176, 1982.

14. Levison ME, Corman LC, Carrington ER, Kaye D: Quantitative microflora of the vagina. Am J Obstet Gynecol 127:80, 1977.

15. Larsen B, Goplerud CP, Petzold CR, Ohm-Smith MJ, Galask RP: Effect of estrogen treatment on the genital tract flora of postmenopausal women. Obstet Gynecol 60:20, 1982.

16. Hemsell D, Hemsell P, Nobles B, Heard M, Bawdon R: Moxalactam versus cefazolin prophylaxis for vaginal hysterectomy. Am J Obstet Gynecol 147:379, 1983.

17. Hemsell DL, Heard ML, Nobles BJ, Hemsell PG: Single-dose cefoxitin prophylaxis for premenopausal women undergoing vaginal hysterectomy. Obstet Gynecol 63:285, 1984.

18. Hemsell DL, Johnson ER, Bawdon RE, Hemsell PG, Heard ML, Nobles BJ: Cefoperazone and cefoxitin prophylaxis for abdominal hysterectomy. Obstet Gynecol 63:467, 1984.

19. Grossman JH III, Adams RL, Hierholzer WJ Jr, Andriole VT: Endometrial and vaginal cuff bacteria recovered at elective hysterectomy during a trial of antibiotic prophylaxis. Am J Obstet Gynecol 130:312, 1978.

20. Hemsell DL, Obregon VL, Heard MC, Nobles BJ: Endometrial bacteria in asymptomatic nonpregnant women. J Reprod Med 34:872, 1989.

21. Osborne NG, Wright RC: Effect of preoperative scrub on bacterial flora of the endocervix and vagina. Obstet Gynecol 50:148, 1977.

22. Monif GR, Thompson JL, Stephens HD, Bear H: Quantitative and qualitative effects of povidone-iodine liquid and gel on the aerobic and anaerobic flora of the female genital tract. Am J Obstet Gynecol 137:432, 1980.

23. Amstey MS, Jones AP: Preparation of the vagina for surgery: A comparison of povidone-iodine and saline solution. JAMA 245:839, 1981.

24. Ledger WJ, Gee C, Lewis WP: Guidelines for antibiotic prophylaxis in gynecology. Am J Obstet Gynecol 121:1038, 1975.

25. Ohm MJ, Galask RP: The effect of antibiotic prophylaxis on patients undergoing vaginal operations: II. Alterations of microbial flora. Am J Obstet Gynecol 123:597, 1975.

26. Ohm MJ, Galask RP: The effect of antibiotic prophylaxis on patients undergoing total abdominal hysterectomy: II. Alterations of microbial flora. Am J Obstet Gynecol 125:448, 1976.

27. Hemsell DL, Heard MC, Hemsell PG, Nobles BJ, Bawdon RE: Alterations in lower reproductive tract flora after single-dose piperacillin and triple-dose cefoxitin at vaginal and abdominal hysterectomy. Obstet Gynecol 72:875, 1988.

28. Swenson R, Michaelson T, Daly M, Spaulding E: Anaerobic bacterial infections of the female genital tract. Obstet Gynecol 42:538, 1973.

29. Sweet RL: Anaerobic infections of the female genital tract. Am J Obstet Gynecol 122:891, 1975.

30. Bartlett JG: Anaerobic infections of the pelvis. Clin Obstet Gynecol 21:351, 1979.

31. Martens MG, Faro S, Hammill HA, Riddle GD, Smith D: Transcervical uterine sampling methods in postpartum endometritis. Obstet Gynecol 74:273, 1989.

32. Webster's Ninth Collegiate Dictionary. Springfield, Mass: Merriam-Webster, 1989.

33. Miller BF, Keane CB; Anderson DA, ed: The Encyclopedia and Dictionary of Medicine, Nursing, and Allied Health, 4th ed. Philadelphia: WB Saunders, 1987.

34. Stedman TL, Hensyl WR, Cady B, Felscher H (eds): Stedman's Medical Dictionary, 25th ed. Baltimore: Williams & Wilkins, 1990.

35. Berkeley AS, Freedman KS, Ledger WJ, et al: Comparison of cefotetan and cefoxitin prophylaxis for abdominal and vaginal hysterectomy. Am J Obstet Gynecol 158:706, 1988.

36. Allen JL, Rampone JF, Wheeless CR: Use of prophylactic antibiotic in elective major gynecologic operations. Obstet Gynecol 39:218, 1972.

37. Shapiro M, Schoenbaum SC, Tager IB, Munoz A, Polk BF: Benefit-cost analysis of antimicrobial prophylaxis in abdominal and vaginal hysterectomy. JAMA 249:1290, 1983.

38. Classen DC, Evans RS, Pestotnik SL, Horn SD, Menlove RL, Burke JP: The timing of prophylactic administration of antibiotics and the risk of surgical-wound infection. N Engl J Med 326:281, 1992.

39. Sinei SKA, Schulz KF, Lamptey PR, et al: Preventing IUCD-related pelvic infection: The efficacy of prophylactic doxycycline at insertion. Br J Obstet Gynaecol 97:412, 1990.

40. Ladipo OA, Farr G, Otolrin E, et al: Prevention of IUD-related pelvic infection: The efficacy of prophylactic doxycycline at IUD insertion. Adv Contracept 7:43, 1991.

41. Jovanovic R, Barone CM, Van Natta FC, Congema E: Preventing infection related to insertion of an intrauterine device. J Reprod Med 33:347, 1988.

42. Stumpf PG, March CM: Febrile morbidity following hysterosalpingography: Identification of risk factors and recommendations for prophylaxis. Fertil Steril 33:487, 1980.

43. Pyper RJD, Ahmet Z, Houang ET: Bacterial contamination during laparoscopy with dye injection. Br J Obstet Gynaecol 95:367, 1988.

44. Pittaway DE, Winfield AC, Maxon W, Daniell J, Herbert C, Wentz AC: Prevention of acute pelvic inflammatory disease after hysterosalpingography: Efficacy of doxycycline prophylaxis. Am J Obstet Gynecol 147:623, 1983.

45. Heisterberg L, Petersen K: Metronidazole prophylaxis in elective first trimester abortion. Obstet Gynecol 65:371, 1985.

46. Darj E, Strålin E-B, Nilsson S: The prophylactic effect of doxycycline on postoperative infection after first-trimester abortion. Obstet Gynecol 70:755, 1987.

47. Levallois P, Rioux J-E: Prophylactic antibiotics for suction curettage abortion: Results of a clinical controlled trial. Am J Obstet Gynecol 158:100, 1988.

48. Layman LC, Sanfilippo JS: Febrile and infectious morbidity after laparotomy for ectopic pregnancy: Potential for antibiotic prophylaxis. J Gynecol Surg 6:161, 1990.

49. Berenson A, Hammill H, Martens M, Faro S: Bacteriologic findings with ectopic pregnancy. J Reprod Med 36:118, 1991.

50. Cartwright PS, Pittaway DE, Jones JW III, Entman SS: The use of prophylactic antibiotics in obstetrics and gynecology: A review. Obstet Gynecol Surv 39:537, 1984.

51. Bhatia NN, Karram MM, Bergman A: Role of antibiotic prophylaxis in retropubic surgery for stress urinary incontinence. Obstet Gynecol 74:637, 1989.

52. Stiver HG, Binns BO, Brunham RC, et al: Randomized, double-blind comparison of efficacies, costs, and vaginal flora alterations with single-dose ceftriaxone and multidose cefazolin prophylaxis in vaginal hysterectomy. Antimicrob Agents Chemother 34:1194, 1990.

53. Turner SJ: The effect of penicillin vaginal suppositories on morbidity in vaginal hysterectomy and on the vaginal flora. Am J Obstet Gynecol 60:806, 1950.

54. Wright VC, Lanning NM, Natale R: Use of a topical antibiotic spray in vaginal surgery. Can Med Assoc J 118:1395, 1978.

55. Smith CV, Gallup DG, Gibbs RL, Labudovich M, Phelan JP: Oral doxycycline vs. parenteral cefazolin: Prophylaxis for vaginal hysterectomy. Infec Surg 99:64, 1989.

56. Swartz WH, Tanaree P: Suction drainage as an alternative to prophylactic antibiotics for hysterectomy. Obstet Gynecol 45:305, 1975.

57. Swartz WH, Tanaree P: T-tube suction drainage and/or prophylactic antibiotics: a randomized study of 451 hysterectomies. Obstet Gynecol 47:655, 1976.

58. Galle PC, Urban RB, Homesley HD, Jobson VS, Wheeler AS: Single dose carbenicillin versus T-tube drainage in patients undergoing vaginal hysterectomy. Surg Gynecol Obstet 153:351, 1981.

59. Wijma J, Kauer FM, van Saene HKF, van de Wiel HBM, Janssens J: Antibiotics and suction drainage as prophylaxis in vaginal and abdominal hysterectomy. Obstet Gynecol 70:384, 1987.

60. Osborne NG, Wright RC, Dubay M: Preoperative hot conization of the cervix: A possible method to reduce postoperative morbidity following vaginal hysterectomy. Am J Obstet Gynecol 133:374, 1979.

61. Richards RW: An evaluation of the local use of sulfonamide drugs in certain gynecological operations. Am J Obstet Gynecol 46:541, 1944.

62. Soper DE, Bump RC, Hurt WG: Bacterial vaginosis and trichomoniasis vaginitis risk factors for cuff cellulitis after abdominal hysterectomy. Am J Obstet Gynecol 163:1016, 1990.

63. Larsson P-G, Platz-Christensen J-J, Forsum U, Pahlson C: Clue cells in predicting infections after abdominal hysterectomy. Obstet Gynecol 77:450, 1991.

64. Poulsen HK, Borel J, Olsen H: Prophylactic metronidazole or suction drainage in abdominal hysterectomy. Obstet Gynecol 63:291, 1984.

65. Nelson KJ, Gallup DG, Gibbs R, Paulk W: Intraoperative antibiotic irrigation as prophylaxis in abdominal hysterectomy: A preliminary report. South Med J 77:700, 1984.

66. Beresford JM, MacKenzie AMR: Bacterial contamination at abdominal hysterectomy: A comparison of staple closure with regular suture closure of the vaginal vault. J Gynecol Surg 7:233, 1991.

67. Zakut H, Lotan M, Bracha Y: Vaginal preparation with povidone-iodine before abdominal hysterectomy. Clin Exp Obstet Gynecol 14:1, 1987.

68. Dicker RC, Greenspan JR, Strauss LT, et al: Complications of abdominal and vaginal hysterectomy among women of reproductive age in the United States: The collaborative review of sterilization. Am J Obstet Gynecol 144:841, 1982.

69. Hemsell DL, Johnson ER, Bawdon RE, Hemsell PG, Nobles BJ, Heard ML: Ceftriaxone and cefazolin prophylaxis for hysterectomy. Surg Gynecol Obstet 161:197, 1985.

70. Regallo M, Scalambrino S, Negri L, Landoni F, Mangioni C: Cefotetan versus piperacillin in the prophylaxis of abdominal and vaginal hysterectomy: A prospective randomized study. Drugs Exp Clin Res 15:315, 1989.

71. Hemsell DL, Bernstein SG, Bawdon RE, Hemsell PG, Heard MC, Nobles BJ: Preventing major operative site infection after radical abdominal hysterectomy and pelvic lymphadenectomy. Gynecol Oncol 35:55, 1989.

72. Orr JW Jr, Sisson PF, Patsner B, et al: Single-dose prophylaxis for patients undergoing extended pelvic surgery for gynecologic malignancy. Am J Obstet Gynecol 162:718, 1990.

73. van Lindert ACM, Giltaij AR, Derksen MD, Alsbach GPJ, Rozenberg-Arska M, Verhoef J: Single-dose prophylaxis with broad-spectrum penicillins (piperacillin and mezlocillin) in gynecologic oncological surgery with observation on serum and tissue concentrations. Eur J Obstet Gynecol Reprod Biol 36:137, 1990.

74. Sevin B-U, Ramos R, Gerhardt RT, Guerra L, Hilsenbeck S, Averette HE: Comparative efficacy of short-term versus long-term cefoxitin prophylaxis against postoperative infection after radical hysterectomy: A prospective study. Obstet Gynecol 77:729, 1991.

75. Hemsell DL, Hemsell PG, Nobles BJ: Doxycycline and cefamandole prophylaxis for premenopausal women undergoing vaginal hysterectomy. Surg Gynecol Obstet 161:462, 1985.

76. diZerega G, Yonekura L, Roy S, Nakamura RM, Ledger WJ: A comparison of clindamycin/gentamicin and penicillin/gentamicin in the treatment of post-cesarean section endomyometritis. Am J Obstet Gynecol 134:238, 1979.

77. Sweet RL, Ledger WJ: Cefoxitin: Single-agent treatment of mixed aerobic-anaerobic pelvic infections. Obstet Gynecol 54:193, 1979.

78. Duff P, Keiser JF, Strong SL: A comparative study of two antibiotic regimens for the treatment of operative site infections. Am J Obstet Gynecol 142:996, 1982.

79. Hager WD, McDaniel PS: Treatment of serious obstetric and gynecologic infections with cefoxitin. J Reprod Med 28:337, 1963.

80. Sweet RL, Gall SA, Gibbs RS, et al: Multicenter clinical trials comparing cefotetan with moxalactam or cefoxitin as therapy for obstetric and gynecologic infections. Am J Surg 155(5A):56, 1988.

81. Pastorek JG, Aldridge KE, Cunningham GE, et al: Comparison of ticarcillin plus clavulanic acid with cefoxitin in the treatment of female pelvic infection. Am J Med 79(S5B):161, 1985.

82. Poindexter AN, Sweet R, Ritter M: Cefotetan in the treatment of obstetric and gynecologic infections. Am J Obstet Gynecol 154:946, 1986.

83. Hemsell DL, Wendel GD, Gall SA, et al: Multicenter comparison of cefotetan and cefoxitin in the treatment of acute obstetric and gynecologic infections. Am J Obstet Gynecol 158:722, 1988.

84. Sweet RL, Robbie MO, Ohm-Smith M, Hadley WK: Comparative study of piperacillin versus cefoxitin in the treatment of obstetric and gynecologic infections. Am J Obstet Gynecol 145:342, 1983.

85. Hemsell DL, Cunningham FG: Combination antimicrobial therapy for serious gynecological and obstetrical infections: Obsolete? Clin Ther 4(suppl A):82, 1981.

86. Strausbaugh LJ, Lorrens AS: Cefoperazone therapy for obstetric and gynecologic infections. Rev Infect Dis 5:S154, 1983.

87. Gilstrap LC III, St. Clair PJ, Gibbs RS, Maier RC: Cefoperazone versus clindamycin plus gentamicin for obstetric and gynecologic infections. Antimicrob Agents Chemother 30:808, 1986.

88. Gilstrap LC III, Maier RC, Gibbs RS, Connor KD, St. Clair PJ: Piperacillin versus clindamycin plus gentamicin for pelvic infections. Obstet Gynecol 64:762, 1984.

89. Hemsell DL, Hemsell PG, Heard MC, Nobles BJ: Piperacillin and a combination of clindamycin and gentamicin for the treatment of hospital and community acquired acute pelvic infections including pelvic abscess. Surg Gynecol Obstet 165:223, 1987.

90. Crombleholme WR, Ohm-Smith M, Robbie MO, DeKay V, Sweet RL: Ampicillin/sulbactam versus metronidazole-gentamicin in the treatment of soft tissue pelvic infections. Am J Obstet Gynecol 156:507, 1987.

91. Giamarellou H, Trouvas G, Avlami A, Aravantinos D, Daikos GK: Efficacy of sulbactam plus ampicillin in gynecologic infections. Rev Infect Dis 8(suppl 5):S579–581, 1986.

92. Berkeley AS, Freedman K, Hirsch J, Ledger WJ: Imipenem/cilastatin in the treatment of obstetric and gynecologic infections. Am J Med 78(suppl 6A):79, 1985.

93. Sweet RL: Imipenem/cilastatin in the treatment of obstetric and gynecologic infections: A review of worldwide experience. Rev Infect Dis 7(suppl 3):S522, 1985.

94. Thadepalli H, Mathai D, Scotti R, Bansal MG, Savage E: Ciprofloxacin monotherapy for acute pelvic infections: A comparison with clindamycin plus gentamicin. Obstet Gynecol 78:698, 1991.

95. Gall SA, Kohan AP, Ayers OM, Hughes CE, Addison WA, Hill GB: Intravenous metronidazole or clindamycin with tobramycin for therapy of pelvic infections. Obstet Gynecol 57:51, 1981.

96. Blanco JD, Gibbs RS, Duff P, Castaneda YS, St. Clair PJ: Randomized comparison of ceftazidime versus clindamycin-tobramycin in the treatment of obstetrical and gynecological infections. Antimicrob Agents Chemother 24:500, 1983.

97. Faro S, Sanders CV, Aldridge KE: Use of a single-agent antimicrobial therapy in the treatment of polymicrobial female pelvic infections. Obstet Gynecol 60:232, 1982.

98. Dodson MG, Faro S, Gentry LO: Treatment of acute pelvic inflammatory disease with aztreonam, a new monocyclic β-lactam antibiotic, and clindamycin. Obstet Gynecol 67:657, 1986.

99. Horan T, Culver D, Jarvis W, et al: Pathogens causing nosocomial infection: Preliminary data from the National Nosocomial Infections Surveillance System. Antimicrob Newslett 3:65, 1988.

100. Komshian SV, Uwaydah AK, Sobel JD, Crane LR: Fungemia caused by *Candida* species and *Torulopsis glabrata* in the hospitalized patient: Frequency, characteristics, and evaluation of factors influencing outcome. Rev Infect Dis 11:379, 1989.

101. Solomkin JS, Flohr AM, Simmons RL: Indications for therapy for fungemia in postoperative patients. Arch Surg 117:1272, 1982.

102. Gaines JD, Remington JS: Diagnosis of deep infection with *Candida*. Arch Intern Med 132:699, 1973.

103. Fraser VJ, Jones M, Dunkel J, Storfer S, Medoff G, Dunagan WC: Candidemia in a tertiary care hospital. Epidemiology, risk factors, and predictors of mortality. Clin Infect Dis 15:414, 1992.

104. Roilides E, Pizzo PA: Modulation of host defenses by cytokines: Evolving adjuncts in prevention and treatment of serious infections in immunocompromised hosts. Clin Infect Dis 15:508, 1992.

105. Bone RC: A critical evaluation of new agents for the treatment of sepsis. JAMA 226:1686, 1991.

106. Styrt B, Gorbach SL: Recent developments in the understanding of the pathogenesis and treatment of anaerobic infections: Part 1. N Engl J Med 321:240, 1989.

107. Styrt B, Gorbach SL: Recent developments in the understanding of the pathogenesis and treatment of anaerobic infections: Part 2. N Engl J Med 321:298, 1989.

Complications in Gynecologic Surgery: Prevention, Recognition, and Management,
edited by James W. Orr, Jr., and Hugh M. Shingleton.
J. B. Lippincott Company, Philadelphia, © 1994.

Chapter 9

Neurologic Injury

Ravinder Tikoo
Walter B. Jones

Neurologic sequelae including stroke, seizure, and altered mental states are potential complications of any operative procedure. Fortunately, neurologic complications related to pelvic surgery are relatively rare, are usually transient, and resolve spontaneously with minimal intervention. However, long-term disability occasionally occurs. Many neurologic injuries are preventable, and pelvic surgeons should recognize their causes and use preventive measures when possible.

This chapter briefly reviews the pelvic neuroanatomy and the mechanisms of nerve injury. Specific neuropathies involving the femoral, sciatic, obturator, and peroneal nerves and procedures to decrease the risk of injury are described. The mechanisms implicated in nerve entrapment and compartment syndromes and their management are summarized. The specific vascular events causing neuropathy are outlined, with an illustrative case report. Finally, autonomic nervous system injury resulting in postoperative bladder and bowel dysfunction is discussed. Recent developments in urodynamic studies have made it possible to more precisely identify potential sites of surgical trauma. Similarly, new insights into the mechanisms of nervous control of bowel function have made it possible for surgeons to minimize disruption of sympathetic and parasympathetic innervation of the bowel.

Anatomy

The relevant anatomy must be reviewed to more completely understand the mechanisms of various neuropathies associated with pelvic surgery.[1] Components of the lumbosacral plexus (Fig. 9–1) and the associated visceral nerves (Fig. 9–2) are the structures most likely to be injured during pelvic operations. The sensory and motor innervation of the nerves of the lumbosacral plexus is varied (Table 9–1).

The lumbar plexus overlies the quadratus lumborum, iliacus, and psoas muscles. The major nerves of interest that emanate from this plexus include the iliohypogastric, ilioinguinal, lateral cutaneous, genitofemoral, femoral, and obturator nerves. The iliohypogastric nerve, the first nerve of the plexus, originates from the T12 and L1 nerve roots, courses over the quadratus lumborum, and finally supplies sensory fibers to the suprapubic region. The lateral femoral cutaneous nerve of the thigh develops from the posterior divisions of the L2 and L3 nerve roots, passes under the psoas muscle for most of its course, and supplies sensory fibers to the majority of the lateral thigh. The genitofemoral nerve, also a sensory nerve, coalesces from the anterior divisions of the nerve roots of L1 and L2, continues anterior to the psoas muscle, and ultimately innervates the skin overlying the labia (the genital branch) and a small region in the superior thigh (the femoral branch).

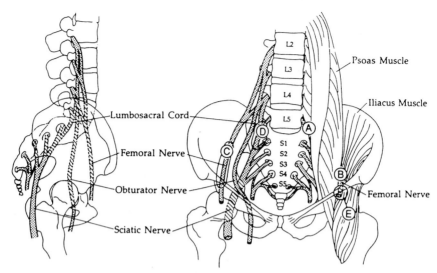

FIGURE 9–1. The lumbosacral plexus showing sites of potential retractor-induced injury to the femoral nerve (*B*) and stretch injury of the femoral nerve during improper lithotomy positioning (*E*). (Reproduced by permission from Donaghy M: Lumbosacral plexus lesions. In Dyck PJ (ed): Peripheral Neuropathy, p 952. Philadelphia: WB Saunders, 1993.)

The femoral nerve, the largest of the lumbosacral plexus, is derived from the posterior divisions of the L2, L3, and L4 nerve roots. The nerve pierces the psoas muscle, continues inferolaterally within the muscle, emerges inferiorly between the iliacus and psoas muscle, and then courses under the inguinal ligament to enter the femoral sheath lateral to the femoral artery. The femoral nerve has both motor and sensory components supplying motor fibers to the iliacus, quadriceps femoris group, sartorius, and pectineus. The primary functions of these muscles are hip flexion and leg extension. Three major sensory nerves emerge from the femoral nerve in the thigh: the intermediate and medial cutaneous nerves of the thigh and the saphenous nerve (supplying sensation to the medial leg). The final major nerve of the lumbar plexus is the obturator nerve, which originates from the anterior L2, L3, and L4 nerve roots, descends through the body of the psoas muscle, emerges medially at the brim of the pelvis, and passes through the obturator foramen into the thigh. This nerve ultimately supplies motor fibers to

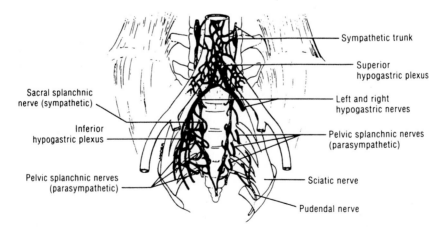

FIGURE 9–2. Autonomic nerves of the pelvis. Diagram shows the superior and inferior hypogastric plexuses and the pudendal nerve. (Reproduced by permission from Agur AMR, Lee MJ (eds). Grant's Atlas of Anatomy, 9th ed, p 178. Baltimore: Williams & Wilkins, 1991.)

TABLE 9–1. **Sensory and Motor Innervation of the Lumbosacral Plexus**

Nerve	Innervation	
	Sensory	*Motor*
Ilioinguinal	Superior medial thigh, pubis	None
Iliohypogastric	Pubis, lateral gluteal	None
Genitofemoral	Inguinal, labial	None
Lateral, femorocutaneous	Lateral thigh	None
Femoral	Anterior and medial thigh	Hip flexion and knee extension
Saphenous branch	Medial leg	None
Obturator	Upper medial thigh	Hip adduction
Sciatic		
Tibial	Plantar surface of foot	Knee flexion
		Ankle plantarflexion
Sural	Lateral ankle	None
Peroneal		
Superficial branch	Dorsum of foot	Ankle dorsiflexion
Deep branch	Area between toes 1 and 2	Ankle eversion

the adductor muscles of the thigh (gracilis, obturator, and adductor longus, brevis, and magnus). In addition, sensory innervation to a small portion of the upper medial thigh is derived from this nerve.

The lumbosacral trunk is the final component of the lumbar plexus which joins to constitute the sacral plexus. The sacral plexus eventually forms the superior gluteal, inferior gluteal, sciatic, posterior cutaneous, and pudendal nerves. The superior and inferior gluteal nerves are both motor nerves that supply the gluteus medius and minimus and the gluteus maximus, respectively. The posterior cutaneous nerve of the thigh (originating from the anterior divisions of the S1, S2, and S3 nerve roots) supplies sensation to the area from which its name derives.

The sciatic nerve, the largest in the body, is composed of two distinct components, the tibial and the common peroneal divisions. The nerve coalesces from the L4, L5, S1, S2, and S3 nerve roots, with the common peroneal division forming from the posterior roots and the tibial division forming from the anterior roots. The sciatic nerve coalesces anterior to the piriformis muscle, passes below it through the greater sciatic foramen, and courses down the posterior thigh. In the thigh, the tibial division of the sciatic nerve supplies motor fibers to the hamstring group of muscles which flex the leg and extend the thigh. Immediately superior to the popliteal fossa the two components divide. The common peroneal nerve then continues anteriorly around the fibular head to supply motor fibers to the dorsiflexor (deep branch) and the evertors (superficial branch) of the foot. Branches of the peroneal nerve also supply sensation to the lateral leg and dorsum of the foot. The tibial nerve descends down the posterior leg, supplying motor fibers to the plantar flexors of the foot, intrinsic foot flexors, and also sensation to the toes and plantar surface of the foot.

The pudendal nerve, a major component of the sacral plexus, originates from the S2, S3, and S4 nerve roots and provides sensory and motor fibers to the perineal region. It exits the pelvis between the piriformis and the coccygeus muscles, bends around the sacrospinous ligament, and enters the perineum via the lesser sciatic notch. Here it divides into several sensory branches: the inferior hemorrhoidal and perineal nerves, which innervate the perineal region, and the dorsal nerve of the clitoris. The perineal nerve also supplies motor innervation to the external urethral sphincter and the deep transverse perineal muscle.

The autonomic nervous system also makes an important contribution to the innervation of the pelvic viscera and is intimately involved in bowel and bladder function.[2,3] The sympathetic and parasympathetic nerve trunks are all located near the lumbosacral plexus.

Parasympathetic innervation originates from S2–4 spinal cord segments and provides the major excitatory input to the urinary bladder. The preganglionic neurons are located in the intermediolateral cell columns in the spinal cord and send fibers, via the pelvic nerves, to ganglion cells in the pelvic plexus and the bladder wall. The ganglion cells are responsible for bladder smooth muscle contraction and micturition.

The sympathetic preganglionic neurons are located in the T11 and L2 spinal cord segments. They send fibers to the sympathetic chain ganglia, hypogastric nerve, hypogastric plexus, pelvic plexus, and finally the bladder and urethra. Postganglionic sympathetic nerves provide excitatory input to the smooth muscle of the urethra and bladder base, where they act via α-adrenergic receptors to constrict these sphincters and stop the flow of urine. Another subset of sympathetic nerves sends inhibitory input to the parasympathetic bladder ganglia by β-adrenergic receptors, which act to inhibit contraction of the bladder. Thus, the sympathetic system has a predominant urinary storage function.

Afferent impulses from the bladder are carried centrally by both sets of autonomic nerves. Those afferent fibers that signal bladder distention and result in reflex constriction of the detrusor muscle travel through the pelvic nerves to the sacral spinal cord. Fibers that transmit pain impulses travel through the pelvic and hypogastric plexuses to reach the sacral and thoracolumbar spinal cord, respectively.

The pudendal nerve provides somatic motor fibers that innervate the external urethral sphincter. This nerve also carries proprioceptive information and supplies sensation to the urethra.

Basic Mechanisms of Nerve Injury

Nerve injury during pelvic surgery is usually the result of physical trauma: from either compression, traction, or transection of a peripheral nerve. The underlying mechanisms of injury can be classified into three types: neurapraxia, axonotmesis, and neurotmesis.[4]

When compressed, a nerve is prone to a first-degree injury termed *neurapraxia,* which is commonly associated with pelvic surgery. This type of injury blocks impulse conduction through the nerve at the site of injury. This is thought to result from mechanical deformation of a myelinated nerve with associated focal demyelination. Axonal and nerve sheath continuity are preserved. Nerves that are already subclinically damaged from an underlying medical cause (i.e., diabetes, malnutrition, uremia, alcoholism) are more susceptible to compressive damage. Common symptoms include weakness, numbness, and paresthesia in the distribution of the injured nerve. Typically, complete recovery occurs several weeks to 4 months after injury.

When a nerve is crushed, the axons of the nerve are severed but the endoneurial sheath usually remains intact. This is designated a second-degree injury, or *axonotmesis.* Failure of impulse conduction across the damaged area occurs immediately following injury, leading to weakness and numbness in the distribution of the nerve. The distal nerve fibers degenerate and become unexcitable 4 to 7 days after the injury. Loss of motor nerve fibers leads to atrophy and electromyographic (EMG) evidence of muscle denervation (positive sharp waves and fibrillation potentials) 2 to 3 weeks after the initial injury. Recovery occurs after motor and sensory fibers regenerate, proximally to distally, which occurs at a rate of approximately 6 to 8 mm/day. The prognosis for recovery is excellent.

With a third-degree injury, or *neurotmesis,* the nerve fibers and the endoneurial sheath are severed. Neurotmesis can result from a penetrating wound, stretch injury, or fracture or can occur iatrogenically during surgery. Despite efforts to repair the nerve, regenerating axons may be misrouted, resulting in aberrant regeneration.

The majority of neurologic complications due to surgery involve first-degree or compressive injuries, and resolution of clinical deficits is generally complete. However, in a small but distinct group of patients in whom nerve injury is more severe, recovery is less certain and residual deficits may remain.

Femoral Neuropathy

Although the nerve most commonly injured during or in association with pelvic surgery is the femoral nerve, isolated femoral neuropathy is relatively rare. Of the multiple causes of femoral nerve injury, the most common is compression secondary to entrapment, tumor, or trauma.[4] In pelvic surgery, femoral neuropathy results from direct physical injury as a result of compression by retractor blades, stretch injury, or surgical dissection.

Symptoms of femoral nerve injury include groin pain and weakness of knee extension and thigh flexion. Numbness and paresthesia may be present in the anterior and medial thigh and the medial leg. The knee jerk reflex is usually absent. If femoral nerve injury is suspected, diagnostic studies should include EMG and nerve conduction velocities, which may show prolonged latencies in the femoral nerve and denervation of the quadriceps muscle. Computed tomography of the pelvis may demonstrate a hematoma. Tests for diabetes mellitus should be performed because undiagnosed diabetes may present as a femoral or lumbar plexus neuropathy or may decrease the threshold for physical injury to the nerve.

The association of femoral neuropathy with gynecologic surgery has been recognized since the 1800s.[5] However, the mechanisms of injury have only become understood in this century. Three common factors initially were identified as causes of femoral neuropathy following hysterectomy.[6] They are (1) use of a self-retaining retractor, (2) use of a transverse or Pfannenstiel incision, and (3) a thin body habitus. The self-retaining retractor may impinge on the femoral nerve directly or indirectly through the overlying psoas muscle, resulting in a compressive nerve injury (Fig. 9–3). The transverse incision is thought to predispose the patient to nerve compression, as the retractor blades are placed in closer proximity to the femoral nerve. Similarly, a thin body habitus predisposes the patient to femoral nerve injury because the retractor blades in the absence of abdominal wall resistance are more likely to rest on the psoas muscle and compress the femoral nerve. Cadaver studies indicate that the segment of the femoral nerve most prone to retractor injury lies 4 cm proximal to the inguinal ligament. Direct femoral nerve injury is uncommon, as the nerve is protected by the psoas muscle throughout most of its pelvic course. Although most patients ultimately achieve complete recovery after femoral nerve injury, residual sensorimotor deficits may persist for several years.

The type of incision, pelvic pathology, and type of hysterectomy are now not thought to be independent risk factors for femoral neuropathy. Stretch injury also is unlikely to lead to neuropathy because of the unusually high forces (> 32 kg) required to produce symptoms.[5] The strong association of neuropathy with the use of self-retaining retractors is in most cases the result of constant pressure, causing ischemic damage to the nerve either by obstructing the vasa nervorum or by compressing the external iliac artery. Careful selection and placement of retractor blades to avoid psoas muscle compression and palpation of the external iliac artery during retractor placement are simple measures to ensure proper positioning. It is worth noting, however, that nerve injury can occur despite intact external iliac pulses and that palpation of the external iliac vessel is of itself an inadequate test and does not ensure safe retractor positioning.

Patients with a thin abdominal wall, poorly developed rectus muscles, and a narrow pelvis are at increased risk for developing femoral neuropathy when long retractor blades are used for hysterectomy.[7] The prudent surgeon selects the appropriate retractor on an individual basis to decrease these risks.

Although the incidence of femoral neuropathy is low, it is not insignificant. In one series of 147 patients who underwent total abdominal hysterectomy,[8] 17 (11.6%) women developed femoral neuropathy. The authors indicated that the use of large self-retaining retractors was in part causal, while incision type, body weight, and procedure length appeared to be unrelated. At 2 months' follow-up, 15 of 17 patients had recovered from their sensorimotor deficits.

Femoral neuropathy occurred in 7.5% and 0.7%, respectively, of patients in a prospective randomized study who underwent abdominal hysterectomy and laparotomy with and without the use of self-retaining retractors.[9] In the latter group, abdominal towels were used to assist with exposure. In "bulky" patients, only hand-held flexible blades were used. These findings clearly implicate self-retaining retractors as a primary cause of femoral nerve injury and argue for careful retractor placement, the use of short blades, and placement of pads under the blades to decrease the incidence of femoral nerve injury.

Patients undergoing lengthy abdominopelvic op-

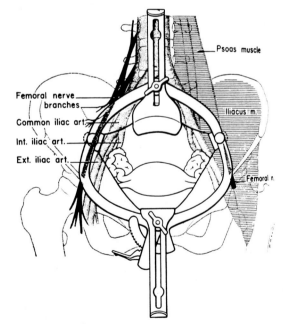

FIGURE 9–3. The relationship between the femoral nerve and the psoas muscle, iliac vessels, and the retractor. (Reproduced by permission from Vosburgh LF, Finn W: Femoral nerve impairment subsequent to hysterectomy. Am J Obstet Gynecol 82:931–937, 1961.)

erations, such as tubal microsurgery, during which self-retaining retractors with large blades and wide abdominal incisions (Pfannenstiel) are used are particularly at risk for nerve injury as a result of prolonged retractor compression of the psoas muscle and femoral nerve.[10,11]

Vaginal hysterectomy is less commonly associated with femoral neuropathy than is abdominal hysterectomy. In one report of 46 cases of femoral neuropathy, only two (4.4%) were associated with vaginal hysterectomy.[5] However, femoral neuropathy following vaginal hysterectomy is frequently bilateral, whereas in abdominal procedures unilateral involvement is the rule. During vaginal surgery positioning in stirrups or movement during the procedure contributes to the potential for neuropathy. Specifically, hip flexion, abduction, and external rotation should be avoided, as they predispose to the development of femoral neuropathy (Fig. 9–4). Lateral thigh supports can prevent the development of excessive hip abduction and external rotation and decrease the risk of nerve injury.[12] Cadaver studies indicate that it is impossible to compress the femoral nerve with a vaginal retractor; however, flexing, abducting, and externally rotating the thighs in the lithotomy position can cause an 80- to 90-degree angulation of the femoral nerve at the inguinal ligament.[13] Therefore, prolonged procedures in such a position can cause compression neuropa-

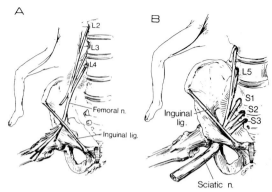

FIGURE 9–5. Femoral and sciatic neuropathy from stretch injury related to improper lithotomy positioning. **A.** The femoral nerve is compressed against the rigid inguinal ligament. **B.** The sciatic nerve is compressed between the sciatic notch and the neck of the fibula. (Reproduced by permission from Flanagan WF, Webster GD, Brown MW, Massey EW: Lumbosacral stretch injury following the use of modified lithotomy position. J Urol 134:567–568, 1985.)

thy by the continuous pressure of the inguinal ligament on the femoral nerve (Fig. 9–5). Although recovery of function usually occurs after several months in the majority of patients, it emphasizes the need for proper positioning as well as the possible role of repositioning in lengthy operations to avoid sustained pressure on a single segment of nerve.

A popular model of lithotomy stirrups (Skytron, Grand Rapids, Mich.) used at Memorial Hospital (Fig. 9–6) locks the patient's ankle and knee in position, eliminating undue pressure at the popliteal fossa. The boots are designed for maximum support

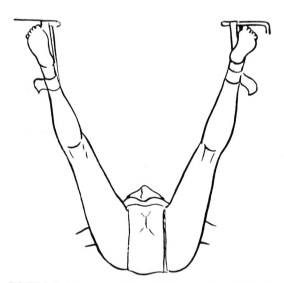

FIGURE 9–4. Lithotomy position with knees and hip joint flexed and with maximum external rotation of thighs, predisposing the patient to stretch injury of the sciatic nerve or its peroneal branch. (Reproduced by permission from Burkhart FL, Daly JW: Sciatic and peroneal nerve injury: A complication of vaginal operations. Obstet Gynecol 28:99–102, 1966.)

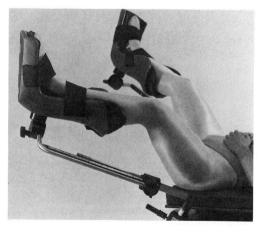

FIGURE 9–6. Lithotomy stirrups designed to limit excessive abduction of the hips and external rotation of the legs. (Courtesy of Skytron, Grand Rapids, Mich.)

with limit stops for rotation, adduction, and abduction.

Sciatic and Peroneal Neuropathy

The most common causes of sciatic nerve injury are fracture dislocations, hematomas, inadvertent sciatic nerve injection, and complications of hip replacement surgery. Rarely, direct compression can occur during coma, anesthesia, tumors, or gluteal artery aneurysms.[4] The mechanism of injury to the sciatic nerve and its divisions during pelvic surgery is most commonly the result of stretching of the nerve.[14] The common peroneal division of the sciatic nerve is more likely to be injured than the tibial division because its position is fixed at two sites in its course, at the sciatic notch and again at the neck of the fibula. Additionally, the nerve descends in a more oblique manner than the tibial division. It has been reported that the sciatic nerve can be stretched up to 1.5 inches before injury occurs.[15] With mild stretching ischemic changes occur, but prompt regeneration and recovery can be anticipated. With more severe injuries, perineurial damage may result, and regeneration is less likely to occur. Overall, the prognosis for sciatic and peroneal nerve damage during pelvic surgery is excellent, with complete resolution of sensorimotor deficits being the rule. In the leg, the common peroneal nerve is the most frequently compressed nerve. Its superficial position at the lateral fibular neck renders it exquisitely sensitive to trauma. During pelvic surgery improper use of the lithotomy position is a common cause of nerve compression.

Injury to the sciatic nerve can produce a variety of signs and symptoms, depending on the level of injury. The sciatic nerve consists of two separate divisions throughout its course, the tibial and common peroneal divisions. Lesions or injuries involving the entire sciatic nerve trunk cause weakness in the hamstrings (knee flexion) and in all muscles below the level of the knee. Sensation may be lost in the foot and lateral aspect of the leg. The peroneal component of the sciatic nerve is thought to be more sensitive to injury than the tibial component.[14] Injury to the peroneal division may occur selectively above or below the bifurcation from the tibial division. Injury to the peroneal division causes weakness in dorsiflexion (foot drop), eversion, and extension of the toes and can result in sensory loss in the dorsal foot and lateral aspect of the leg. Lesions above the bifurcation may result in weakness in knee flexion, plantar flexion, and flexion of the toes. EMG and nerve conduction velocity studies can aid in the diagnosis and better delineate the level of injury.

Positioning and body habitus are recognized factors predisposing to sciatic nerve injury, particularly in association with the semilithotomy position utilizing free-hanging stirrups.[16] In tall or heavy patients, there is a tendency for the hip joint to rotate externally in free-hanging stirrups. In short patients there may not be enough flexion at the knee joint, which may predispose to stretch injury.

Gynecologic procedures performed with the patient in the lithotomy position rarely result in sciatic nerve injury. In a report on more than 2,000 vaginal operations, including vaginal hysterectomy, vulvectomy, colpotomy, colpectomy, vaginal repair, dilation and curettage, radium insertion, and cervical conization, only five patients (0.2%) sustained nerve injury. Three had peroneal nerve involvement and two had sciatic nerve damage.[17] These findings are similar to those in a group of 1,000 patients who underwent only vaginal hysterectomy; the frequency of sciatic nerve injury was 0.3%.[18] Awareness of the fact that maximal tension on the sciatic nerve occurs as a result of hip flexion and knee extension or of external hip rotation and knee flexion has played a role in avoiding injury. The optimal lithotomy position consists of flexion and abduction of the thigh with minimal external rotation. Excessive external rotation, as occurs with inadvertent leaning on the inner aspect of the thigh or leg, will stretch the nerve and increase the chance of injury. Lack of leg flexion, which may occur in a short patient, also increases the probability of stretch injury. Excessive, sudden movement and extension of the legs in the lithotomy position should be avoided. It becomes important, therefore, to maintain adequate anesthesia during the operation.

In an unusual case of peroneal neuropathy following pelvic exenteration performed with the patient in "low stirrups," the injury was attributed to compression of the nerve between the low stirrups and the fibula.[19] In this case, no improvement in the neuropathy was apparent during the first 2 postoperative years.

Control of surgical hemorrhage may also result in sciatic or femoral nerve injury. In these instances, the use of large mattress sutures deep in the lateral pelvis may directly injure the nerves. Similarly, control of hemorrhage by means of constant pressure applied with gauze packs or surgical clamps may result in permanent nerve injury if significant pressure is applied for prolonged periods of time.

Thus, in addition to attention during lithotomy positioning, it is important that surgeons continually minimize the risk of compressive injury to sciatic or peroneal nerves by appropriate stirrup selection and avoiding direct nerve trauma.

Obturator Neuropathy

Obturator nerve compression is also rare, but injury may occur at the point where the nerve passes through the obturator canal as a result of obturator hernia, intrapelvic tumors, or pressure from the fetal head during childbirth.[20] In gynecologic surgery, obturator neuropathy is usually associated with radical pelvic surgery or pelvic lymphadenectomy. The obturator nerve is formed from the lumbar plexus within the psoas muscle by fibers from the L2–L4 spinal nerve roots. It descends within the psoas muscle into the pelvis, leaving the pelvis through the obturator foramen. It supplies the adductor muscles of the thigh and a small area of skin on the upper inner thigh.[21] Injury to the nerve therefore manifests as weakness in the hip adductors and sensory loss in the upper medial thigh (Fig. 9–7). Radical hysterectomy with bilateral pelvic lymphadenectomy for the treatment of cervical carcinoma requires complete removal of fibrovascular and lymph-bearing tissues of the pelvis and distal aorta, including nodal tissue in the obturator fossa. The node-bearing tissues of the obturator space may obscure the location of the obturator nerve and predispose it to injury. Gentle medial or lateral traction on the external iliac artery and vein permits access to the obturator space and decreases the risk of obtur-

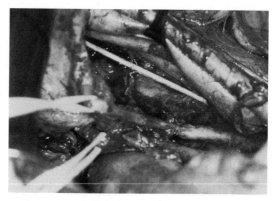

FIGURE 9–8. Obturator nerve as seen during radical hysterectomy and pelvic lymphadenectomy. Retraction of the iliac vessels during the operation can decrease the risk of injury.

ator nerve injury (Fig. 9–8). Inadvertent transection of the obturator nerve should be immediately repaired, if possible, to prevent the possibility of impaired adduction of the leg. However, complete recovery of function can be expected even in the patient in whom the transection is unrecognized if the patient undergoes postoperative physiotherapy.

Indirect obturator nerve trauma may also result in injury, as in the report of left leg weakness on the third postoperative day in a patient who had undergone radical hysterectomy with pelvic and aortic lymphadenectomy for carcinoma of the cervix.[19] In that case, both obturator nerves were visualized at the completion of the lymphadenectomy, suggesting that excessive traction or compression of the nerve may have been the cause of the obturator nerve palsy. The impairment resolved in 4 months.

Ilioinguinal and Iliohypogastric Neuropathy

Ilioinguinal and iliohypogastric neuropathies related to scar formation and nerve entrapment occur following lower abdominal wall surgical incisions (Fig. 9–9). These nerves can also be injured by direct suturing during wound closure. The ilioinguinal nerve supplies sensation to a small area of the inguinal region, an area over the symphysis, the proximal labia majora, and a small segment of the medial thigh. The iliohypogastric nerve supplies sensation to the groin and symphysis (Fig. 9–10). Pain in the inguinal region after a surgical procedure requires careful evaluation of the patient in order to arrive at the correct diagnosis.

Ilioinguinal or iliohypogastric nerve entrapment syndromes may be suggested by pain occurring im-

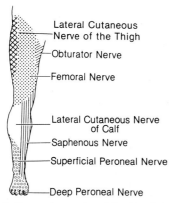

FIGURE 9–7. Sensory innervation of the skin of the upper inner thigh supplied by the obturator nerve. (Reproduced by permission from Stewart JD: Compression and entrapment neuropathies. In Dyck PJ (ed). Peripheral Neuropathy, p 971. Philadelphia: WB Saunders, 1993.)

Lateral Cutaneous Nerve of the Thigh
Obturator Nerve
Femoral Nerve
Lateral Cutaneous Nerve of Calf
Saphenous Nerve
Superficial Peroneal Nerve
Deep Peroneal Nerve

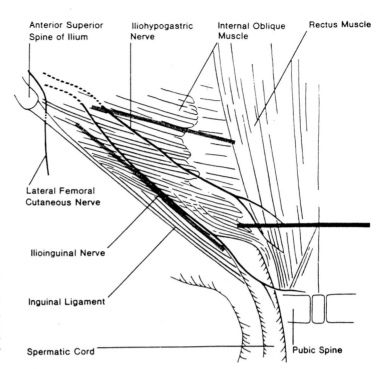

Anterior Superior
Spine of Ilium

Iliohypogastric
Nerve

Internal Oblique
Muscle

Rectus Muscle

Lateral Femoral
Cutaneous Nerve

Ilioinguinal Nerve

Inguinal Ligament

Spermatic Cord

Pubic Spine

FIGURE 9–9. Common incisions (in this case, in a male) that can result in iliohypogastric and ilioinguinal neuropathies. (Reproduced by permission from Stulz P, Pfeiffer KM: Peripheral nerve injuries resulting from common surgical procedures in the lower abdomen. Arch Surg 117:324–327, 1982.)

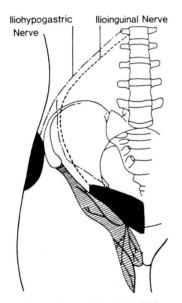

Iliohypogastric
Nerve

Ilioinguinal Nerve

FIGURE 9–10. Sensory innervation of the iliohypogastric and ilioinguinal nerves. The genitofemoral nerve sensory distribution is indicated by the hatched area. (Reproduced by permission from Stulz P, Pfeiffer KM: Peripheral nerve injuries resulting from common surgical procedures in the lower abdomen. Arch Surg 117:324–327, 1982.)

mediately after operation or after a delay of up to 6 months. The diagnostic triad for the syndrome of nerve entrapment consists of (1) sharp, burning pain, (2) paresthesias over the appropriate nerve distribution, and (3) pain relief following infiltration of a local anesthetic.[22] Treatment may require surgical resection of the involved nerve(s), as medical treatment may afford only temporary relief. Immediate and complete relief of pain can be obtained by resection in more than 70% of patients.

Compartment Syndrome

Compartment syndrome is most commonly associated with trauma or vascular procedures; however, it may occur following long gynecologic procedures in the lithotomy position such as tubal reanastomosis and lysis of adhesions.[23] The patient complains of severe leg cramps in the immediate postoperative period, followed later by numbness, burning, and difficulty moving the legs. Pulses may remain intact, but foot drop and decreased sensation over both feet may be present. On follow-up, foot drop and hypoesthesia may persist.

The pathogenesis of the compartment syndrome is thought to be related to an inflammatory process that results in an acute increase in pressure in a limited anatomic compartment. The pressure-related compromise of the neurovascular structures can lead to decreased blood flow, tissue necrosis, and further edema, all of which increase the compartmental pressures and initiate a destructive cycle. Factors contributing to the development of the syndrome include (1) passive dorsiflexion of the ankle joint, increasing compartmental pressures, (2) the weight of the leg itself on an underlying surface such as a stirrup, increasing compartmental pressures, and (3) elevation of the leg above the heart, decreasing arterial blood flow. Symptoms typically include pain, hypoesthesia, and weakness in the distribution of the nerve in the affected compartment. These symptoms can be elicited by passive stretch of the affected muscles. The risk of this complication can be reduced by avoiding prolonged lithotomy positioning and frequently repositioning the patient if the lithotomy position is unavoidable.

Vascular Events Involving the Lumbosacral Plexus

Transcatheter embolization is an established procedure for the control of bleeding in patients with pelvic trauma and pelvic malignancies. The procedure is also used to control hemorrhage in women with benign gynecologic conditions, as indicated in a recent report on five patients with massive vaginal hemorrhage following curettage (1), cesarian section (2), and total abdominal hysterectomy (3) who underwent embolization of both internal iliac arteries with Gelfoam, alone or in combination with stainless steel coils.[24] The bleeding stopped immediately in all of the patients. Four of them recovered completely without neurologic deficits and one died of disseminated intravascular coagulation and multi-organ failure.

It is important to remember that in association with pelvic surgery, embolization and infarction of arteries supplying the lumbosacral plexus can result in severe morbidity. Ischemic plexopathy resulting from pelvic arterial embolization is demonstrated in the following case report of a patient who underwent an embolization procedure designed to control hemorrhage after surgery and radiation therapy for cervical cancer.

Autonomic Nervous System Injury

Abnormal bladder and bowel function resulting from disruption of sympathetic and parasympathetic nerve fibers has received less attention than

CASE REPORT. A 51-year-old woman referred to Memorial Hospital with a confirmed diagnosis of infiltrating squamous cell carcinoma was found to have tumor replacing the entire cervix and upper vagina and extending to the lower one third of the anterior vaginal wall. The tumor extended to both parametria and to the left pelvic side wall. Involvement of the cul-de-sac peritoneum was found, and pelvic washings were cytologically positive for squamous cell carcinoma.

The patient was treated initially with external beam radiation therapy and then by Syed template interstitial implantation in the cervix with adequate dosing. Six months later rectal bleeding developed. Sigmoidoscopy revealed severe radiation proctitis. Treatment consisted of hydrocortisone enemas and multiple blood transfusions.

Two months later, the patient underwent a sigmoid colostomy with a Hartmann pouch but continued to have monthly episodes of acute rectal bleeding refractory to conservative measures. Three months later a chest radiograph revealed a 4-cm nodular density in the left lung. Percutaneous biopsy revealed an adenocarcinoma thought to represent a primary lung cancer. A radical resection was performed.

The woman continued to experience rectal bleeding, and 9 months after the thoracotomy she underwent pelvic arteriography and bilateral hypogastric artery embolization. Postembolization digital films demonstrated nonfilling of distal portions of most of the left hypogastric vessels, occlusion of the distal right hypogastric vessels, and stasis in the proximal portion of the right hypogastric artery. Approximately 1 hour after completion of the left hypogastric embolization and immediately after completion of the right hypogastric embolization, the patient complained of numbness in the left lower leg with pain and tingling. Assessment indicated normal left lower extremity pulses with decreased sensation along the medial and lateral aspects of the left calf to the level of the ankle as well as decreased muscle strength and voluntary movement of the left lower leg. Neurologic examination revealed bilateral leg weakness, much more marked on the left, especially in the muscles innervated by L5–S1 nerve roots. There was an absent ankle jerk reflex with brisk knee reflexes present. Embolization and infarction of the lower lumbosacral plexus with ischemic lumbosacral plexopathy and neuropathic pain syndrome were diagnosed. After the embolization procedure, the patient continually demonstrated clinical improvement.

More than 33 months after the diagnosis of cervical cancer, 16 months after thoracotomy for lung cancer, and 7 months after embolization, the patient was clinically free of cancer and the rectal bleeding had ended. She has a neurogenic bladder as a result of the lumbosacral plexopathy and performs self-catheterization. Continued effort with occupational therapy has resulted in increased mobility using a roller walker.

focal neuropathies, perhaps as a result of underreporting due to the wide range and severity of symptoms that may accompany autonomic nerve injury. Normal micturition and absence of residual urine may occur even with severe neurogenic paresis.[25] On the other hand, significant voiding dysfunction, a decrease in bladder sensation, and continence problems, as well as functional bowel obstruction, can follow a variety of pelvic operations.

The physiology of urinary function is complex and not completely understood. However, several general concepts are clear. The sympathetic, parasympathetic, and somatic nervous system fibers innervate the bladder, urethra, and sphincters in a coordinated fashion to provide for urine storage and elimination. During storage, a low level of afferent activity in the pelvic nerve activates reflexive efferent firing of the sympathetic and somatic pathways, resulting in detrusor inhibition and sphincter constriction. During micturition, a high level of pelvic nerve afferent activity results in activation of the parasympathetic pathways and inhibition of the sympathetic and somatic pathways, resulting in the elimination of urine.[2]

The reported frequency of urinary tract dysfunction following nonradical gynecologic operations is quite variable. Storage function of the lower urinary tract after nonradical and vaginal hysterectomy, studied by comparing pre- and postoperative urodynamic parameters, is characterized by a significant reduction in maximum cystometric capacity and a decline in bladder compliance. Both findings have been attributed to a decrease in the musculoelastic properties of the detrusor muscle caused by edema and surgical injury. In one study, however, neither a decrease in bladder capacity nor a decrease in compliance resulted in clinical sequelae. Urodynamic studies of changes in evacuation function failed to show any significant changes in detrusor contractility and suggested in a similar study that lower urinary tract evacuation function remained unaltered by either total abdominal or vaginal hysterectomy.[26,27]

One recent study evaluated the role of preexisting urinary tract dysfunction in women treated by total abdominal hysterectomy for benign conditions who lacked urinary symptoms. Urodynamic evaluation was performed preoperatively and again at 4 weeks and 4 months postoperatively. These studies failed to demonstrate operation-related urinary frequency, nocturia, urgency, or stress incontinence. It was concluded that urinary dysfunction should not be a consequence of an uncomplicated total hysterectomy for benign conditions in women who were previously free of urinary symptoms.[28] Indeed, it has been suggested that urinary tract symptoms should be no more common after hysterectomy than after curettage.[29]

In contrast, the incidence of vesicourethral dysfunction after simple hysterectomy, as determined by urodynamic studies and sacral reflex latencies (SRLs) (i.e., sensory thresholds measured as the conduction latencies from the dorsal nerve of the clitoris to the urethral and anal sphincters and from the urethral to the anal sphincter), has been reported to be as high as 30%, with approximately 70% of patients having some evidence of pelvic neuropathy as detected by SRLs.[30] In these studies, injury to the pelvic plexus was attributed to (1) division of the lateral ligaments of Mackenrodt where the principal branches of the plexus pass beneath the uterine arteries, (2) blunt dissection of the bladder, uterus, and cervix, as the major portion of the vesical innervation enters at the bladder base before innervating the remaining bladder, and (3) extensive dissection of the paravaginal tissues, which may injure nerve fibers near the lateral aspects of the vagina. In fact, cadaver studies indicate that plexus injury occurs only if the cardinal ligaments are excised or an unusually long cuff of the upper vagina is removed.[31] The symptoms associated with this nerve injury include detrusor instability and urethral obstruction. Therefore, during total hysterectomy dissection should remain close to the uterus with minimal vaginal mobilization or excision. Careful, sharp separation of the bladder base from the uterus and cervix is also recommended.

The findings observed after radical hysterectomy differ significantly from those observed after total hysterectomy. In these cases, a significant reduction in detrusor contractility and considerable abdominal straining are often required to empty the bladder.[32] Severe urinary dysfunction after radical pelvic surgery occurs in as many as 30% to 70% of patients.[33,34] Following radical hysterectomy, two phases of bladder dysfunction have been described: a hypertonic phase and a hypotonic phase.[35] The first phase occurs immediately postoperatively and is characterized by a high filling pressure and reduced capacity of the bladder. It is generally ascribed to postoperative changes such as edema and hematoma affecting the elastic properties of the bladder, but sympathetic denervation may also be involved. This phase generally resolves spontaneously, but in a small group of patients it may progress to the hypotonic phase. If improper urinary drainage and bladder overdistention occur, the detrusor muscle decompensates, resulting in alteration of bladder function characterized by a large capacity and low filling pressure. This results in urinary retention and high susceptibility to urinary tract infections. In a study of urinary dysfunction in 64 patients before and after radical hysterectomy, neurogenic bladder dysfunction was observed in 70% of patients.[35] All patients received early rehabilitative treatment consisting of kinesitherapy and/or pharmacologic therapy, with significant (91%) recovery of bladder function.

The effect of division of the cardinal ligaments on urinary dysfunction appears to be significantly more important following radical hysterectomy than following total hysterectomy. For example, in a study of 22 women who were serially evaluated by history and CO_2 cystourethroscopy after radical hysterectomy, 11 had the inferior 1 to 2 cm of these ligaments spared.[36] Satisfactory voiding occurred significantly earlier (20 vs. 51 days) in women who underwent incomplete transection of the ligaments. Vesical sensation was diminished in all patients, and although the magnitude of the sensory deficit was no greater in those with a complete transection, stress incontinence was significantly more frequent in the patients who had complete cardinal ligament transection. Hypertonic cystometric measurements and decreased intraurethral pressure were common postoperative findings, suggesting that sympathetic denervation was responsible for both alterations. Some authors recommend modification of the surgical technique of radical hysterectomy by limiting the dissection to the anterior part of the cardinal ligament, if feasible, which may eliminate postoperative voiding dysfunction.

The Wertheim hysterectomy with removal of pelvic lymph nodes, it should be remembered, includes clearance of fat, lymphatics, and lymph nodes from the common iliac vessels above to the pelvic floor below, and extends from the rectum posteriorly to the obturator foramen anteriorly (see Fig. 9–10). Surgical pathologic studies show considerable numbers of nerve fibers in excised specimens from the region lateral to the cervix, in the vesicovaginal septum, and in the area between the uterine artery and the pelvic floor in which the vesical autonomic nerves are located. It is clear that extensive dissection below and lateral to the uterine artery causes bladder denervation.[37] The depth of the web containing the plexus of nerves differs when the patient is in the supine position and undisturbed (Fig. 9–11) compared to that in the patient in whom the uterus is under traction, where a portion of the plexus is usually excised during radical hysterectomy (Fig. 9–12).[38]

A review of the late effects of radical hysterectomy indicates that 50% of patients report severe urinary symptoms on direct questioning, and there is a similar incidence of abnormally high residual urine volumes.[39] Bladder management in these situations consists of conservative measures, such as bladder training by means of transurethral resection of the bladder neck to reduce residual urine and operations on the urethra to abolish stress incontinence. It cannot be overemphasized that adequate urinary drainage must be maintained during the hypertonic phase by catheterization or pharmacologic therapy if long-term disability following radical hysterectomy is to be reduced. This is apparent from a study of 110 consecutive patients treated by radical hysterectomy, in whom urinary tract dys-

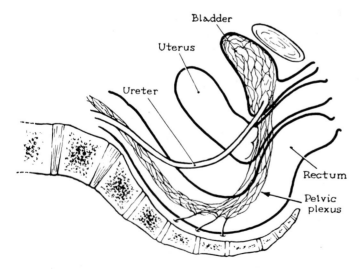

FIGURE 9–11. Location of the pelvic nerve plexus from the junction of the parasympathetic and sympathetic nerves to the distribution on the surface of the bladder. (Reproduced by permission from Twombly GH, Landers D: The innervation of the bladder with reference to radical hysterectomy. Am J Obstet Gynecol 71:1291–1300, 1956.)

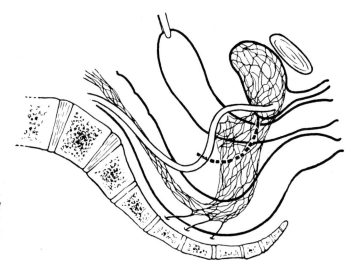

FIGURE 9–12. Portion of the pelvic plexus usually excised during radical hysterectomy (*dotted lines*). (Reproduced by permission from Twombly GH, Landers D: The innervation of the bladder with reference to radical hysterectomy. Am J Obstet Gynecol 71:1291–1300, 1956.)

function was not associated with tumor volume, operative blood loss, or the type of radical hysterectomy performed. However, inability to remove a suprapubic catheter before the 21st postoperative day was associated with a significant increase in urinary tract dysfunction at 3 months.[40]

Several recent studies have provided new insight into the mechanisms of nervous control of large bowel function and thus a more complete understanding of large bowel dysfunction after hysterectomy. In a study designed to investigate anorectal and urethral physiology following total abdominal hysterectomy, 26 women were studied before and 6 weeks and 6 months after surgery.[41] There was a postoperative increase in both rectal and vesical sensitivity, irrespective of the type of hysterectomy performed. In this study, no significant changes in rectal or bladder compliance were noted, no change in whole gut transit time, and anal pressure and urethral pressure and length were unchanged after surgery. Urinary symptoms occurred in 6 of 26 women and gastrointestinal symptoms in 2 of 26 women. The authors concluded that significant changes in rectal and vesical sensitivity occur after hysterectomy for benign disease and may persist for at least 6 months postoperatively, but are not always associated with urinary or gastrointestinal symptoms.

Varma studied the motility of the human distal bowel by physiologic investigation involving electrical stimulation of sacral parasympathetic outflow in patients with high spinal injuries and in patients with intractable constipation following pelvic surgery.[42] Women with intractable constipation after hysterectomy had significantly increased rectal vol-

ume and compliance, together with deficits in rectal sensory function. After stimulation with Prostigmin (neostigmine), a colorectal motility gradient was paradoxically reversed in these patients, thus constituting a functional obstruction. Denervation supersensitivity was demonstrated in two patients tested with carbachol provocation but not in control subjects. It was concluded that dysfunction of the autonomic innervation of the hindgut occurs after hysterectomy in some patients, resulting in severe constipation. It should be noted that the parasympathetic fibers may be directly injured during dissection of the anterolateral aspect of the lower rectum, and indirectly may be stretched during mobilization of the rectum during radical pelvic surgery. As with the potential for urinary dysfunction, the possibility of operative disruption of rectal autonomic innervation should not be allowed to compromise an appropriate cancer operation.

Summary

Neurologic complications associated with gynecologic surgery are uncommon. The current literature indicates that three major factors in patients undergoing gynecological surgical procedures predispose to neurologic injury. These factors are (1) the use of self-retaining retractors, particularly those with deep retractor blades, (2) stirrup selection and positioning of patients in the lithotomy position, and (3) radical dissection resulting in autonomic nerve disruption.

Fortunately, most cases of neurologic injuries are

transient and require little intervention. However, surgeons should be aware of the potential for injury and thus avoid complications that may result in long-term morbidity.

References

1. Moore KL: Clinically Oriented Anatomy. Baltimore: Williams & Wilkins, 1985.
2. de Groat WC, Booth AM: Autonomic systems to the urinary bladder and sexual organs. In Dyck PJ (ed): Peripheral Neuropathy. Philadelphia: WB Saunders, 1984.
3. Bradley WE: Autonomic regulation of the urinary bladder. In Low PA (ed): Clinical Autonomic Disorders: Evaluation and Management. Rochester, Minn: Mayo Foundation, 1993.
4. Bosch EP, Mitsumoto H: Disorders of peripheral nerves. In Bradley WG (ed): Neurology in Clinical Practice. Boston: Butterworth-Heinemann, 1989.
5. Rosenblum J, Schwarz GA, Bendler E: Femoral neuropathy: A neurological complication of hysterectomy. JAMA 195:409–414, 1966.
6. Vosburg LF, Finn W: Femoral nerve impairment subsequent to hysterectomy. Am J Obstet Gynecol 82:931–937, 1961.
7. Georgy FM: Femoral neuropathy following abdominal hysterectomy. Am J Obstet Gynecol 23:819–822, 1975.
8. Kvist-Poulsen H, Borel J: Iatrogenic femoral neuropathy subsequent to abdominal hysterectomy: Incidence and prevention. Obstet Gynecol 60:516–520, 1982.
9. Goldman JA, Feldberg D, Dicker D, Samuel N, Dekel A: Femoral neuropathy subsequent to abdominal hysterectomy: A comparative study. Eur J Obstet Gynecol Reprod Biol 20:385–392, 1985.
10. Meldrum DR: Femoral nerve compression injury and tubal microsurgery. Fertil Steril 32:345–346, 1979.
11. Hassan AA, Reiff RH, Fayez JA: Femoral neuropathy following microsurgical tuboplasty. J Fertil Steril 45:889–911, 1986.
12. Roblee MA: Femoral neuropathy from the lithotomy position: Case report and new leg holder for prevention. Am J Obstet Gynecol 97:871–872, 1967.
13. Hopper CL, Baker JB: Bilateral femoral neuropathy complicating vaginal hysterectomy: Analysis of contributing factors in 3 patients. Obstet Gynecol 32:543–547, 1968.
14. Sunderland S: The relative susceptibility to injury of the medial and lateral popliteal divisions of the sciatic nerve. Br J Surg 41:300–302, 1953.
15. Denny-Brown D: Effects of transient stretching of peripheral nerves. Arch Neurol Psychiatry 54:116–129, 1945.
16. Batres F, Barclay DL: Sciatic nerve injury during gynecologic procedures using the lithotomy position. Obstet Gynecol 62:92–94, 1983.
17. Burkhart FL, Daly JW: Sciatic and peroneal nerve injury: A complication of vaginal operations. Obstet Gynecol 28:99–102, 1966.
18. McQuarrie HG, Harris JW, Ellsworth HS, Stone RA, Anderson AE 3d: Sciatic neuropathy complicating vaginal hysterectomy. Am J Obstet Gynecol 113:223–232, 1972.
19. Hoffman MS, Roberts WS, Cavanagh D: Neuropathies associated with radical pelvic surgery for gynecologic cancer. Gynecol Oncol 31:462–466, 1988.
20. Donaghy M: Lumbosacral plexus lesions. In Dyck PJ (ed): Peripheral Neuropathy. Philadelphia: WB Saunders, 1993.
21. Stewart JD: Compression and entrapment neuropathies. In Dyck PJ (ed): Peripheral Neuropathy. Philadelphia: WB Saunders, 1993.
22. Stulz P, Pfieffer KM: Peripheral nerve injuries resulting from common surgical procedures in the lower abdomen. Arch Surg 117:324–327, 1982.
23. Adler LM, Loughlin JS, Morin CJ, Haning RV Jr: Bilateral compartment syndrome after a long gynecologic operation in the lithotomy position. Am J Obstet Gynecol 162:1271–1272, 1990.
24. Finnegan MF, Tisnado J, Bezirdjian DR, Cho SR: Transcatheter embolotherapy of massive bleeding after surgery for benign gynecologic disorders. Can Assoc Radiol J 39:172–177, 1988.
25. Glahn BE: The neurogenic factor in vesical dysfunction following radical hysterectomy for carcinoma of the cervix. Scand J Urol Nephrol 4:107–116, 1970.
26. Vervest HA, van Venrooij GE, Barents JW, Haspels AA, Debruyne FM: Non-radical hysterectomy and the function of the lower urinary tract: I. Urodynamic quantification of changes in storage function. Acta Obstet Gynecol Scand 68:221–229, 1989.
27. Vervest HA, van Verooij GE, Barents JW, Haspels AA, Debruyne FM: Non-radical hysterectomy and the function of the lower urinary tract: II. Urodynamic quantification of changes in evacuation function. Acta Obstet Gynecol Scand 68:231–235, 1989.
28. Langer R, Neuman M, Ron-el R, Golan A, Bukovsky I, Caspi E: The effect of total abdominal hysterectomy on bladder function in asymptomatic women. Obstet Gynecol 74:205–207, 1989.
29. Griffith-Jones MD, Jarvis GJ, McNamara HM: Adverse urinary symptoms after total hysterectomy: Fact or fiction: Br J Urol 67:295–297, 1991.
30. Parys BT, Haylen BT, Hutton JL, Parsons KF: The effects of simple hysterectomy on vesicourethral function. Br J Urol 64:594–599, 1989.
31. Mundy AR: An anatomical explanation for bladder dysfunction following rectal and uterine surgery. Br J Urol 54:501–504, 1982.
32. Vervest HA, Barents JW, Haspells AA, Debruyne FM: Radical hysterectomy and the function of the lower urinary tract: Urodynamic quantification of changes in storage and evacuation function. Acta Obstet Gynecol Scand 68:331–340, 1989.
33. Kadar N, Nelson JH: The frequency, causes and prevention of severe urinary dysfunction after radical hysterectomy. Br J Obstet Gynecol 90:858–863, 1983.
34. Fishman IJ, Shabsigh R, Kaplan AL: Lower urinary tract dysfunction after radical hysterectomy for carcinoma of cervix. Urology 28:462–468, 1986.
35. Zanolla R, Monzeglio C, Campo B, Ordesi G, Balzarini A, Martino G: Bladder and urethral dysfunction after radical abdominal hysterectomy: Rehabilitative treatment. J Surg Oncol 28:190–194, 1985.
36. Forney JP: The effects of radical hysterectomy on bladder physiology. Am J Obstet Gynecol 138:374–382, 1980.
37. Smith PH, Ballantyne B: The neuroanatomical basis for denervation of the urinary bladder following major pelvic surgery. Br J Surg 55:929–933, 1968.
38. Twombly GH, Landers D: The innervation of the bladder with reference to radical hysterectomy. Am J Obstet Gynecol 71:1291–1300, 1956.

39. Fraser AC: The late effects of Wertheim's hysterectomy on the urinary tract. J Obstet Gynaecol Br Commonw 73:1002–1007, 1966.

40. Buller RE, Tamir IL, DiSaia PJ, Berman ML: Early evaluation of the urinary tract following radical hysterectomy: Structure and function relationships. Obstet Gynecol 78:840–844, 1991.

41. Prior A, Stanley K, Smith AR, Read NW: Effect of hysterectomy on anorectal and urethrovesical physiology. Gut 33:264–267, 1992.

42. Varma JS: Autonomic influences on colorectal motility and pelvic surgery. World J Surg 16:811–819, 1992.

Complications in Gynecologic Surgery: Prevention, Recognition, and Management,
edited by James W. Orr, Jr., and Hugh M. Shingleton.
J. B. Lippincott Company, Philadelphia, © 1994.

Chapter 10

The Lymphatic System

Hugh M. Shingleton
Barry S. Siller

History

Thomas Bartholin's *Vasa Lymphatica,* published in 1653, is credited with being the first to delineate the significance of the human lymphatic system.[1] In the next hundred years the lymphatic valves were described, as was the lymphatic system of the uterus.[2] William Cruikshank[3] in 1768 established the foundation of modern knowledge concerning the lymphatic system. The anatomic atlas of Paolo Mascagni,[4] published in 1787, contained engravings of the lymphatics. Jean Cruveilhier's two-volume work on pathologic anatomy,[5] published in 1829 and 1842, contained illustrations of the lymphatic system, while Henry Savage's *Female Pelvic Organs,*[6] published in 1880, described and diagramed the pelvic lymphatic system. In *Cancer of the Uterus,* published in 1900, Thomas Cullen cited the work of Poirier in regard to the pelvic lymphatics.[7]

Lymphatics were first described as a site for metastases from a breast primary cancer by Henri Francois Le Dran, in 1757.[8] John M. Scudder's *Diseases of Women,*[9] published in 1877, described uterine cancer spread to adjacent tissues and pelvic lymphatics. Works by Mann, Winter, and Cullen published between 1888 and 1895 further documented pelvic lymph gland involvement in the late stages of uterine cancer.[7,10,11]

In 1895 Emil Reis, a surgeon in Chicago described a radical operation with pelvic lymph node dissection for cervical cancer. He performed the operation only on dogs and human cadavers.[12]

Rumpf in Germany described an operation similar to Reis's. In 1895 John G. Clark in Baltimore included partial lymphadenectomy in a number of extended operations for cervical cancer. In 1913 Clark abandoned extensive pelvic node dissection because it added to the hazards and did not raise the percentage of permanent cures.[13] In *Operative Gynecology,* published in 1906, Howard Kelly stated, "Each of these operators (Reis, Rumpf, Clark), wishing to establish a parallel between the wide operations upon cancerous breasts associated with the removal of the axillary glands and cancer of the uterus, proposed as far as possible to remove the pelvic glands and in this way to make the operation more thorough and to reduce the percentage of relapses."[14] In 1898 Ernst Wertheim reported on a series of radical operations for cancer of the cervix but never advocated complete lymphadenectomy. He believed that the pelvic retroperitoneal spaces should be opened to palpate nodal areas. They were only removed if enlarged. In 1912 he stated, "Against the demand . . . to remove all of the lymphatic system is the fact that, first of all, this could not be accomplished, and second, it is not necessary to do so."[15] In 1944 Joe Vincent Meigs reintroduced the radical operation for cervical cancer in the United States and stated, "Without doubt node dissection as it is done in the radical operation is at best a crude dissection of the pelvic nodes."[16]

In the past half century, gynecologic surgeons worldwide have performed lymphadenectomy as a part of operations on women with female genital

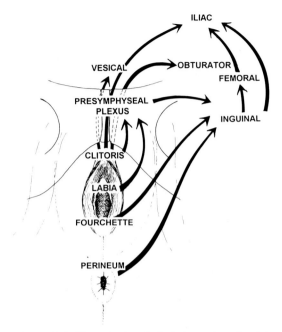

FIGURE 10–1. The major lymphatic drainage channels of the vulva. (Adapted from Plentl AA, Friedman EA: Lymphatic System of the Female Genitalia, p 25. Philadelphia: WB Saunders, 1971.)

cancers of all types. Despite this vast experience, it is still unclear how often lymphadenectomy is therapeutic. However, when regional lymph nodes are involved, the prognosis is altered.

Lymphatic Anatomy and Drainage

The lymphatic drainage of the vulva, the vagina, the cervix, the uterine corpus, and adnexal structures is well established. Dissection entails requisite surgery to remove primary as well as secondary routes of lymphatic spread during treatment for malignant disease involving these structures. Although many systems of nomenclature exist, we have used the terminology suggested by Mangan et al.[16a] in 1986 in our modifications of drawings from Plentl's[17] 1971 monograph (Figs. 10–1 through 10–5). For completeness, lymphatic drainage of the abdominal wall, the abdominal contents (small and large bowel, omentum), the rectum, the anal canal, and the perineum is also listed (Table 10–1). Knowledge of the locations of the lymph nodes relevant to gynecologic cancers is essential for surgeons treating these disease entities (Fig.10–6).

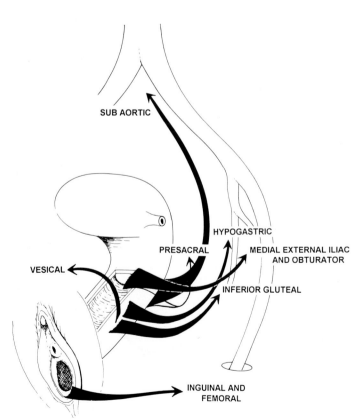

FIGURE 10–2. The major lymphatic drainage channels of the vagina. (Adapted from Plentl AA, Friedman EA: Lymphatic System of the Female Genitalia, p 55. Philadelphia: WB Saunders, 1971.)

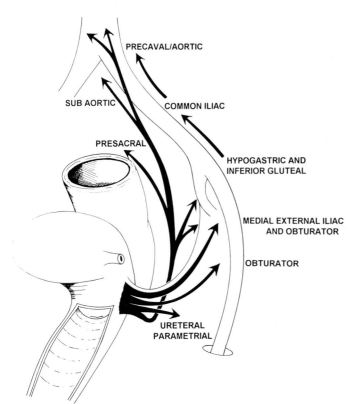

FIGURE 10–3. The major lymphatic trunks of the cervix. (Adapted from Plentl AA, Friedman EA: Lymphatic System of the Female Genitalia, p 83. Philadelphia: WB Saunders, 1971.)

Nonsurgical Evaluation of the Pelvic and Para-aortic Lymph Nodes

Although pathologic examination remains the reference standard in the detection of pelvic and para-aortic lymph node metastases, appropriate imaging techniques in specific clinical settings can provide valuable information. The three main noninvasive studies used to evaluate the retroperitoneal lymph nodes are computed tomography (CT), lymphangiography, and magnetic resonance imaging (MRI). The diagnostic capabilities and inherent limitations of these imaging techniques differ and will be discussed.

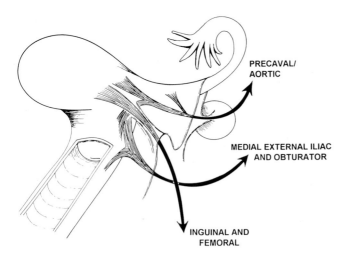

FIGURE 10–4. The major lymphatic channels draining the uterus. (Adapted from Plentl AA, Friedman EA: Lymphatic System of the Female Genitalia, p 122. Philadelphia: WB Saunders, 1971.)

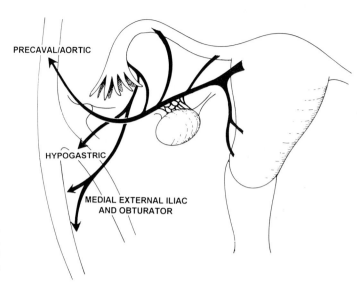

PRECAVAL/AORTIC

HYPOGASTRIC

MEDIAL EXTERNAL ILIAC
AND OBTURATOR

FIGURE 10–5. The major lymphatic channels draining the ovaries. (Adapted from Plentl AA, Friedman EA: Lymphatic System of the Female Genitalia, p 172. Philadelphia: WB Saunders, 1971.)

Computed Tomography

CT permits demonstration of the cross-sectional anatomy of the retroperitoneal lymph nodes in the pelvic and para-aortic areas. CT can be used to distinguish normal from abnormal nodal morphology based strictly on size. Lymph nodes greater than 20 mm in diameter are considered abnormal (Fig. 10–7); however, smaller lymph nodes with micro-metastases would be considered normal. Occasionally bulky enlarged nodes are obscured, especially in the pelvic area, because of the proximity of

TABLE 10–1. **Lymphatic Drainage (Primary)**

Site	Lymph Nodes Drained
Abdominal wall (upper)	Pectoral group of axillary nodes
	Parasternal nodes
Abdominal wall (lower)	External iliac nodes (or most caudal portion)
	Superficial inguinal nodes
Omentum	Presence of lymphatic vessels not established; if present, may drain into gastroepiploic nodes
Small bowel	
Duodenum (upper)	Pyloric nodes (front) and biliary nodes (behind)
(lower)	Superior mesenteric nodes
Ileum	Mesenteric nodes
Jejunum	Mesenteric nodes
Large bowel	
Ascending colon	Right colic nodes
Transverse (right flexure and right 2/3)	Middle colic nodes
Transverse (left flexure and left 1/3)	Inferior mesenteric nodes
	Superior mesenteric nodes
Descending and sigmoid colon	Inferior mesenteric nodes
Rectum	
Upper	Inferior mesenteric nodes
Lower	Internal iliac nodes
Other routes	Sacral and median common iliac nodes
	Small anorectal lymph nodes
	Pararectal nodes
Anal canal (greater part)	Vessels run across ischiorectal fossa or upward with those of the rectum
(below pectinate line)	Superior inguinal nodes
Perineum	Superficial inguinal nodes

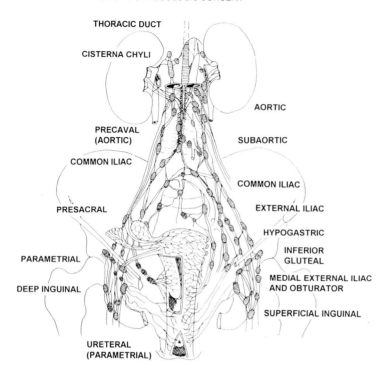

FIGURE 10–6. The lymphatic system of the female genital organs. (Adapted with permission from Meigs JV (ed): Surgical Treatment of Cancer of the Cervix, p 90. New York: Grune & Stratton, 1954.)

major pelvic vessels and the relative paucity of fat. CT evaluation of the pelvis is associated with false positive and false negative rates of approximately 20% each (Table 10–2). Its sensitivity ranges from 9% to 26%. CT evaluation of the para-aortic nodes has been associated with false negative and false positive rates of approximately 5% and 15%, respectively. The overall accuracy is approximately 82% (Table 10–3) but varies considerably between institutions. The specificity of CT in the detection of disease metastatic to the para-aortic and pelvic nodes is approximately 90%; however, the sensitivity is slightly higher in the para-aortic area, where the large amount of fat and the simple architecture facilitate distinction of lymph nodes from major vessels (Table 10–3).

Lymphangiography

Bipedal lymphangiography, first described by Kinmouth et al. in England, is an imaging technique that provides useful information on the status of the pelvic and retroperitoneal lymph nodes.[18] Currently it is the only imaging technique that demonstrates the internal architecture of the lymph nodes and shows smaller, potentially involved nodes (Fig. 10–8). Lymphangiography does have diagnostic limitations: metastatic disease of less than 3 to 5 mm may go undetected. Additionally, completely replaced lymph nodes or incomplete visualization of the lymph node may result in a false negative study.[19,20] For these reasons, the sensitivity and specificity of lymphangiography in evaluating the pelvic lymph nodes are approximately 25% to 30% and 80% to 90%, respectively (Table 10–4). The sensitivity of lymphangiography in evaluating

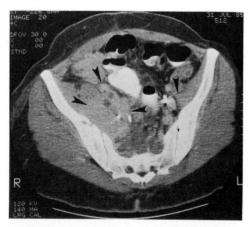

FIGURE 10–7. Pelvic CT scan of a patient with advanced cervical cancer. Pathologically enlarged nodes are present (*arrows*). (Reproduced with permission from Shingleton HM, Orr JW Jr: Cancer of the Cervix: Diagnosis and Treatment, 2nd ed, p 111. New York: Churchill Livingstone, 1987.)

TABLE 10–2. **CT Demonstration of Pelvic Lymph Node Metastases**

Study, Year	No. of Pts.	Results		Accuracy (%)	Sensitivity (%)	Specificity (%)
		False Negative (%)	*False Positive (%)*			
Grumbine et al., 1981[110]	24	25	4	72	0	94
Walsh and Joblerud, 1981[133]	75	30	22	74	—	—
Brenner et al., 1982[111]	10	0	20	80	100	75
Whitley et al., 1982[112]	7	0	14.5	66	100	83
Engelshoven et al., 1984[113]	20	57	7	75	43	92
Vas et al., 1985[134]	59	—	—	—	62	78
King et al., 1986[114]	25	9	9	82	85	80
Newton et al., 1987[115]	50	—	—	—	9.1	97.4
Vercamer et al., 1987[116]	55	—	—	—	18	95
Camilien et al., 1988[117]	61	50	18	80	25	97
Matsukama et al., 1989[118]	44	3	55	96.2	26.3	98.8
Mean		*22*	*19*	*78*	*47.0*	*89.0*

the pelvic aortic nodes is slightly higher, ranging from 67% to 83%, but the specificity is slightly lower, ranging from 47% to 76%.[21–23]

Magnetic Resonance Imaging

MRI has been used to evaluate the pelvic and para-aortic lymph nodes and, like CT, differentiates normal from abnormal lymph nodes based strictly on size, not nodal architectural features. Currently, microscopic tumor deposits in normal-sized lymph nodes cannot be identified, and malignant enlargement cannot be differentiated from benign or reactive hyperplasia. In a study performed by Brodman et al.[24] in 60 women with cervical cancer, the sensitivity and specificity of MRI in evaluating the pelvic and para-aortic lymph nodes were 28% and 64%, respectively. The overall accuracy was 62%. Greco et al.[25] reported similar results in 46 cervical cancer patients, with an overall accuracy rate of 75%. Although the clinical experience using MRI to evaluate the pelvic and para-aortic lymph nodes is limited, it appears comparable to that seen with CT and lymphangiography.

TABLE 10–3. **CT Demonstration of Para-aortic Node Metastases**

Study, Year	No. of Pts.	Results		Accuracy (%)	Sensitivity (%)	Specificity (%)
		False Negative (%)	*False Positive (%)*			
Photopulos et al., 1979[119]	17	24	0	76	60	100
Brenner et al., 1982[111]	20	10	5	85	67	93
Whitley et al., 1982[112]	16	6	6	88	80	92
Villasanta et al., 1983[120]	42	7	10	83	77	86
Bandy et al., 1985[121]	44	7	7	86	75	91
Vas et al., 1985[134]	59	—	—	—	50	79
King et al., 1986[114]	25	21	12	68	50	79
Newton et al., 1987[115]	50	—	—	—	66.7	94
Camilien et al., 1988[117]	61	—	—	—	67	100
Matsukama et al., 1989[118]	70	—	—	—	71.4	96.8
Heller et al., 1990[21]	264	—	—	—	34	95.8
Mean		*12.5*	*7*	*81*	*63.4*	*91.5*

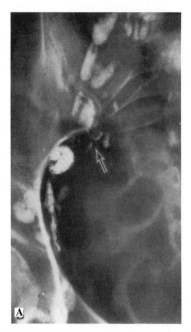 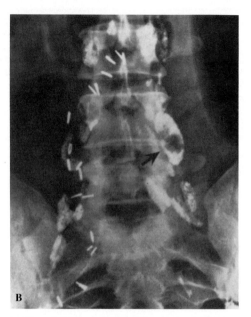

FIGURE 10–8. Pelvic lymphangiogram of a patient with metastatic carcinoma of the cervix. **A.** The two small nodes containing metastatic carcinoma are crescent in configuration (*arrow*). **B.** The single metastatic node (*arrow*) was beyond the reach of the surgeon. Postoperative radiographs were necessary to confirm the biopsy of the nodes in question. (Reproduced with permission from Wallace S, Jing B-S: Carcinoma. In Clouse ME (ed): Clinical Lymphangiography, pp 188, 211. Baltimore: Williams & Wilkins, 1977.)

The finding of enlarged nodes on any of these imaging techniques—CT, lymphangiography, or MRI—indicates a high probability of nodal metastatic disease, but the absence of an enlarged node correlates poorly with disease status. In general, these imaging studies appear to be of most clinical benefit in the evaluation of women with advanced stage disease. Results are too unreliable for routine use in the diagnostic staging of malignant conditions of the pelvis, especially in women with apparently early stage gynecologic cancer.

TABLE 10–4. **Lymphangiography Demonstration of Lymph Node Metastases**

Node Group/ Study, Year	No. of Pts.	Sensitivity (%)	Specificity (%)
Pelvic			
Muylder et al., 1984[19]	100	28	100
Feigan et al., 1987[20]	36	25	82
Vercamer et al., 1987[116]	43	29	86
Para-aortic			
Brown et al., 1979[23]	21	83	47
Ashraf et al., 1982[22]	39	67	76
Heller et al., 1990[21]	264	79	73
Para-aortic and pelvic			
Averette et al., 1966[122]	83	77	90
Piver et al., 1971[123]	103	77	98
Berman et al., 1977[104]	65	56	86
Mean		*58*	*82*

Fine Needle Aspiration of Lymph Nodes

Fine needle aspiration (FNA) can be used to obtain tissue samples for cytologic diagnosis (Fig. 10–9). FNA is especially useful to confirm the presence of metastatic disease in suspicious or enlarged lymph nodes demonstrated on CT, lymphangiography, or MRI. The technique is generally performed with local anesthesia and CT guidance, which offers the best direct imaging of the depth and path of the biopsy needle.[26] A 20 cc syringe with a 22 to 23 gauge needle of appropriate length is used. Once the needle has entered the target area, suction is applied, released, and the needle removed. Three to five passes in each target area will increase the chance of successful aspiration. The cytologic material is fixed immediately and stained by the Papanicolaou method. The finding of malignant cells confirms metastatic disease. However, if the sample is inadequate or if the test is negative, further studies are necessary for definitive diagnosis. Kline and Neal[27] performed over 3,000 FNAs, with an overall accuracy of 90%. Others have reported comparable results (Table 10–5).[28–30] FNA is inexpensive, can be performed on an outpatient basis, and has the potential of avoiding the morbidity and cost of major surgery. The principal disadvantages of FNA include a small risk of introducing infection or of causing internal bleeding.

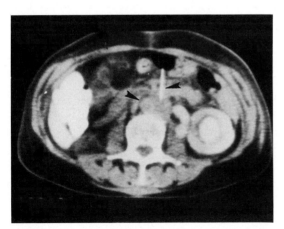

FIGURE 10–9. Computed tomogram (CT) demonstrating a needle (*upper arrow*) inserted into an enlarged para-aortic node (*lower arrow*). The path of the needle is only partially in the plane of the tomogram. (Courtesy of Peyton T. Taylor, MD, University of Virginia Medical Center, Charlottesville, Virginia. Reproduced with permission from Shingleton HM, Orr JW Jr: Cancer of the Cervix: Diagnosis and Treatment, 2nd ed, p 106. New York: Churchill Livingstone, 1987.)

TABLE 10–5. Fine Needle Aspiration of Enlarged or Suspicious Lymph Nodes

Study	No. of Pts.	Accuracy (%)
McDonald et al.[29]	37	74
Kline and Neal[27]	3,267	90
Sevin et al.[30]	73	94.5
Zornoza et al.[28]	72	82.9
Mean		*89.9*

Indications for Lymphadenectomy

Lymphadenectomy is an important part of curative therapy for cancers of the vulva, cervix, endometrium, and ovary.

Cancer of the Vulva

Surgery for microscopically invasive vulvar lesions routinely involves the unilateral or bilateral dissection of the superficial groin nodes above the level of the cribriform fascia. With more extensive lesions the deep inguinal (femoral) nodes are also dissected. In the era of ultraradical surgery for vulvar cancer, ca. 1950–1975, extraperitoneal or transperitoneal techniques allowing comprehensive dissection of the pelvic nodes were employed for all invasive vulvar lesions. A subsequent tendency toward conservatism has resulted in sampling or dissection of only the groin nodes, with postoperative pelvic radiation therapy prescribed for the dissected area (if involved) and for the next higher chain (pelvic) of nodes, which are usually left undissected. Extensive routine bilateral groin and pelvic node dissections, as performed by Way of Newcastle and Collins of New Orleans, have been replaced by dissection of only the ipsilateral groin in the case of small unilateral vulvar lesions.[31,32] The practice of creating large transverse abdominal incisions for en bloc node dissections and vulvectomy, often with removal of much skin overlying the groin nodes and pubis, has been modified so that now multiple incisions are made, each groin incision separate from the vulvar dissection, without a significant increase in local recurrence rates.[33,34] Pelvic node dissections are rarely performed now except for the most advanced lesions.

Cervical Cancer

Modern therapeutic operations for cancer of the cervix include comprehensive dissection of the pelvic and common iliac nodes and frequently dissection or extensive sampling of the lower para-aortic precaval nodes. After the abdomen is opened, surgical attention is directed to the secondary nodal drainage. If the common iliac or aortic nodes contain metastatic tumor, a radical hysterectomy is usually abandoned in favor of radiation therapy delivered to the pelvis and the affected node groups.

A decade of information obtained from surgical staging of all stages of cervical cancer has delineated the frequency and patterns of cervical cancer spread. However, surgical staging has been abandoned, for surgical staging alone has not been shown to contribute to long-term patient survival.[35]

Endometrial Cancer

In recent years, interest has focused on the spread of uterine cancer to regional lymphatics. Whereas U.S. gynecologic oncologists extensively sample nodes in the pelvis, this dissection is usually not as comprehensive as that performed for early stage cancer of the cervix. Although aortic node sampling is also advocated as part of a curative operation for uterine cancer, the majority of dissections are not extended as far cephalad as the lymphatic drainage along the ovarian vessels might require. Additionally, the nodes above, on either side of, or below the aorta and vena cava have not been consistently evaluated. To date, lymphadenectomy in the treatment of cancer of the endometrium has frequently consisted of random node sampling, prognostic in intent, rather than therapeutic node dissection as such. However, the nodal information obtained at lymphadenectomy may eliminate the need for use of pelvic radiation in high-risk stage I uterine lesions.[36]

Cancer of the Ovary

Ovarian cancer is thought to be an intraperitoneal disease, and, as a result of its pattern of spread and the advanced stage at diagnosis, routine pelvic lymphadenectomy has not played an important part in many primary operations. In some cases of extensive tumor debulking at the time of primary operations and in conjunction with second-look operations to determine the presence of any residual tumor following chemotherapy, both pelvic and aortic nodes are routinely sampled. As in endometrial cancer, however, the role of lymphadenectomy in ovarian cancer is not yet established or thought to be as important as in the surgical treatment of cancers of the cervix or vulva.

Cancer of the Vagina

Vaginal cancers are rarely treated surgically. In the event of primary operations or operations for radiorecurrent tumors, lesions involving the upper two thirds of the vagina are known to drain to the pelvic nodes and must be dissected as part of a curative surgical procedure. Invasive lesions involving the lower half of the vagina drain to the inguinal nodes, which may also require dissection if surgery is the primary or secondary mode of therapy.

Cancer of the Fallopian Tube

Fallopian tube cancers are often encountered incidentally during abdominal operations for other indications. The pattern of spread of fallopian tumors and their management parallel that of cancer of the ovary. Routine pelvic lymphadenectomy is not an established part of treatment but may occasionally be employed by cancer surgeons as a diagnostic (early stage) or therapeutic (bulky nodes) approach.

Technique of Lymphadenectomy

The standard pelvic and para-aortic lymphadenectomy is usually performed through a transperitoneal incision. However, similar node sampling can be performed by a laparoscopic or extraperitoneal approach, which is used primarily to assess the status of the para-aortic nodes in patients with cervical cancer. Inguinal node dissection may be necessary in the treatment of lower vaginal or vulvar cancers.

Pelvic Node Dissection

Pelvic lymph node dissection is usually begun by dividing the round ligaments and developing the pararectal and paravesical spaces. After the ureters are identified, the common and external iliac nodes are dissected caudally to the circumflex iliac vein. The genital femoral nerves, located laterally on the psoas muscle, are usually identified and spared. The obturator nodes are exposed by lateral retraction of the external iliac vein (over the obturator space). The obturator nerve is identified in its entirety and the fat pad containing the obturator nodes is dissected off the pelvic side wall. Usually clips are placed caudally and the nodes are dissected cephalad to the hypogastric artery, where clips are usually placed to prevent bleeding.

Para-aortic Node Dissection

Before performing a para-aortic lymphadenectomy, the operator packs the intestinal tract to expose the peritoneum overlying the right common iliac artery. This peritoneum is incised, and a retractor is then placed retroperitoneally to expose the right para-aortic node group (supracaval fat pad) (Fig. 10–10). These nodes are carefully dissected off the vena cava, with hemoclips applied to perforators and the lateral aspects of the dissection for hemostasis. The left para-aortic nodes are palpated but generally not excised for histologic evaluation unless they are suspiciously fixed or enlarged. If a left para-aortic node dissection is performed, the nodes can be approached through the same incision, or if necessary they can be exposed by reflecting the sigmoid and descending colon medially.

Groin Node Dissection

An elliptical incision is placed approximately 2 cm lateral to the pubic tubercle and 2 cm inferior to the iliac crest along the length of the inguinal ligament. The incision is extended through the subcutaneous tissue to the superficial fascia. This tissue above the fascia lata contains the superficial nodes. During this dissection the saphenous vein is usually identified and ligated at the apex of the femoral triangle and again at its origin at the femoral vein. The fas-

cia lata is incised and the fat pad overlying the femoral vessels and containing the femoral nodes is removed during a deep groin dissection.

Special Operative Considerations

Completeness of Dissection

The techniques used for lymphadenectomy vary according to surgical training and experience. Two techniques used in recent years to provide a more complete dissection and greater yield of nodes are intraoperative lymphangiography and nodal radionuclide incorporation. Both allow intraoperative identification of remaining nodes in the dissection field. Using lymphangiography, Kjorstad et al.[37] in 1984 established that a more complete dissection was possible in patients with cervical cancer. However, this did not result in improved long-term survival, and one in every five patients who underwent "complete" pelvic dissections developed significant lower extremity edema. Gitsch et al.,[38] also in 1984, used intraoperative lymph node scintigraphy to increase node yield and reported reduced recurrence rates in patients with stage I cervical cancer, but the survival rates in patients with surgically staged stage II carcinomas were not improved. Despite the clinical potential, neither of these methods has gained general acceptance.

Ligation of Afferent Lymphatics and Use of Drains

Some authors suggest that the afferent lymphatics should be ligated, which is often accomplished by applying surgical clips prior to division. Proponents of ligation believe it reduces postoperative drainage and lowers the risk of pelvic (or groin) lymphocysts. Others do not ligate lymphatic trunks since they have not observed problems as a consequence of nonligation. Drainage of the operative site, both for groin dissections and for pelvic lymph node dissections, has shifted from rubber drains of the Penrose type to closed suction drains. Many investigators believe that such drains cut down on lymphocyst formation and pelvic infection; however, Clarke-Pearson et al.[39] in a study of almost 500 patients undergoing lymphadenectomy for various gynecologic indications, were not convinced that closed suction drainage was of benefit, and in fact suggested that it could introduce infection into these areas, with concomitant increases in febrile

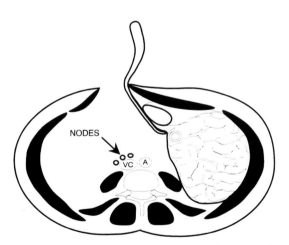

FIGURE 10–10. Extraperitoneal approach to the para-aortic node area. The abdominal contents are displaced to the patient's left, allowing dissection of the nodes between the renal vessels and the bifurcation of the iliac vessels. vc, vena cava; a, aorta. (Reproduced with permission from Shingleton HM, Orr JW Jr: Cancer of the Cervix: Diagnosis and Treatment, 2nd ed, p 106. New York: Churchill Livingstone, 1987.)

morbidity, pulmonary embolism, and urinary fistula formation. A recent retrospective, controlled evaluation of drain usage following radical hysterectomy came to the same conclusion.[40] The preponderance of available evidence does not support the use or benefit of prophylactic pelvic drainage following lymphadenectomy.

Laparoscopic Lymphadenectomy (Investigational)

Recent literature reports evince an interest in a laparoscopic approach to lymphadenectomy and lymph node sampling. The first description in the American literature of an endoscopic pelvic lymphadenectomy was that by Reich et al.[41] in 1990. Reich's group described the care of a patient with ovarian cancer found incidentally at laparoscopy (Table 10–6). Since then a number of other reports have appeared. Gersham et al.[42] described a laparoscopic technique for pelvic lymphadenectomy, which they performed in 20 pigs. Querleu et al.[43] developed and performed a similar technique on 39 patients with cervical cancer. The average operative time for lymphadenectomy was 90 minutes and the mean number of nodes removed was 8.7. Querleu's group described no significant morbidity, and 97% of their patients were discharged on the first postoperative day. Schuessler et al.[44] in 1991 performed pelvic lymphadenectomy endoscopically on 12 patients with prostatic cancer. No major complications were reported, and all patients were discharged the following day.

TABLE 10–6. **Laparoscopic Lymphadenectomy**

	Type of Lymphadenectomy	
Study, Year	*Pelvic (n)*	*Para-aortic (n)*
Reich et al., 1990[41]	1	0
Gersham et al., 1990[42*]	20	0
Querleu et al., 1991[43]	39	0
Schuessler et al., 1991[44†]	12	0
Herd et al., 1992[45*]	0	2
Childers et al., 1992[46§]	10	7
Childers et al., 1992[47‡]	2	2
Dargent et al., 1992[48‖]	176	0

Note: Numbers under Type of Lymphadenectomy are numbers of patients.
*Performed on swine.
†Patients with prostate cancer.
‡Patients with endometrial cancer.
§Patients with cervical cancer.
‖Panoramic retroperitoneal pelviscopy.

Sampling the para-aortic nodes was not initially attempted laparoscopically, predominantly because of technical difficulties. Recently, however, a laparoscopic approach to evaluating the para-aortic nodes has been described by several authors (Table 10–6). Herd et al.[45] in 1992 reported a way to visualize and sample the para-aortic nodes in pigs. In the same year Childers et al.[46] reported the first successful para-aortic node dissection in two postmenopausal women with stage I endometrial cancer. The procedure performed was very similar to that described in 1991 by Querleu's group. Childers et al.[47] subsequently reported successful para-aortic node dissections in seven patients with cervical cancer, without significant complications.

Dargent et al.[48] in 1992 reported a new technique, panoramic retroperitoneal pelviscopy, for performing pelvic lymphadenectomy for gynecologic malignancies. A retropneumoperitoneum was created to gain access to the pelvic wall via a suprapubic route. The procedure was completed in 176 (88%) patients; in 24 (12%) it was abandoned because of technical difficulties. The average procedure duration was 55 minutes, with an average of 5.2 nodes removed. The hospital stay averaged 3.2 days.

A laparoscopic approach appears to offer the advantage of completing pelvic and para-aortic lymph node dissection without a major incision, thus decreasing morbidity and length of hospital stay. However, this technique does not have clearly defined indications in patients with pelvic malignancy. The procedure is not simple and demands an understanding of pelvic anatomy, pelvic dissection, and laparoscopic technique. We conclude that until further short-term and long-term experience is available, it might be considered investigational.

Complications Associated with Lymphadenectomy

Intraoperative Complications

Arterial Injury

Acute injury to one of the major groin, pelvic, or abdominal arteries can result in significant hemorrhage. Fortunately, these thick-walled arteries are resistant to trauma, and injuries associated with dissection of adjacent lymph nodes are quite rare. Simple lacerations are repaired with fine (5-0), interrupted, nonabsorbable vascular sutures. Repair of a major artery such as the aorta, common iliacs, or their major branches may require clamping the afferent and efferent limb of the injured vessel with vascular clamps. Consultation with a vascular surgeon is appropriate if arterial transection or complex injuries occur, as grafting may be appropriate.

Injuries to specific major vessels can have very different consequences. Occlusion of the hypogastric artery rarely results in significant postoperative morbidity. However, ligation of the external iliac artery will result in a 10% to 15% risk of ipsilateral limb loss. Complete occlusion of the common iliac artery will always result in ipsilateral limb loss.[49] Although ligation of the femoral artery during groin dissection is exceedingly rare, it can result in significant postoperative morbidity. There is generally no significant consequence if the inferior mesenteric artery (IMA) requires ligation during para-aortic node dissection. Postoperative ischemia of the descending or sigmoid colon can occur if a previous partial colectomy has been performed, particularly if there is no arterial anastomosis between the middle and left colic arteries. In this situation, reimplantation of the IMA is recommended.

Venous Vascular Injuries

Venous injuries occur more commonly than arterial injuries during lymphadenectomy and are more difficult to repair, owing to the thin less resistant walls of the venous system. Small venous injuries can be initially managed by tamponade of the injured area with a sponge stick. If hemostasis does not occur, the injury may be repaired with hemostatic clips or fine sutures placed with an interrupted mattress or running technique. Repair of large venous defects may be facilitated by occluding the distal and proximal segments of the vein. Vascular clamps on major veins should be avoided if possible, as their use may worsen the defects.

Extensive venous injuries create difficult intraoperative problems. Not only are these injuries associated with excessive blood loss, but attempts at repair, with or without graft placement, are plagued with subsequent thrombosis and secondary thromboembolism. If necessary, occlusion of the infrarenal portion of the vena cava can be performed with minimal sequelae; however, ligation of the suprarenal cava is associated with significant mortality.[50] Communicating venous systems make ligation of the left renal vein minimally morbid, but occlusion of the right renal vein usually results in loss of the right kidney. Thus, right renal vein injury must be repaired. Occasionally extensive injury occurs to the iliac venous system and requires ligation. If the common iliac or external iliac vein is ligated, post-

operative edema of the ipsilateral extremity should be expected. Ligation of the internal iliac vein is generally associated with minimal morbidity. Ligation of the saphenous vein, part of a routine groin node dissection, does not contribute significantly to leg edema. However, occlusion of the femoral vein can result in significant postoperative edema, the degree of which is highly dependent on the proximity of the occlusion and the amount of collateral circulation remaining.

Nerve Injuries

The genitofemoral and the obturator nerves are the two nerves most commonly encountered during pelvic lymphadenectomy. Transection of the genitofemoral nerve results in loss of sensation or paresthesia in the skin of the medial thigh. Therefore, a transected genitofemoral nerve need not be repaired. The obturator nerve affects adduction of the ipsilateral extremity and repair should be considered if this nerve is transected. Even without repair, however, the majority of patients will have significant recovery of ipsilateral limb function if they undergo postoperative physiotherapy.[49]

No major nerves should be encountered in a routine groin node dissection. However, if the dissection is extended inferior to the cribriform fascia, the femoral nerve may be transected. This nerve, which supplies the quadriceps responsible for leg extension, should be repaired if injured.

Ureteral Injuries

Injury to the pelvic ureter is uncommon, occurring in 0.1% to 1.5% of major pelvic surgical procedures.[51] The majority of information related to ureteral injury during pelvic and para-aortic lymph node dissection is derived from series of extended or radical hysterectomies. Recent reports of such operations cite a 1% to 2% risk of ureteral injury.[52] Ureteral injuries during radical pelvic surgery are most likely secondary to the dissection of the pelvic ureter performed during uterine removal. In fact, pelvic node dissection contributes little to the risk of ureteral injury.

Intestinal Injuries

Gastrointestinal injuries are also uncommon complications of pelvic or para-aortic node dissection. Theoretically, the bowel segment most likely to be injured is the duodenum, which lies retroperitoneally and potentially could be injured during retraction for a para-aortic node dissection. Repair of bowel injuries is discussed in Chapter 7.

Postoperative Complications

Because pelvic and inguinal lymphadenectomy is usually performed as part of a radical procedure for cancer treatment, the independent contribution of node dissection to postoperative complications is unknown. There are, however, two complications thought to be specific for patients undergoing pelvic lymphadenectomies—lymphocyst and lower extremity lymphedema.

Pelvic Lymphocysts Following Pelvic Node Dissection

A lymphocyst or lymphocele, a lymph-filled space without a distinctive epithelial lining, is a postoperative complication primarily seen after pelvic lymphadenectomies for gynecologic and urologic malignancies. It is related to accumulation of retroperitoneal fluid at the dissection site.

The lymphocyst that develops after pelvic lymphadenectomy was first described by Kobayashi and Inoue[53] in 1950 and later redescribed by Gray and associates[54] in 1958. The incidence of pelvic lymphocysts detected clinically (since 1980) is 3% to 5% but varies widely in the literature, ranging from 1% to 58% (Table 10–7). There appears to have been a significant decrease in lymphocysts over the past several decades. This may be attributed to improved operative techniques, the use of prophylactic antibiotics, and the decreased frequency with which pelvic lymphadenectomy is performed after pelvic irradiation.[39,55] Recent data fail to confirm the protective effect of closed suction drainage. The preponderance of information known about the pelvic lymphocyst has been obtained in patients with cervical cancer; few reports deal with the incidence associated with other gynecologic cancers. Even fewer studies have systematically evaluated the presence of lymphocysts by radiologic means. Petru et al.[56] in 1989 reported lymphocyst formation in 135 patients with ovarian malignancy treated by tumor debulking and pelvic and periaortic lymphadenectomy. Petru's group evaluated all patients with postoperative CT and found a 32% rate of lymphocyst formation. Paraaortic lymphocysts appear to be extremely rare, with only a few cases reported in the literature.[57]

RISK FACTORS. Many risk factors for lymphocyst formation following pelvic lymphadenectomy

TABLE 10–7. **Incidence of Pelvic Lymphocysts Following Radical Abdominal Hysterectomy and Pelvic Lymphadenectomy**

Study, Year	No. of Pts.	Lymphocysts (%)
Kobayashi and Inoue, 1950[53]	156	14
Mori, 1955[58]	140	49
Gray et al., 1958[54]	55	16.4
Ferguson and MacIyre, 1961[59]	95	12.6
Byron et al., 1966[72]	79	5
Dodd et al., 1970[63]	453	28.9
Jonsson et al., 1977[124]	15	20
Benedet et al., 1980[125]	241	2
Choo et al, 1986[70]	108	5.6
Shingleton and Orr, 1987[126]	444	1
Artman et al., 1987[135]	153	1
Ilancheran and Monaghan, 1988[62]	221	25
Fuller et al., 1989[127]	418	1.4
Kenter et al., 1989[128]	213	6.7
Mann et al., 1989[71]	124	2
Petru et al., 1989[56]	173	20*
Conte et al., 1990[68]	36	22†
Massi et al., 1992[129]	228	0.4
	3,352	*11.5*

*Diagnosis by computed tomography.
†Diagnosis by ultrasonography.

have been advanced in the literature. None have been established as causes. The risk factor most often reported is the extent of operative interference with lymphatic drainage. Theoretically, the more extensive the lymphadenectomy, the more leakage of lymph in the area of dissection, and the higher is the risk of lymphocyst formation.[58,59] Prior radiation therapy has also been suggested as a risk factor by several studies[29,54,58]; however, a direct relationship between previous radiation therapy and lymphocysts has not been proved.

The use of minidose heparin is also reported to be associated with lymphocyst formation.[60] Lymphocytic fluid contains clotting factors but is deficient in platelets. Anticoagulation may prolong lymph drainage by preventing the sealing of several lymph vessels by fibrin. Diuretics[61] may also increase the risk of lymphocyst formation by increasing the flow of lymph. Other suggested risk factors that have been noted in isolated cases include pregnancy,[59] poorly differentiated cancers,[62] and the finding of positive lymph nodes.[57,62a]

CLINICAL PRESENTATION. The symptoms attributed to lymphocysts are generally related to the size and location of the cyst. The majority of lymphocysts are small, and most patients remain asymptomatic. The lymphocysts generally produce minimal or no sequelae. However, large lymphocysts can cause considerable discomfort secondary to their space-occupying effect (Fig. 10–11). Symptoms usually do not become evident until the immediate postoperative discomfort has subsided and the patient is ambulatory.[63] The onset of symptoms varies; however, symptoms generally manifest within 3 weeks postoperatively.[62,64] In a series of 453 patients Dodd et al.[63] in 1970 reported that 80% of patients with lymphocysts were diagnosed between 2 and 12 months after the surgical procedure. Symptoms included lower abdominal fullness, urinary frequency, and constipation.

Common findings include an oval nontender mass in the iliac fossa paralleling the inguinal ligament. The mass is generally appreciated on bimanual examination with the abdominal hand; however, a small lymphocyst may easily be missed on examination because of its location. Lymphocysts are thought to occur bilaterally in about 50% of cases,[65] though some studies have suggested a left-sided predominance.[58,59] Edema of the external genitalia and lower extremities may occur and is thought to be secondary to compression of the pelvic veins. Tenderness, erythema, and warmth are uncommon and generally suggest an inflammatory component.

Most lymphocysts resolve spontaneously over several weeks to several months. In the process of reabsorption (presumably as lymphatic channels seal and collaterals develop) the cyst may lose its fluctuance and develop a firm consistency that may be difficult to differentiate from recurrent carcinoma.

DIAGNOSTIC EVALUATION. As with any disease process, the diagnosis of a lymphocyst should be made in the appropriate clinical setting while attempting to differentiate from other common disease entities such as hematoma, pelvic abscess, thrombophlebitis, seroma, urinoma, adnexal masses, or carcinoma. The most commonly used diagnostic tests are ultrasonography (US) and CT. The finding of a unilocular or multilocular pelvic mass on US or CT in a patient who has recently undergone a lymphadenectomy can be suggestive of, but not specific for, a lymphocyst. A definitive diagnosis generally requires needle aspiration, which includes gross inspection as well as chemical and cytologic examination of the fluid to exclude urinoma, infection, and tumor.

TREATMENT. Conservative management is the treatment of choice for lymphocysts as the great majority are asymptomatic and resolve spontaneously. Several indications exist for immediate drainage, the most common of which is the development of progressive ureteral obstruction with secondary pyelonephritis. If indicated, drainage may be attained by a variety of alternatives. Relief of symptoms from the ureteral obstruction may be achieved by needle aspiration. This technique is convenient and easy to perform; however, the lymphocyst usually refills in 24 to 48 hours, often necessitating multiple aspirations. Because multiple aspirations may predispose to secondary infection and abscess formation, this technique is primarily used to establish a diagnosis and as a one-time therapeutic procedure.

Recurrent lymphocysts are probably best managed by placement of a percutaneous 7 to 14 French pigtail catheter inserted under US, CT, or fluoroscopy guidance with prolonged drainage or drainage and sclerosis. This method is successful in preventing recurrence of lymphocysts in most cases. The disadvantage of this technique is that it may require long-term catheter drainage, averaging 14 to 18

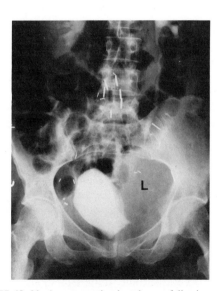

FIGURE 10–11. A postoperative lymphocyst following radical hysterectomy. The lymphocyst (L) displaces the bladder and the left ureter medially. (Reproduced with permission from Shingleton HM, Orr JW Jr: Cancer of the Cervix: Diagnosis and Treatment, 2nd ed, p 147. New York: Churchill Livingstone, 1987.)

days (range, 4–120 days).[66–68] Larger lymphocysts, especially those greater than 10 cm, tend to need a longer drainage time. Patients managed with long-term indwelling catheters are at risk for infection, and it is recommended that periodic flushing (three or four times a day) with 10 mL of sterile saline be performed to prevent plugging of the catheter.[66–71]

As an alternative to long-term percutaneous catheter drainage, a sclerosing agent such as tetracycline may be introduced. One gram of tetracycline is mixed in 500 mL of sterile saline. This fluid is instilled as long as flow is easy. After clamping for 1 hour, the fluid is withdrawn. Prior to injection of the tetracycline mixture, a radiographic dye is instilled to ensure that there is no direct venous or arterial communication within the cavity; the presence of such a communication is a contraindication to this type of treatment.[71]

If conservative methods fail, exploration with cyst cavity marsupialization may be indicated. This procedure removes the anterior wall of the cyst cavity, providing a "window" for the internal drainage of lymphocyst fluid into the pelvic cavity. Modifications of this technique have included suturing the sigmoid and cecum[72] and omentum[63,73] into the cavity of the lymphocyst. The efficacy of open marsupialization has not been compared with percutaneous catheter drainage.

PREVENTION. Theoretically, any technique that decreases lymphatic leakage should decrease the incidence of lymphocyst formation. Therefore, lymphatic vessel ligation at the periphery of the dissection by hemoclip or cautery should decrease the risk of lymphocyst formation.

There is little question that a significant amount of fluid will be removed if closed suction drainage is used after lymphadenectomy.[36] Symmonds and Pratt[74] in 1961 first suggested that postoperative closed suction drainage of the retroperitoneal space after radical hysterectomy and pelvic lymphadenectomy could decrease the frequency of lymphocyst formation. Since then several authors have demonstrated similar findings.[57,75–77] Interestingly, some have suggested that suction drains do not prevent lymphocysts but in fact may increase their frequency by stimulating lymph drainage.[54,62,63] Advocates believe that closed suction allows the pelvic peritoneum to lie against the pelvic side wall, where it remains until fixed or until the possibility of fluid accumulation has passed. If used, suction drains are usually removed 3 to 6 days after surgery, depending on the amount of drainage.

Another technique employed to decrease lymphocyst formation involves nonreperitonealization following pelvic lymphadenectomy. Other possible factors that may be involved in decreasing the frequency of lymphocyst formation include better surgical techniques, avoiding the excessive use of cautery, and discontinuing the use of heparin and diuretics.[60] Prophylactic antibiotics have never been shown to affect the incidence of lymphocyst formation. However, no study has evaluated the difference in lymphocyst formation after an extraperitoneal versus a transperitoneal lymphadenectomy.

Lymphocysts and Seromas Following Groin Dissections

Lymphocysts are mentioned as a complication of groin node dissection. Unfortunately, distinguishing inguinal seromas and lymphocysts is difficult, and the two may in fact be the same entity—no study has documented a seroma and a lymphocyst in the same patient. The incidence of lymphocyst is approximately 10% in the few studies (Table 10–8) that have described lymphocyst formation following groin dissection.[78–82]

Piver et al.[81] 1983 suggested an association between minidose heparin and the incidence of inguinal lymphocyst formation. In their study, 43% (8/19) of patients who received minidose heparin and underwent an en bloc procedure developed lymphocysts, compared to 2% of patients who were not given heparin. This association has not been demonstrated in other studies.

Seroma formation occurs in approximately 10% to 20% (Table 10–8) of patients undergoing groin dissection, regardless of the type of incision used.[33,34,65,83–85] The high prevalence of inguinal seromas following node dissection is thought to be secondary to the decreased vascularity of the wound edges and to the large amount of dead space created with this operative procedure. Two techniques proposed to aid in decreasing seroma formation with subsequent infection and wound breakdown include refraining from thinning the skin flaps[33] and using suction drainage.[83,84] The suction drains are left in the groin for approximately 10 to 14 days, or until the drainage has ceased. If a seroma occurs, periodic sterile aspirations are often adequate treatment. Postoperative pressure dressings or ice packs on the groin may decrease blood supply and are not recommended.

The prevention and treatment of inguinal lymphocysts are similar to that described for

TABLE 10–8. **Frequency of Seroma (S) and Lymphocyst (L) Formation Following Groin Node Dissection**

Study, Year	No. of Pts.	Type of Complication	Frequency (%)
Rutledge and Smith, 1970[65]	151	S	20
Hacker et al., 1981[33]	100	S	13
Podratz et al., 1983[85]	175	S	11
Helm and Shingleton, 1992[34]	64	S	25
Ballon and Lamb, 1975[78]	18	L	11
(Morley, 1976[79])	(278)	(L)	("Rare")
Piver et al., 1983[81]	115	L	9
Berman et al., 1985[82]	50	L	12
Mean			14*

*Excluding Morley, 1976

seroma formation. Should a lymphocyst occur, it usually responds to periodic sterile aspirations.

Chronic Lymphedema Following Pelvic Lymphadenectomy

Lymphedema of the lower extremity attributed to interruption of lymphatic drainage occurs in 10% or less of patients following ordinary pelvic lymph node dissections (Table 10–9). The most common risk factor thought to increase the incidence of chronic lymphedema is an extensive radical lymphadenectomy[86] or a combination of pelvic lymph node dissections and external groin irradiation. Some studies have been able to demonstrate this relationship between radiation treatment and lymphedema.[76] However, Soisson et al.[87] in 1990 reviewed the cases of 320 patients with stage Ib and IIa cervical cancer treated with radical hysterectomy; 77 (22%) also received adjuvant external pelvic irradiation. Chronic lymphedema occurred in 22% of the patients who received adjuvant radiation therapy, compared to 5.2% of patients who were treated with surgery alone. This statistically significant difference was apparent even after patients with recurrent cancer were excluded.

Most instances of lymphedema are usually mild and transient, although elephantiasis may occur (Fig. 10–12). In persistent cases the limb weight of the affected extremity may significantly compromise function. Chronic edema tends to occur bilaterally in about 50% of cases and is equally divided

TABLE 10–9. **Lymphedema of the Lower Extremities Associated with Pelvic Lymphadenectomy**

Study, Year	No. of Pts.	Lymphedema	
		No.	*(%)*
Symmonds, 1966[130]*	101	8	(7.9)
Parker et al., 1967[131]	265	6	(2.3)
Martimbeau et al., 1978[86†]	402	94	(23.4)
Sall et al., 1979[132]	349	5	(1.4)
Webb and Symmonds, 1979[76]	610	61	(10.0)
Soisson et al., 1990[87‡]	320	29	(9.0)
Shingleton, 1992[§]	401	12	(3.0)
Mean			8.8

*Only two patients with real clinical significance.
†Only 5% with severe clinical lymphedema.
‡16/29 patients received adjuvant radiation treatment.
§Unpublished data.

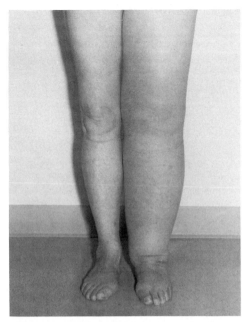

FIGURE 10-12. Elephantiasis of a permanent type in a patient who has undergone pelvic lymphadenectomy and postoperative radiation.

This method and others[89] appear beneficial in reducing large accumulations of lymphedema, including those in patients who are resistant to pressure elastic (Jobst type) stockings.[90,91]

Surgery has been recommended for severe refractory lymphedema. The chief method involves excision of the edematous subcutaneous tissue of the affected extremity as initially described by Charles[92] in 1912. Approximately 30% of patients benefit from this procedure. Its use is generally limited to those with massive edema.[93] Corrective surgery is associated with significant postoperative morbidity and tends to substitute one deformity for another; American gynecologic oncologists do not advocate its use.

Other surgical techniques to improve lymphatic drainage in patients with chronic lymphedema have been described. Thompson[94] in 1962 attempted to drain the subcutaneous tissue of the affected extremity into a deep muscle compartment utilizing a dermal flap. Goldsmith and Delos Santos[73] in 1967 transposed an omental flap into the affected extremity to act as a new conduit of lymph drainage. Interestingly, both operative procedures require the excision of a significant amount of subcutaneous tissue; therefore, success using those techniques may be secondary to the removal of the subcutaneous tissue rather than to improved drainage.

Lymphedema Following Groin Dissections

Lymphedema related to the interruption of lymphatic drainage from the lower extremities, either transient or chronic, occurs in about 40% of women following groin node dissections (Table 10–10). Fortunately, most instances are transient, with chronic lymphedema reported in only 11% of cases.

between the right and left lower extremities.[86] Common complications associated with lymphedema include recurrent episodes of cellulitis or lymphangitis.

Mild or moderate lymphedema often responds to conservative treatment, including leg elevation and graded compression stockings.[87] In refractory or severe cases, intermittent compression devices have been successfully used. Zelikouski et al.[88] in 1980 developed a method for intermittent high-pressure sequential compression that induces a physiologic milking action of the lymphedematous extremity.

TABLE 10–10. **Incidence of Lower Extremity Edema Following Groin Node Dissection**

Study, Year	No. of Pts.	Type of Incision*	Lymphedema (Transient and Chronic) (%)	Chronic Lymphedema (%)
Rutledge and Smith, 1970[65]	151	SI	32	20
Ballon et al., 1975[95]	18	TI	55	22
Hacker et al., 1981[33]	100	TI	20	14
Podratz et al., 1983[85]	175	SI	69	4.5
Berman et al., 1989[82]	50	TI	—	6
Burke et al., 1990[96]	32	TI	—	6
Cavanagh et al., 1990[99]	415	SI	—	8.6
Stehman et al., 1992[98]	155	TI	19	8.6
Mean			*39*	*11.2*

*TI, triple incision (some patients may have had an ipsilateral groin dissection only); SI, single incision (en bloc radical vulvectomy with bilateral groin node dissection).

Numerous risk factors have been suggested to increase the incidence of lymphedema following inguinal dissection. Although none have been established as causes, a common belief is that the incidence of lymphedema is related to the radicality of the groin node dissection, especially when performed simultaneously with pelvic lymphadenectomy. Some authors report a 15% to 20% incidence of chronic lymphedema.[33,65,95] In the early 1990s, studies of superficial groin node dissections alone have reported a lower incidence of lymphedema, ranging from 6% to 8%.[96–98]

Inguinal irradiation following node dissection may contribute to lower extremity edema. However, there are essentially no convincing data to substantiate this belief. Homesley et al.[99] in 1986 reported a Gynecologic Oncology Group prospective randomized trial that found no evidence of major morbidity associated with the addition of radiation therapy to the groins after bilateral groin node dissection. In that series, lymphedema occurred in 19% of the irradiated group and in 11% of the nonirradiated group, a difference that was not statistically significant.

Postoperative groin infection may result in increased rates of peripheral edema. Hacker et al[33] in 1981 reported that 28.6% of patients with major groin wound breakdown developed chronic lower extremity edema, compared to 11.6% of patients who did not have a major wound breakdown. This difference was not statistically significant. Prophylactic antibiotics[65] and the prompt treatment of cellulitis with antibiotics[100] are also considered beneficial in preventing lymphedema, although there are no prospective randomized studies to support this thought.

Other potential risk factors include saphenous vein ligation and the performance of preoperative lymphangiography of the lower extremities, which may contribute to postoperative lymphatic obstruction.

Management of lower extremity lymphedema includes bed rest, leg elevation, the use of compression devices or stockings, and prompt antibiotic treatment should cellulitis occur. Unfortunately, management of severe cases of chronic lower extremity edema is frequently not successful.

Pelvic Infection Following Pelvic Node Dissection

Retroperitoneal space infection may complicate routine gynecologic surgery and may vary in severity from a localized minor cellulitis to an infected hematoma or abscess. Pelvic lymphadenectomy has been considered by some to be associated with an increased risk of pelvic infection. However, Webb and Simmons[76] in 1979 and Powell et al.[101] in 1986 each reported an incidence of pelvic infection or abscess formation (4%–5%) following lymphadenectomy comparable to that seen in other gynecologic procedures not including lymphadenectomy.

Recurrent Lymphangitis, Cellulitis, and Phlebitis

Recurrent lymphangitis, cellulitis, or phlebitis occurs in some patients following groin node dissection.[85] Patients with chronic lower extremity edema appear to be at increased risk. Management usually consists of leg elevation and the institution of nonsteroidal anti-inflammatory agents and antibiotics. Oral erythromycin is usually sufficient therapy.

Wound Infection and Other Complications Following Groin Dissection

The most common complication related to groin node dissection is wound infection, which often results in necrosis and breakdown (Table 10–11). Such wound complications occurred in over 50% of cases in series in which en bloc (single incision) radical vulvectomy and bilateral groin node dissection was performed, with the majority of breakdowns occurring in the groin area. The separate incision technique, which leaves a skin bridge between the vulva and groin, has regained popularity because of an improved rate of primary healing. This procedure, thought to significantly decrease the risk of wound breakdown because the closure is not under tension, was popularized by Taussig[102] in 1940 and later by Byron et al.[83] in 1965. Several more recent studies using the triple incision technique have reported wound breakdown occurring in approximately 20% to 25% without compromising long-term outcome. These risks represent a significant improvement when compared to the single en bloc incision technique.

Helm et al.[97] in 1992 compared the standard en bloc radical vulvectomy and bilateral inguinal-femoral lymphadenectomy with a bilateral groin node dissection performed using a triple incision technique. Each of the study groups contained 32 patients with vulvar cancer, matched for stage, lymph node status, and size and location of vulvar lesion. Nineteen percent of the patients in the single incision group had major wound breakdown in the groin, compared to only 3% in the triple incision

TABLE 10–11. Groin Node Dissection Using Single Incision (SI) or Triple Incision (TI) and Associated Incidence of Wound Infection, Necrosis, and Breakdown

Study, Year	No. of Pts.	Type of Incision	Wound Infection, Necrosis, Breakdown (%)
Rutledge and Smith, 1970[65*]	151	SI	>50
Morley, 1976[79]	278	SI	>50
Podratz et al., 1983[85‡]	175	SI	85
Cavanagh et al., 1990[100]	415	SI	54
Helm et al., 1992[97†]	32	SI	<u>35</u>
Mean			>50
Hacker et al., 1981[33*]	100	TI	44
Berman et al., 1989[82]	50	TI	12
Burke et al., 1990[96]	32	TI	15.5
Stehman et al., 1992[98]	155	TI	23
Helm et al., 1992[97§]	32	TI	<u>19</u>
Mean			22.7

*Fourteen percent major breakdown.
§3 percent major breakdown.
†Nine percent major breakdown.
‡Nineteen percent major breakdown.

group. It appears that multiple incisions offer the benefit of improved healing.

The contribution of dissection of the deep femoral nodes to the morbidity of wound breakdown is unknown. The 1990 report from Burke's group suggests it may contribute to wound complications.[96] They reviewed the cases of 32 patients with early stage vulvar cancer, 27 of whom were treated with a triple incision technique and superficial node dissection, five of whom were treated with a triple incision technique and a superficial and deep groin node dissection. Eighty percent of both the acute and the late complications occurred in patients who had undergone the deep groin node dissection, suggesting that dissection of the deep groin (or femoral) nodes may also increase wound complications.

Daly and Pomerance[80] left the groin incisions open in 13 of 29 patients after en bloc radical vulvectomy and bilateral groin node dissection. No major wound breakdown occurred in the open incision group, compared to a 35% incidence of wound breakdown in the closed incision group. The disadvantage to this technique is that it requires approximately 7 weeks for complete epithelialization; therefore, no one currently advocates use of this technique.

Various other methods have been suggested to improve wound healing in groin dissections. Transplantation of the sartorius muscle over the femoral vessel following an inguinal/femoral node dissec-

tion was advocated to protect the major vessels from infection (and subsequent hemorrhage), which is reported to occur in 1% of groin dissections. No prospective study of this technique has proved its benefit,[85,97,100] and it is rarely performed today.

After surgery, bed rest is advisable for 3 to 5 days to allow immobilization of the wound to assist healing. When the patient is fully mobilized, sitz baths or whirlpool treatments are helpful and soothing. Should necrosis, infection, and wound breakdown occur, debridement and frequent wound dressing changes are recommended. The denuded groin area will granulate over several weeks and may be managed with home nursing care.

Femoral Hernias Following Groin Dissection

Femoral hernias are a rare complication following groin node dissection, with an incidence ranging from 0 to 5%.[82,85,97,98] Femoral hernias may be prevented by closing the femoral canal intraoperatively with sutures from the inguinal ligament to Cooper's ligament (although this is not routinely performed). Treatment for late femoral hernia following this procedure generally requires surgery.

Mortality of Groin Dissection

The perioperative mortality associated with a radical or modified radical vulvectomy and bilateral groin node dissection ranges from 0 to 6%.[33,85,98,100,103] The mortality associated with the operation is usually a result of such things as cardiac arrest, pulmonary thromboembolism, and respiratory failure. Theoretically, the mortality should be decreased in patients with a less radical and/or separate incision technique because of the lower incidence of wound complications. It should be remembered that most patients undergoing groin node dissection for vulvar cancer are elderly and often obese, with multiple medical problems such as diabetes (10%–14%), hypertension (40%), and cardiovascular diseases (30%).[65,85]

Complications of Surgical Staging Procedures for Cervical Cancer

Selective sampling of the pelvic and para-aortic lymph nodes can be performed by either a transperitoneal or extraperitoneal approach.[95,104–106] Staging operations are intended to assess the para-aortic node status in patients with cervical cancer, as these nodes are out of the routine radiation treatment field and metastases to aortic nodes carry significant prognostic implications. The extraperitoneal approach and the transperitoneal approach are equal in sensitivity in detecting para-aortic nodal metastasis and show no significant difference in perioperative surgical complications.[104–106] The most commonly reported morbidities are vascular injuries and infection; less frequent complications include ureteral and bowel injuries and lymphocyst formation. The reported frequency of these complications ranges from 2% to 16%.[104–106]

Para-aortic (extended-field) radiation therapy following staging operations using a transperitoneal approach is associated with an increased incidence of small bowel complications, including fistula formation, obstruction, radiation enteritis, and even death.[104–106] This has been attributed to the development of extensive intra-abdominal small bowel adhesions overlying the aorta or pelvic vessels. Extraperitoneal approaches were developed to minimize these adhesions. In earlier reports[107,108] the prevalence of small bowel complications due to radiation treatment to the para-aortic area following a transperitoneal node dissection was approximately 30%, with mortality ranging from 6% to 22%. The prevalence of small bowel complications was significantly decreased with the extraperitoneal approach, ranging from 2% to 5%.[95,104,106,109] A major factor contributing to the excessive morbidity in the transperitoneal group was the high radiation dose (6,000 rads) to the para-aortic area, a dose that is not well tolerated regardless of the approach used.

More recent studies using lower doses of radiation to the para-aortic area (4,000–5,000 rads) have reported a decrease in small bowel morbidity. The incidence of complications with these lower doses, regardless of approach, is approximately 2% to 10%, a notable improvement over rates reported in earlier studies. Open surgical staging is rarely performed today, however, having been largely replaced by less invasive methods (CT with FNA of enlarged para-aortic nodes).

References

1. Bartholin T: Vasa Lymphatica 1653. In Norman JM (ed): Morton's Medical Bibliography, 5th ed, p 178. Aldershot, England: Scolar Press, 1991.
2. de Graaf, cited in Le Clerc D: Histoire de la Médecine, p 216. I. van der Kloot: A La Haye, 1729.
3. Cruikshank W, cited in Norman JM (ed): Morton's Medical Bibliography, 5th ed, p 178. Aldershot, England: Scolar Press, 1991.
4. Mascagni P, (1787), cited in Norman JM (ed): Morton's Medical Bibliography, 5th ed, p 179. Aldershot, England: Scolar Press, 1991.
5. Cruveilhier (1829, 1842), cited in Norman JM (ed): Morton's Medical Bibliography, 5th ed, p 360. Aldershot, England: Scolar Press, 1991.
6. Savage H: The Surgery, Surgical Pathology and Surgical Anatomy of the Female Pelvic Organs, 3rd ed., rev. and greatly extended. New York: William Wood, 1880.
7. Cullen TS: Cancer of the Uterus, p 15. New York: D Appleton, 1900.
8. Le Dran, cited in Norman JM (ed): Morton's Medical Bibliography, 5th ed, p 416. England: Scolar Press, 1991.
9. Scudder JM: A Practical Treatise on the Diseases of Women, 8th ed. Cincinnati: Medical Publishing Co, 1877.
10. Mann MD (ed): A System of Gynecology. Philadelphia: Lea Bros, 1888.
11. Winter, cited in Cullen TS: Cancer of the Uterus. New York: D Appleton, 1900.
12. Reis E: Eine neue Operation: Methode des Uterus Carcinoma. Geburtsh Gynakol 32:266, 1895.
13. Clark JG: The radical abdominal operation for cancer of the uterus. Surg Gynecol Obstet 16:255, 1913.
14. Kelly HA: Operative Gynecology. New York: D Appleton, 1906.
15. Wertheim E: The extended abdominal operation for carcinoma uteri (transl H Grad). Am J Obstet Dis Women Child 66:169, 1912.
16. Meigs JV: Carcinoma of the cervix: The Wertheim operation. Surg Gynecol Obstet 78:195, 1944.
16a. Mangan CE, Rubin SC, Rabin DS, Mikuta JJ: Lymph node nomenclature in gynecologic oncology. Gynecol Oncol 23:222, 1986.
17. Plentl AA, Friedman EA: Lymphatic System of the Female Genitalia. Philadelphia: WB Saunders, 1971.
18. Kinmouth JB, Harper RA, Taylor GW: Lymphangiography by radiological methods. J Fac R Coll Radiol 6:217, 1955.

19. Muylder X, Belanger R, Vauclair R, Audex-Lapointe P, Cormier A, Methot U: Value of lymphography in Stage IB cancer of the uterine cervix. Obstet Gynecol 148:610, 1984.

20. Feigen M, Crocker EF, Read J, Crandon AJ: The value of lymphoscintigraphy, lymphangiography and computed tomography scanning in the preoperative assessment of lymph nodes involved by pelvic malignant conditions. Surg Gynecol Obstet 165:107, 1987.

21. Heller PB, Malfetano JH, Bundy BN, Barnhill DR, Okagaki T: Clinical-pathologic study of Stage IIB, III and IVA carcinoma of the cervix: Extended diagnostic evaluation for paraaortic node metastasis. A Gynecologic Oncology Group study. Gynecol Oncol 38:425, 1990.

22. Ashraf M, Elyaderani MK, Gabrielle OF, Krall JM: Value of lymphangiography in the diagnosis of paraaortic lymph node metastases from carcinoma of the cervix. Gynecol Oncol 14:96, 1982.

23. Brown RC, Buchsbaum HJ, Platz CE: Accuracy of lymphangiography in the diagnosis of paraaortic lymph node metastases from carcinoma of the cervix. Obstet Gynecol 54:571, 1979.

24. Brodman M, Friedman F, Dottino P, Janus C, Plaxe S, Cohen C: A comparative study of computerized tomography, magnetic resonance imaging, and clinical staging for the detection of early cervix cancer. Gynecol Oncol 36:409, 1990.

25. Greco A, Mason P, Leyng AWL, Dische S, McIndoe GAJ, Anderson MC: Staging of carcinoma of the uterine cervix: MRI-surgical correlation. Clin Radiol 40:401, 1989.

26. Haaga JR, Alfidi RJ: Precise biopsy localization by computer tomography. Radiology 118:603, 1976.

27. Kline TS, Neal HS: Needle aspiration biopsy: A critical appraisal. JAMA 239:36, 1978.

28. Zornoza JJ, Jonsson K, Wallace S, Lukeman JM: Fine needle aspiration biopsy of retroperitoneal lymph nodes and abdominal masses: An update report. Radiology 125:87, 1977.

29. McDonald TW, Morley GW, Choo YC, Shields JJ, Cordoba RB, Maylor B: Fine needle aspiration of paraaortic and pelvic lymph nodes showing lymphographic abnormalities. Obstet Gynecol 61:383, 1983.

30. Sevin BU, Greening SE, Nadji M, Ng AB, Averette HE, Nordqvist SR: Fine needle aspiration cytology in gynecologic oncology: I. Clinical aspects. Acta Cytol 23:277, 1979.

31. Way S: Carcinoma of the vulva. In Meigs JV, Sturgis SH (eds): Progress in Gynecology, vol III, p 489. New York: Grune & Stratton, 1957.

32. Collins JH, Barclay DL, Collins CG: Vulvectomy. Am J Obstet Gynecol 84:1135, 1962.

33. Hacker NF, Leuchter RS, Berek JS, Castaldo TW, Lagasse LD: Radical vulvectomy and bilateral inguinal lymphadenectomy through separate groin incisions. Obstet Gynecol 58:574, 1981.

34. Helm CW, Shingleton HM: The management of squamous cell carcinoma of the vulva. Curr Obstet Gynaecol 2:31, 1992.

35. Barber HRK: Cervical cancer: Pelvic and para-aortic lymph node sampling and its consequences. Baillières Clin Obstet Gynaecol 2(4):769, 1988.

36. Orr JW Jr, Barter JF, Kilgore LC, Soong S-J, Shingleton HM, Hatch KD: Closed suction pelvic drainage after radical pelvic surgical procedures. Am J Obstet Gynecol 155:867–871, 1986.

37. Kjorstad KE, Kolbenstvedt A, Strickert T: The value of complete lymphadenectomy in radical treatment of cancer of the cervix, Stage IB. Cancer 54:2215, 1984.

38. Gitsch E, Philipp K, Patelsky N: Intraoperative lymph scintigraphy during radical surgery for cervical cancer. Nucl Med 25:486, 1984.

39. Clarke-Pearson DL, Synan JS, Creasman WT: Significant venous thromboembolism caused by pelvic lymphocysts: Diagnosis and management. Gynecol Oncol 13:136, 1982.

40. Jensen JK, DiSaia PJ, Lucci JA III, Manetta A, Berman ML: To drain or not to drain: A retrospective study of closed-suction drainage following radical hysterectomy with pelvic lymphadenectomy (abst). Presented at the 24th annual meeting of the Society of Gynecologic Oncologists. Palm Desert, CA, Feb. 7–10, 1993.

41. Reich H, McGlynn F, Wilkie W: Laparoscopic management of Stage I ovarian cancer: A case report. J Reprod Med 35:601, 1990.

42. Gersham A, Daykhousky L, Chandra M, Danoft D, Grundfes WJ: Laparoscopic pelvic lymphadenectomy. J Laparoendosc Surg 1:3, 1990.

43. Querleu D, Lablanc E, Chastelwin B: Laparoscopic pelvic lymphadenectomy in the staging of early carcinoma of the cervix. Am J Obstet Gynecol 164:579, 1991.

44. Schuessler WW, Vancailler TG, Reich H, Griffith DP: Transperitoneal endosurgical lymphadenectomy in patients with localized prostate cancer. J Urol 145:988, 1991.

45. Herd J, Fowler JM, Shenson D, Lacy S, Montz FJ: Laparoscopic para-aortic lymph node sampling: Development of a technique. Gynecol Oncol 44:271, 1992.

46. Childers J, Surwit E, Hatch K: The role of laparoscopic lymphadenectomy in the management of cervical carcinoma (abstr 24). Presented at the 23rd annual meeting of the Society of Gynecologic Oncologists, 1992.

47. Childers JM, Surwit FA: Combined laparoscopic and vaginal surgery for the management of two cases of Stage I endometrial cancer. Gynecol Oncol 45:46, 1992.

48. Dargent D, Arnould P, Roy M: The value and the limits of panoramic retroperitoneal pelviscopy (PRPP) in gynecologic cancer (abstr 23). Presented at the 23rd annual meeting of the Society of Gynecologic Oncologists, 1992.

49. Piver MS, Lele SB: Complications of pelvic and aortic lymphadenectomy. In Delgado G, Smith JP (eds): Management of Complications in Gynecologic Oncology, pp 199–211. New York: John Wiley & Sons, 1982.

50. Duckett JW, Lifland JH, Peters PC: Resection of the inferior vena cava for adjacent malignant diseases. Surg Gynecol Obstet 136:711, 1973.

51. Thompson JD: Operative injuries to the ureter: Prevention, recognition and management. In Thompson JD, Rock JA (eds): TeLinde's Operative Gynecology, 7th ed, p 749. Philadelphia: JB Lippincott, 1992.

52. Shingleton HM, Orr JW Jr: Cancer of the Cervix: Diagnosis and Treatment, p 146. London: Churchill Livingstone, 1987.

53. Kobayashi T, Inoue S: Lymphatic cyst seen after radical hysterectomy for cancer of the uterine cervix and its clinical significance. Clin Gynecol Obstet 4:91, 1950.

54. Gray MJ, Plentl AA, Taylor HC Jr: The lymphocyst: A complication of pelvic lymph node dissections. Am J Obstet Gynecol 75:1059, 1958.

55. Twiggs LB, Potish RA, George RJ, Adcock LL: Pretreatment extraperitoneal surgical staging in primary carcinoma of the cervix uteri. Surg Gynecol Obstet 158:243, 1984.

56. Petru E, Tamussino K, Lahousen M, Winter R, Pickel H, Haas J: Pelvic and paraaortic lymphocysts after radical surgery because of cervical and ovarian cancer. Am J Obstet Gynecol 161:937, 1989.

57. Helmkamp BF, Krebs HB, Jsikoff MB, Poliak SR, Averette HE: Para-aortic lymphocyst. Am J Obstet Gynecol 138:395, 1980.

58. Mori N: Clinical and experimental studies on so-called lymphocyst which develops after radical hysterectomy in cancer of uterine cervix. J Jpn Obstet Gynecol Soc 7:178, 1955.

59. Ferguson JH, Maclyre JG: Lymphocele following lymphadenectomy. Am J Obstet Gynecol 82:783, 1961.

60. Catalona WJ, Kadmon D, Crawe DB: Effect on minidose heparin on lymphocele formation following extraperitoneal pelvic lymphadenectomy. J Urol 123:890, 1980.

61. Szwed JJ, Maxwell DR, Kleit SA, Hamburger RJ: Angiotensin. II. Diuretics and thoracic duct lymph flow in the dog. Am J Physiol 224:705, 1973.

62. Ilancheran A, Monaghan JM: Pelvic lymphocyst: A 10-year experience. Gynecol Oncol 29:333, 1988.

62a. Rutledge F, Dodd GD Jr, Kasilag FB Jr: Lymphocysts: A complication of radical pelvic surgery. Am J Obstet Gynecol 77:1165, 1959.

63. Dodd GD, Rutledge F, Wallace S: Postoperative pelvic lymphocysts. Am J Roentgenol 108:312, 1970.

64. Bassinger GT, Giltes RF: Lymphocyst: Ultrasound diagnosis and urologic management. J Urol 114:740, 1975.

65. Rutledge F, Smith JP, et al: Carcinoma of the vulva. Am J Obstet Gynecol 106:1117, 1970.

66. White M, Mueller PR, Ferrucci JT, et al: Percutaneous drainage of postoperative abdominal and pelvic lymphoceles. AJR 145:1065, 1985.

67. Van Sonnenberg E, Wittich GR, Casola G, et al: Lymphoceles: Imaging characteristics and percutaneous management. Radiology 161:593, 1986.

68. Conte M, Panici PB, Guariglia L, Scambia G, Greggi S, Mancuso S: Pelvic lymphocele following radical paraaortic and pelvic lymphadenectomy for cervical carcinoma: Incidence rate and percutaneous management. Obstet Gynecol 76:268, 1990.

69. Aronowitz J, Kaplan AL: The management of a pelvic lymphocele by the use of a percutaneous indwelling catheter inserted with ultrasonic guidance. Gynecol Oncol 292:16, 1983.

70. Choo YC, Wong LC, Wong KP, Ma HK: The management of intractable lymphocyst following radical hysterectomy. Gynecol Oncol 24:309, 1986.

71. Mann WJ, Vogel F, Pastner B, Chalas E: Management of lymphocysts after radical gynecologic surgery. Gynecol Oncol 33:248, 1989.

72. Byron RL, Yonemoto RH, Davajan V, Townsend D, Bashore R, Morton DG: Lymphocysts: Surgical correction and prevention. Am J Obstet Gynecol 94:20, 1966.

73. Goldsmith HS, Delos Santos R: Omental transposition in primary lymphadenoma. Surg Gynecol Obstet 125:607, 1967.

74. Symmonds RE, Pratt JH: Prevention of fistulas and lymphocysts in radical hysterectomy. Obstet Gynecol 17:57, 1961.

75. van Nagell JR, Schwietz DP: Surgical adjuncts in radical hysterectomy and pelvic lymphadenectomy. Surg Gynecol Obstet 143:715, 1976.

76. Webb MJ, Symmonds RE: Wertheim hysterectomy: A reappraisal. Obstet Gynecol 54:140, 1979.

77. Cavanagh D, Praphat H, Ruffolo EH: Carcinoma of the uterine cervix: Some current views. Obstet Gynecol Annu 10:193, 1981.

78. Ballon SC, Lamb J: Separate inguinal incisions in the treatment of carcinoma of the vulva. Surg Gynecol Obstet 140:81, 1975.

79. Morley GW: Infiltrative carcinoma of the vulva: Results of surgical treatment. Am J Obstet Gynecol 124:874, 1976.

80. Daly JW, Pomerance AJ: Groin dissection with prevention of tissue loss and postoperative infection. Obstet Gynecol 53:395, 1979.

81. Piver MS, Malfetano JH, Lele SB, Moore RH: Prophylactic anticoagulation as a possible cause of inguinal lymphocyst after radical vulvectomy and inguinal lymphadenectomy. Obstet Gynecol 62:17, 1983.

82. Berman ML, Soper JT, Creasman WT, Olt GT, DiSaia PJ: Conservative surgical management of superficially invasive Stage I vulvar carcinoma. Gynecol Oncol 35:352, 1989.

83. Byron RC, Mishell DR, et al: The surgical treatment of invasive carcinoma of the vulva. Surg Gynecol Obstet 121:1243, 1965.

84. Abitbol MM: Carcinoma of the vulva: Improvements in the surgical approach. Am J Obstet Gynecol 117:483, 1973.

85. Podratz KC, Symmonds RE, Taylor WF, Williams TJ: Carcinoma of the vulva: Analysis of treatment and survival. Obstet Gynecol 61:63, 1983.

86. Martimbeau PW, Kjorstad KE, Kolstad P: Stage IB carcinoma of the cervix, the Norwegian Radium Hospital, 1968–1970: Results of treatment and major complications. I. Lymphedema. Am J Obstet Gynecol 131:389, 1978.

87. Soisson AP, Soper JT, Clarke-Pearson DL, Berchuck A, Montana G, Creasman WT: Adjuvant radiotherapy following radical hysterectomy for patients with Stage IB and IIA cervical cancer. Gynecol Oncol 37:390, 1990.

88. Zelikouski A, Manoach M, Giler S, et al: Lympha-press: A new pneumatic device for the treatment of lymphedema of the limbs. Lymphology 13:68, 1980.

89. Ginsberg JS, Edwards PB, Kowalchik G, Hirsh J: Intermittent compression units for the postphlebitic syndrome. Arch Intern Med 149:1651, 1989.

90. Richmond DM, O'Donnell TF, Zelikouski A: Sequential pneumatic compression for lymphadema. Arch Surg 120:1116, 1985.

91. Klein MJ, Alexander MA, Wright JM, Redmond CK, LeGasse AA: Treatment of adult lower extremity lymphedema with the Wright linear pump: Statistical analysis of a clinical trial. Arch Phys Med Rehabil 69:202, 1988.

92. Charles RH: Elephantiasis Scrot.: A System of Treatment, vol III (edited by A Latham and TC English). London: Churchill, 1912.

93. Chilvers AS, Kinmouth JD: Operations for lymphoedema of the lower limbs. J Cardiovasc Surg 16:115, 1975.

94. Thompson NT: Surgical treatment of chronic lymphedema of the lower limb with preliminary report of new operation. Br Med J 2:1566, 1962.

95. Ballon SC, Berman KL, Lagasse LD, Dekilli FS, Caslaloo TW: Survival after extraperitoneal pelvic and paraaortic lymphadenectomy and radiation therapy in cervical carcinoma. Obstet Gynecol 57:90, 1981.

96. Burke TW, Stringer CA, Gershenson DM, Edwards CL, Morris M, Wharton JT: Radical side excision and selec-

tive inguinal node dissection for squamous cell carcinoma of the vulva. Gynecol Oncol 38:328, 1990.

97. Helm CW, Hatch K, Austin JM, Partridge EE, Soong S-J, Elder JE, Shingleton HM: A matched comparison of single and triple incision techniques for the surgical treatment of carcinoma of the vulva. Gynecol Oncol 46:150,1992.

98. Stehman FB, Bundy BN, Dvoretsky PM, Creasman WT: Early Stage I carcinoma of the vulva treated with ipsilateral superficial inguinal lymphadenectomy and modified radical hemivulvectomy: A prospective study of the Gynecologic Oncology Group. Obstet Gynecol 79:490, 1992.

99. Homesley HD, Bundy BN, Sedlis A, Adcock L: Radiation therapy versus pelvic node resection for carcinoma of the vulva with positive groin nodes. Obstet Gynecol 68:733, 1986.

100. Cavanagh D, Fiorica JV, Hoffman MS, et al: Invasive carcinoma of the vulva: Changing trends in surgical management. Am J Obstet Gynecol 163:1007, 1990.

101. Powell MC, Worthington BS, Sokal M, Wastie M, Buckley J, Symonds EM: Magnetic resonance imaging: Its application to cervical cancer. Br J Obstet Gynaecol 93:1276, 1986.

102. Taussig FJ: Cancer of the vulva: An analysis of 155 cases (1911–1940). Am J Obstet Gynecol 40:764, 1940.

103. Goplerud DR, Keettel WC: Carcinoma of the vulva. Am J Obstet Gynecol 100:550, 1968.

104. Berman ML, Lagasse LD, Watring WC, et al: The operative evaluation of patients with cervical carcinoma by an extraperitoneal approach. Obstet Gynecol 50:658, 1977.

105. LaPolla JP, Schlaerth JB, Gaddis O, Morrow SP: The influence of surgical staging on the evaluation and treatment of patients with cervical carcinoma. Gynecol Oncol 24:194, 1986.

106. Weiser EB, Bundy BN, Hoskins W, et al: Extraperitoneal versus transperitoneal selective paraaortic lymphadenectomy in the pretreatment surgical staging of advanced cervical carcinoma (a Gynecologic Oncology Group study). Gynecol Oncol 33:283, 1989.

107. Piver MS, Barlow JJ, Krishnamsetty R: Five year survival (*with no evidence of disease*) in patients with biopsy-confirmed aortic node metastasis from cervical carcinoma. Am J Obstet Gynecol 139:575, 1981.

108. Wharton JR, Jones HW, Day T, Rutledge FN, Fletcher GH: Preirradiation oliotomy and extended field irradiation for invasive carcinoma of the cervix. Obstet Gynecol 49:333, 1977.

109. Potish RA, Twiggs LB, Prem KA, Levitt SH, Adcock LL: The impact of extraperitoneal surgical staging on morbidity and tumor recurrence following radiotherapy for cervical carcinoma. Am J Clin Oncol (CCT) 7:245, 1984.

110. Grumbine FC, Rosenshein NB, Zerhoyni EA, Siegelman SS: Abdomino-pelvic computed tomography in the preoperative evaluation of early cervical cancer. Gynecol Oncol 12:286, 1981.

111. Brenner DE, Whitley NO, Prempree T, Villasanta U: An evaluation of the computed tomographic scanner for the staging of carcinoma of the cervix. Cancer 50:2323, 1982.

112. Whitley NO, Brenner DE, Francis A, Villasanta U, Aisner J, Wiernik PH, Whitley J: Computed tomographic evaluation of carcinoma of the cervix. Radiol 142:439, 1982.

113. Engelshoven JMA, Versteege CWM, Ruys JHJ et al: Computed tomography in staging untreated patients with cervical cancer. Gynecol Obstet Invest 18:289, 1984.

114. King LA, Talledo E, Gallup DG, Gammal FL: Computed tomography in evaluation of gynecologic malignancies: A retrospective analysis. Am J Obstet Gynecol 155:960, 1986.

115. Newton WA, Roberts WS. Marsden DE, Cavanagh D: Value of computerized axial tomography in cervical cancer. Oncol 44:124, 1987.

116. Vercamer R, Jannsens J, Usewills R, Ide P, Baery A, Lauwerijns J, Bork J: Computed tomography and lymphography in the presurgical staging of early carcinoma of the uterine cervix. Cancer 60:1745, 1987.

117. Camilien L, Gordon D, Fruchter RG, Maiman M, Boyce JG: Predictive value of computerized tomography in the presurgical evaluation of primary carcinoma of the cervix. Gynecol Oncol 30:209, 1988.

118. Matsukuma K, Tsukamoto N, Matsuyama T, Ono M, Nakano H: Preoperative CT study of lymph nodes in cervical cancer—its correlation with histological findings. Gynecol Oncol 33:168, 1989.

119. Photopulos G, McCartney WH, Walton LA, Staab EV: Computerized tomography applied to gynecologic oncology. Am J Obstet Gynecol 135:381, 1979.

120. Villasanta U, Whitley NO, Hawes PJ, Brenner D: Computed tomography in invasive carcinoma of the cervix: An appraisal. Obstet Gynecol 62:218, 1983.

121. Bandy LC, Clarke-Pearson DL, Silverman PM, Creasman WT: Computed tomography in evaluation of extrapelvic lymphadenopathy in carcinoma of the cervix. Obstet Gynecol 65:73, 1985.

122. Averette HE, LeMaire WJ, Lecart CJ, Ferguson JH: Lymphography in the preoperative detection of lymphatic metastasis. Obstet Gynecol 27:122, 1966.

123. Piver MS, Wallace S, Castro JR: The accuracy of lymphangiography in carcinoma of the uterine cervix. AJR 111:278, 1971.

124. Jonsson K, Wallace S, Jing BS, Johnson DE, Dodd GD: Changes in the lymphatic dynamics after retroperitoneal lymph node dissection. J Urol 118:814, 1977.

125. Benedet JL, Turko M, Boyes DA, Nickerson KG, Bienkowska BT: Radical hysterectomy in the treatment of cervical cancer. Am J Obstet Gynecol 137:254, 1980.

126. Shingleton HM and Orr JW Jr. Cancer of the Cervix: Diagnosis and Treatment. London: Churchill Livingstone 146, 1987.

127. Fuller AF, Elliott N, Kosloff C, Hoskins WJ, Lewis JL Jr: Determinants of increased risk for recurrence in patients undergoing radical hysterectomy for Stage IB and IIA carcinoma of the cervix. Gynecol Oncol 33:34, 1989.

128. Kenter GG, Ansink AC, Heintz APM, Aartsen EJ, Delemarre JFM, Hart AAM: Carcinoma of the uterine cervix Stage I and IIA: Results of surgical treatment: complications, recurrence and survival. Eur J Surg Oncol 15:55, 1989.

129. Massi G, Savino L, Susini T: Schauta-Amreich's vaginal hysterectomy and Wertheim-Meigs abdominal hysterectomy in the treatment of cervical cancer: A retrospective analysis. Amer J Obstet Gynecol 1992, in press.

130. Symmonds RE: Morbidity and complications of radical hysterectomy with pelvic lymph node dissection. Am J Obstet Gynecol 94:666, 1966.

131. Parker RT, Wilbanks GD, Yowell RK, Carter FB: Radical hysterectomy and pelvic lymphadenectomy with and without preoperative radiotherapy for cervical cancer. Am J Obstet Gynecol 99:933, 1967.

132. Sall S, Pineda AA, Calanog A, Heller P, Greenberg H: Surgical treatment of Stages IB and IIA invasive carci-

noma of the cervix by radical abdominal hysterectomy. Am J Obstet Gynecol 1979; 135:442, 1979.

133. Walsh JW, Goplerud D: Prospective comparison between clinical and CT staging in primary cervical carcinoma. Am J Roentgenol 137:977, 1981.

134. Vas W, Wolverson N, Freel J, Salimi Z, Sundaram

M: Computed tomography in pretreatment assessment of carcinoma of the cervix. J Comput Tomogr 9:359, 1985.

135. Artman LE, Hoskins WJ, Bibro MC, et al: Radical hysterectomy and pelvic lymphadenectomy for stage IB carcinoma of the cervix: 21 years experience (abst). Gynecol Oncol 28(1):8, 1987.

Complications in Gynecologic Surgery: Prevention, Recognition, and Management,
edited by James W. Orr, Jr., and Hugh M. Shingleton.
J. B. Lippincott Company, Philadelphia, © 1994.

Chapter 11

Nutritional Complications

William J. Mann, Jr.

"Starvation does not improve the prognosis of any known disease process."
P.Q. Bessey and M.D. Custer, 1987[1]

Most gynecologic surgery is elective and performed on healthy women. Very infrequently, postoperative complications such as ileus or small bowel obstruction may occur, leading to prolonged periods of starvation. In gynecologic cancer patients interference with normal gastrointestinal tract function may occur with intraperitoneal spread of cancer, complications of radical or ultraradical surgery, or as a direct effect of pelvic or abdominal radiation therapy. Regardless of cause—benign or malignant—when nutritional problems arise enteral or parenteral nutritional support is frequently necessary.

Nutritional preparations are now commercially available in all hospital pharmacies, and the technique of administration has been simplified and become safe. However, judgment of the need to begin a program of enteral or parenteral nutrition requires a solid background in the indications for, complications from, and methods of nutritional support. Practical experience in actual patient management allows the physician or support team to achieve nutritional goals with fewer patient risks.

Assessing the need for nutritional support, or performing a "nutritional assessment," should be within every physician's capability. The gynecologist should also be sufficiently familiar with the clinical aspects of nutrition to assess the efficacy of

a consultant or nutrition team managing one of his or her patients.

This chapter reviews the historical background of nutritional support, describes the clinical situations in gynecology in which nutritional support may play a role, outlines the various aspects of a nutritional assessment, and provides an overview of how enteral and parenteral support is given.

History

The modern era of nutritional support began in 1967 with Stanley J. Dudrick's intravenous (IV) support of a newborn infant girl with nearly complete atresia of the small intestine. He and his colleagues at the University of Pennsylvania School of Medicine were able to demonstrate growth and development over a period of 22 months while she was fed entirely by vein. In 1968, Dudrick's group published their results in six beagle puppies and 30 severely ill humans. Using IV solutions, they demonstrated growth and development, and also demonstrated that a positive nitrogen balance could be achieved.[2] This was accomplished without crystalline amino acid solutions, trace elements, or fat-soluble vitamins, none of which were available. The value of this technique became readily apparent, and improved methods and products came rapidly. Anyone who intends to devote a significant effort to provide nutritional support or who wishes to know more about this area could benefit from reading Dudrick's reminiscences in the 1977 article, "The genesis of intravenous hyperalimentation."[3]

Nutrition was deliberately withheld from the sick until the late 19th century, when Robert Graves began to give his patients sugar water and broths. It was ultimately recognized that fever increased energy needs, and nutrition was given orally, by tube feedings, and rectally.[1] Safe IV administration of medicines and fluids was not accomplished until the late 1800s.[4] It was realized that infusions of glucose could provide nutrition, but the large volumes necessary led to fluid overload and electrolyte abnormalities. When more concentrated solutions were used, thrombophlebitis occurred. The use of concentrated glucose solutions became possible when methods of delivering the fluids through major vessels were developed. Several investigators used these methods to maintain the weight of adult dogs.[3,5] This and other work formed the foundation of knowledge upon which Dudrick and his colleagues built.

Various protein hydrolysates were administered as tube feedings, and casein hydrolysate and dextrose were first successfully given IV to a patient in 1939.[1] Synthetic crystalline amino acid solutions were subsequently developed and progressively refined.

In 1976, Hansen et al. published their results on the use of IV lipids in nutritional support.[6] They reasoned that use of a fat emulsion might prevent peripheral vein irritation and allow a higher caloric intake to be administered in small volumes. They used a 10% soybean solution (Intralipid 10%) that had previously been evaluated in Europe with considerable success and a low rate of associated complications. However, they did not rely on lipids alone, and clearly emphasized the need to combine lipid emulsions with amino acid preparations and glucose.

Vitamin and essential element and mineral requirements were determined, both empirically and with deliberate study. The required components were then available: glucose in high concentrations, amino acid solutions, lipid emulsions, vitamins, and minerals. Administration systems utilizing central lines and automatic delivery systems quickly became available.

It would not be unheard of in 1994 for a supervised first-year house staff physician to insert a central line and write initial total parenteral nutrition (TPN) orders as a matter of routine. A cursory reading of the early articles in the field will suggest the great distance we have traveled in our ability to provide nutritional support. But the current ease of initiation of nutritional support, which has come about with the ready availability of nutrient solutions, improved methods of maintaining central lines, and greater skill in managing the infrequent complications that occur, has also led to a proliferation of the services utilizing TPN. Thus, we are not yet able to define a group of gynecologic patients who would clearly benefit from this expensive care.

Indications for Nutritional Support

One cannot rely on published experience to determine which patients would benefit from nutritional support. The majority of studies are heavily weighted toward male subjects, and the overwhelming majority deal with nongynecologic disease.

Depending on individual study criteria, a significant percentage of hospitalized patients, as many as 40%, could be classified as malnourished. However, the majority of patients on a gynecologic service are admitted for elective surgery and do not have chronic disease. Consequently, the majority of gynecologic patients have no significant nutritional deficits and do well in this arena.

Infrequently, one of these patients will have a fistula or small bowel obstruction that will lead to progressive protein-calorie malnutrition. On an oncology service, intercurrent major medical illnesses are common. Radical and ultraradical surgery carry a recognized risk of major gastrointestinal injury. In addition, radiation therapy and chemotherapy may markedly impair a patient's nutritional balance. The antitumor treatment may further insult an already nutritionally deficient patient.[7] Radiation therapy can cause severe acute, then chronic radiation enteritis. There is a suggestion that TPN can limit weight loss during treatment and possibly decrease gastrointestinal side effects.[8] There are no data on its effect on survival or treatment results.

Chemotherapy may cause nausea and vomiting, generalized malaise, diarrhea, malabsorption, mucositis, and disabling electrolyte imbalances.[7] Although many studies on small groups of patients undergoing chemotherapy and TPN have been reported, there is little evidence that patients benefited from TPN, and there is some suggestion of an increased risk of significant infection.[9] No benefit in survival or response was reported in patients with lymphoma, sarcoma, cancer of the colon, lung cancer, or testicular cancer. A decrease in survival was reported in patients with lung and colon cancer.[10] All of these studies were flawed by a failure to include TPN-related results in patients with known malnutrition and to separate those patients from well-nourished women in the subsequent analysis.

Management of an intestinal fistula is complex and often entails multiple medical and surgical interventions.[11] Initial management usually includes restricting oral input (NPO) to lessen fistula output, localization of the fistula, usually radiographically, and then allowing the patient a chance to heal without surgical intervention. Patients with obstruction distal to the fistula or with an abscess are usually treated surgically. Although TPN is not needed in the management of all patients with fistula, it probably benefits some.[12] It has been proposed that the use of TPN markedly reduces fistula output, particularly if combined with the use of somatostatin; fistula closure was seen in 73% of patients within 14 days.[13] The complexity of the conditions of patients who develop a fistula, the wide number of potential intercurrent diseases, and the severe complications that occur prevent any reasonable attempt to compare two groups of patients with similar fistulas, one group given TPN and the other not, controlled for nutritional status, underlying disease, site of fistula, prior surgery, and so forth. Therefore, it is unlikely that decisions to provide nutritional support for patients with a fistula will be based on any more information than the inadequate clinical material that is available. In these situations and in nutritional assessments, calculation of losses forms the basis for decisions on the need for TPN.

Intraperitoneal cancer or severe radiation damage occasionally requires massive small bowel resection. In this situation, TPN plays an important short-term role in supporting the patient while the bowel recovers and adapts.[14]

Major operative complications are uncommon after benign gynecologic surgery, making risk stratification difficult. On gynecologic cancer services coexisting diseases often result in a "high-risk" surgical patient. Even on oncology services, however, the patient at high risk for complications can only be identified on a statistical basis, which precludes risk assessment in any single patient as opposed to a population of patients with a given disease or undergoing a given procedure. Studies in the surgical literature suggest that TPN probably lowers the postoperative complication rate but does not affect mortality.[15,16] Other studies have found no influence on the complication rate.[17] It may be that the greatest value of TPN is to shorten the postoperative convalescent period.[15,18] The American College of Physicians, after reviewing data from 11 randomized or quasi-randomized studies, concluded that perioperative TPN probably led to fewer postoperative complications and fewer deaths. TPN was considered very safe, but its use in unselected patients was not thought to be justified. TPN was only indicated for severely malnourished patients, select groups of moderately malnourished patients, or nourished patients expected to be in a poor nutritional balance for 10 or more days.[19] It is unlikely that the role of TPN in perioperative patient care will be easily resolved.

Morbidity, not mortality, and convalescence will be the parameters to follow. However, it is fair to note Burns's comments: "Most surgeons remain convinced that technical factors such as ischemia, suture placement, and intraoperative contamination remain the most important causes of postoperative complications. . . . It seems almost unfair to expect nutritional support to compensate for mistakes or inadequacies in technique."[15] An assessment of the value of perioperative TPN suffers from the fact that negative studies, in which no effect is found, are unlikely to be published. Many studies include patients who are not clearly malnourished, a patient population that is too varied with respect to disease state and intercurrent problems, and in which the extent or effects of surgery are not standardized. Moreover, most studies of TPN have been conducted in predominantly male populations with nongynecologic diseases. Clearly, careful prospective clinical trials need to be designed and completed.[20] The existence of malnutrition must be documented using agreed-upon criteria, and complications and outcome must be clearly shown to be related to this malnutrition and not to underlying disease. The use of standard nutritional formulas must be investigated over sufficient periods of time to assess efficacy in reversing malnutrition and then to allow assessment of any change in the incidence of complications.[21]

As the public continues to become better informed and more involved in medical care decisions, situations may arise where ethical considerations might lead to the institution of nutritional support in terminal patients incapable of oral intake whose families cannot face a loved one's death by starvation.[22] These cases will undoubtedly be difficult for all involved.

The most reasonable approach to deciding candidacy for nutritional support was well stated in guidelines published by the American Society of

Parenteral and Enteral Nutrition in 1986.[23] As the society pointed out, variability in clinical situations does not allow the development of absolute criteria. The lack of information from randomized trials cannot be used to support any criteria. The society concluded that health professionals, not always physicians, must balance the benefits and risks of instituting nutritional support and make a decision with input from all involved in each individual clinical situation. TPN should be considered in the care of patients with massive small bowel resection, in those with severe radiation enteritis, in those on high-dose chemotherapy regimens, or in those with a catabolic status lasting 5 to 7 days. TPN is of potential benefit in patients undergoing major surgery that would result in 10 or more days without oral intake, in patients with fistulas, in patients with hyperemesis, in malnourished patients undergoing major surgery, and in patients who will not have oral input for 10 days or longer. Although these guidelines seem logical and reasonable, they are based on the assumption that being well nourished is of benefit. In many situations there is no evidence to support this logical but unproven assumption.

Starvation and Cancer Cachexia

During the first few days of starvation the glycogen stores of the liver and muscle are used. The obligate glucose needs of the brain and red blood cells then force the body to synthesize glucose by breaking down protein into amino acids, which can be converted into glucose. As much as 75 g of protein can be metabolized daily. However, the body later adjusts and uses fat as an energy source by breaking down fatty acids to ketone bodies to meet peripheral and central nervous system demands.[24] This "fat conversion" minimizes protein breakdown, sparing muscle and viscera.

In cancer patients the ability to spare protein by switching to a lipid-derived energy source is absent. Glucose utilization persists, leading to progressive protein breakdown. Other abnormalities of glucose, carbohydrate, lipid, and protein metabolism have been described in cancer patients.[25,26] These abnormalities include glucose intolerance, increased needs for glucose, and recycling of glucose through pathways that lead to energy loss (the Cori cycle). Lipid metabolism is not suppressed by the administration of glucose, and protein breakdown continues. In addition, cancer patients experience anorexia, loss of taste, and complications from antineoplastic therapies. The degree of cancer ca-

chexia does not necessarily correlate with stage or disease extent. Mechanical factors related to intake or absorption rarely play a major role. Patients with inadequate caloric intake are likely to benefit from enteral or parenteral support. Those with metabolic abnormalities may not benefit. Control of the malignant process almost always results in an improved nutritional state.[24]

Nutritional Assessment

A patient's nutritional status is a dynamic process. Consequently it must be evaluated repeatedly during treatment to ascertain the effects of various clinical interventions or diseases. A marginally nourished patient who is subjected to extensive testing that requires intervals of NPO or minimal liquid intake or testing in an environment radically different from home may become frankly malnourished. Major surgery increases metabolic demands at a time when the patient is taking no oral diet. The simplest means of assessing nutritional status only requires a history and physical examination (Table 11–1).

Recent weight loss suggests potential nutritional problems, particularly if the amount lost exceeds 10% of the patient's normal weight.[27] In addition,

TABLE 11–1. **Assessment of Nutritional Status**

History/interview with family and friends
  Current weight, recent weights, recalled weight loss, change in clothes size
  Is patient following "special" diet?
  Record typical day's diet (confirm with family)
  Prior photos
  Recent medical treatment: surgery, chemotherapy, radiation therapy
  Occupation
  Sports/hobbies/exercise patterns
Physical examination
  Appearance (muscle wasting, decreased subcutaneous tissue)
  Weight and height
  Triceps skin fold
  Midarm muscle circumference
Laboratory evaluation
  Absolute lymphocyte count (WBC count × % lymphocytes in differential)
  Creatinine (serum and urinary)
  Albumin (urinary if spilling protein)
  Total protein
  Transferrin
  Prealbumin
  Retinol-binding globulin
  Vitamin levels
  Skin tests

one can suspect inadequate diet if the patient relates a history of frequent nausea and vomiting, recent surgery, radiation therapy or chemotherapy, or a history of drug or alcohol abuse. Recalled weights are probably quite inaccurate.[28] A patient's relatives or friends may provide important observations or facts related to weight loss or inadequate diet. Prior medical records, if available, may contain previous weights for comparison if the patient fails to recognize or denies significant losses. A recent photograph may also be valuable. A useful historical tool involves eliciting what the patient considers typical daily meals. Peculiar diet habits or "tea and toast" diets may be described by the patient as normal eating habits while actually providing inadequate protein and calories. Occasionally an occupational history (i.e., dancing, modeling) may suggest a strict calorie-depriving diet despite a patient's statement that she is eating normally. A patient with dentures who has problems talking because of loss of soft tissue and poor denture fit may also have problems maintaining an adequate caloric intake. These abnormalities should be noted and their onset determined.

The physical examination may reveal wasting of subcutaneous tissues such as facial thinning and loss of subcutaneous tissue from the arms, intercostal areas, and legs. These losses result in marked prominence of the underlying musculature, producing a drawn and sallow appearance. A profile view may disclose flaccid muscles, a concave abdomen and prominent mons, atrophic breasts, and well-defined muscles in the extremities. The buttocks may appear muscular. The rib cage, clavicles, and bony protuberances of the long bones are visible, and the skin is often dry and easily lifted from the underlying tissues. In extreme cases the patient needs assistance to rise or stand. The head may rest to the side with the chin on the chest.

Recording the patient's weight is an important initial step. Weight is an easily obtained value of great import. Ideally, weight is measured daily and at the same time of day. The patient's hydration status, use of diuretics, or the presence of ascites, effusions, masses, or edema may spuriously raise weights into the normal range even in severely malnourished patients.[29] Trends in weight over many days or weeks may offer a crude assessment of nutritional status, although on a surgical service they are more likely to reflect the adequacy or excess of fluid replacement. In outpatients who are on a stable medical regimen, serial weight determinations may be of use in assessing nutritional status, particularly if these determinations are made over several months. Usually a height is recorded. Asking the patient her height is unacceptable since the answer is frequently inaccurate. Moreover, height diminishes in the menopause without the patient's cognizance. Reference to standard tables is mentioned only to disparage it. The most commonly used references are decades old and often include smokers in the "normal" groups. Smokers weigh less than their nonsmoking counterparts and have smaller skin folds and arm circumferences than their nonsmoking counterparts.[30,31] This difference between smokers and nonsmokers is not apparently related to caloric intake, activity, illness, or socioeconomic status.

Attempts can be made to directly measure subcutaneous fat stores and muscle mass by obtaining anthropometric measurements to assess nutritional status. The most commonly used measurements are the triceps skin fold thickness and the midarm muscle circumference. These measurements are easily taken using calipers and the process is not painful to the patient. The triceps skin fold is measured by elevating the skin over the posterior aspect of the muscle and measuring the thickness of the skin fold with calipers. Approximately 50% of fat stores in the human are subcutaneous fat, hence the rationale for using this measurement. The value obtained is then compared with similar values in standard tables. Unfortunately, standardization in technique is not easy, and significant error can be introduced, particularly if multiple individuals are taking the measurements.[32,33] The midarm muscle circumference is intended to be a measurement of body protein stores, since skeletal muscle comprises 60% of total body protein. The technique is simple, requiring only the measurement of the circumference of the middle portion of the upper arm. The midarm muscle circumference can then be determined by the formula: midarm muscle circumference = measured arm circumference − (0.341 × triceps skin fold).[33,34] Errors in standardization again are a problem, and the formula assumes the mid-upper arm is circular. Standard anthropometric measurements as well as suggestions for ways to standardize the measurements can be found in Grant's *Handbook of Parenteral Nutrition*. I have not found anthropometric measurements to be of benefit in patient management, but they do provide useful points of departure for discussions on rounds with students and house staff. I have also observed that serial measurements by a serious dietician or nutritionist often seem more reliable than those made by house staff or faculty.

A wide variety of substances found in the blood

have been advocated as markers of nutritional status. Although the values of many markers can be readily determined, some are available only through reference laboratories. All have confounding factors that may negate their value in any given situation (Table 11–2).

From the commonly ordered complete blood cell count and differential, an absolute lymphocyte count can be determined by multiplying the percent lymphocytes in the differential by the total white blood cell count. Values below 1,500 suggest malnutrition and possible immunocompromise. Values below 1,000 suggest severe malnutrition. The absolute lymphocyte count is easy to obtain but is of little value in patients who are infected, on chemotherapy, or receiving radiation therapy. Drug-related alterations in the total WBC count also invalidate this measurement. However, as a single test, the absolute lymphocyte count is valuable in suggesting whether further evaluation is needed.

Immunocompetence, an indication of adequate nutrition or perhaps of the absence of severe malnutrition, can be evaluated with skin testing against common antigens (mumps, candida). However, this is a time-consuming test that is not easily used serially. Further, anergy is common in patients with cancer or who are receiving chemotherapy. When detected, anergy is too nonspecific a marker to follow during assessment of subsequent interventions.

Creatinine is produced by muscle metabolism and excreted in the urine, assuming that renal function is normal and the patient has not been placed on drugs that interfere with renal function.[32] Urinary creatinine excretion over a 24-hour period can be compared with values in standard tables based on height and sex to assess lean body mass. The data in these tables are over 15 years old. In addition, there appears to be a decrease in creatinine

clearance with advanced age, although data for women are scarce.[5] The accuracy of the urine collection is vital. Some emphasize that accurate assessment requires the patient to be on a meat-free diet and in a normocatabolic state.[33]

Serum total protein and albumin have been used to estimate the adequacy of visceral protein stores. Serum protein and albumin levels reflect a balance between synthesis, volume distribution, and catabolism. Therefore, clinical situations that alter volume, such as diuresis or fluid overload, or that lead to increased catabolism, such as surgery or sepsis, may alter protein and albumin levels and cloud their usefulness in assessing malnutrition.[33] These values are easily obtained and the normal range is well established. An albumin level below 3 g/dL or a serum protein concentration below 6 g/dL suggests malnutrition. Lower values are associated with a worse nutritional status.[27] Serial measurements must be carefully evaluated to be sure the patient is not experiencing changes in volume status or "stress" that could account for the changes noted. Administration of fresh frozen plasma, blood, or albumin preparations invalidates the use of serum protein and albumin levels for assessing nutritional status. As long as these limitations are recognized, serum albumin and protein levels may be helpful in identifying the patient with kwashiorkor. This type of malnutrition develops even though skeletal muscle and subcutaneous fat distribution and overall appearance may not suggest malnutrition. In affected patients, low serum albumin and protein levels alert the clinician to reduced visceral protein stores. The half-life of albumin is approximately 20 days; thus, low levels reflect long-term malnutrition, and when nutritional support is given there will be a considerable time lag before higher levels are achieved.[34]

TABLE 11–2. **Nutritional "Markers"**

Marker	Half-Life	Confounding Factors
Total lymphocyte count	—	Sepsis, chemotherapy, radiation therapy
Skin tests	—	Chemotherapy, cancer
Urinary creatinine excretion	—	Renal disease, diuretics, must be on meat-free diet, advanced age
Albumin	20 days	Renal disease, ascites, volume shifts, blood products
Transferrin	8–9 days	Iron deficiency, transfusions
Prealbumin	2 days	Liver disease, renal disease
Retinol-binding globulin	12 hours	Liver disease, renal disease, hyperthyroidism, deficiency of vitamin A, zinc deficiency

Other serum proteins including transferrin, retinol-binding globulin, and prealbumin have been used to assess the need for and the efficacy of nutritional support. Transferrin transports iron in the serum and has a half-life of 8 to 9 days. In addition to nutritional status, transferrin levels also reflect iron stores. Therefore, serum transferrin levels may be elevated in iron deficiency and low in patients who have received multiple transfusions.[24] Prealbumin carries thyroxine and has a half-life of approximately 2 days. Levels are reduced in patients with cirrhosis and hepatitis and elevated in the presence of renal disease. Retinol-binding globulin has a half-life of 12 hours and carries vitamin A in serum. Low levels are seen with hyperthyroidism, liver disease, vitamin A and zinc deficiency, and like prealbumin elevated levels are seen with renal disease.[35]

In the absence of confounding factors, one could interpret serum levels of these proteins as follows: acute malnutrition lowers retinol-binding protein, while a slightly longer period of stress also lowers prealbumin. Only malnutrition of several weeks' duration or longer would be expected to lower transferrin and then serum albumin levels. From these observations the duration of diagnosed malnutrition can be estimated, and this may suggest how long the underlying disease has been present. More important, when nutritional therapy is instituted in a malnourished patient with depressed serum protein levels, serial measurement of these proteins may determine the adequacy of the replacement regimen. Although it may take weeks for transferrin to begin to rise or to normalize, twice weekly measurement of prealbumin levels can aid in assessing the adequacy of treatment. Unfortunately, the reality of clinical medicine is such that confounding factors are almost always present and no one laboratory study can be used to determine the need for or adequacy of therapy.

It has been argued that malnutrition is difficult to define and that if everyone admitted to the hospital were assessed, all would have at least one abnormal laboratory value consistent with malnutrition and many would have more than one abnormality.[33,36] If one believes that malnourished patients suffer more surgical complications than well-nourished patients and that nutritional intervention is beneficial to malnourished patients, then clearly those at risk of major problems need to be identified preoperatively.[37,38] "Panels" including various combinations of serum values or anthropometric measurements do not clearly improve our ability to detect malnourished patients and probably do not yield a clinically relevant measure of the success of a given supportive intervention. If malnourished patients suffer more complications, an opinion that is certainly not unanimous, then the true measure of adequate nutritional support is the demonstration of a lack of complications.[17,39,40] If TPN is given to allow a patient to be kept NPO for a prolonged time to allow a fistula to heal, then closure of the fistula is proof of adequate support. Similarly, if poor wound healing is feared, then lack of dehiscence would indicate adequate nutritional support. It is not certain that measuring serum protein levels, following serial weights, or anthropometric measurements correlate with clinically desired outcomes, particularly since many other nonnutritional factors may interact. Undoubtedly, part of the problem in determining whether nutritional assessments are successful relates to the complexity of the conditions of the patients involved, the wide variety or intensity of clinical interventions unrelated to TPN that occur in those patients, and intercurrent medical diseases.

Probably the major determinant of whether nutritional support is needed for a given patient is the seasoned judgment of an experienced clinician. In a review of one small series of patients, clinical assessments by two physicians agreed closely with laboratory and anthropometric measurements in detecting the presence of malnutrition.[41] The subjective clinical evaluation, which was in good agreement between physicians, also predicted complications. In a larger series, 202 patients scheduled to undergo major gastrointestinal surgery were evaluated by a clinical team consisting of three physicians, a nurse practitioner, and a research nurse at two major teaching hospitals in Canada. Transferrin levels, creatinine excretion, percent ideal weight, percent body fat, and total lymphocyte count were not helpful in predicting the risk of major complications. However, a subjective evaluation and serum albumin levels were predictive.[42] Interestingly, in this series there was a low (10%) incidence of nutrition-associated complications.

The current state of the art is such that the clinician must maintain a high index of suspicion for the presence of malnutrition, particularly in the elderly or the oncology patient. They must be fully aware of the stress a proposed intervention, especially surgery, will place on an individual patient. If a patient is NPO and maintained on a standard 5% glucose IV solution in a low-stress situation, the patient would be expected to lose at least 10 g of nitrogen each day. At best, TPN can replace 3 to 5 g of nitrogen a day. Thus, it takes at least 3 days of nutritional support to "catch up" for 1 day of being NPO on dextrose 5% in water (D5W).[23] A thorough history and physical examination and "routine admitting tests" will occasionally yield an unsuspected abnormal laboratory or physical finding. With abnormal results, a more thorough assessment of nutritional status, including a directed history, physical examination, and laboratory evaluation that includes total lymphocyte count and multiple serum protein levels, should be considered. Infrequently, the clinician may order anthropometric measurements and apply skin testing to assess the presence or absence of anergy. Intercurrent medical problems, medical therapies, and fluid shifts can confuse the clinical situation. No double-blind, randomized, controlled studies will be available to confirm or refute the use of TPN in a given situation.

Against this complex, confusing, and unclear background the seasoned clinician will consult with appropriate colleagues, including nutritionists, nurses, and pharmacists, and decide whether the patient is well nourished, malnourished, or severely malnourished. If the proposed intervention is thought to have minimal impact on the patient's nutritional state, the physician may proceed without nutritional intervention but should plan to intervene postoperatively. With procedures that may further worsen the patient's nutritional status by leading to a period of 5 to 7 days of inadequate nutrition, TPN will probably be used in malnourished patients. When adequate calories cannot be ingested for 7 or more days, TPN will probably be prescribed in all patients.[43] All cancer patients may need support if major surgery is planned.

To have a measurable response, TPN needs to be administered for 7 to 10 days.[44] However, it is not necessary to delay intervention that long if time is of the essence. Even if started immediately preoperatively, TPN may still be helpful, since the beneficial effects can be expected to occur in the postoperative period. The patient will at least be spared further starvation and will begin to have desired changes in measurable laboratory parameters in the postoperative period.

The Team Approach

Although there are physicians whose practice is heavily weighted toward the management of nutritional deficits, most doctors encounter malnourished patients infrequently and seldom institute TPN. It has been argued that most physicians are inadequately trained in the principles of nutrition and are not able to diagnose and treat malnutrition.[34] Consequently, a consult service or nutritional support service may be created and function as a consultation service with expertise in assessing nutritional needs, suggesting types of intervention, and instituting and monitoring therapies. Usually this team will consist of one or more physicians, a nutritionist, and nurses familiar with administering solutions and caring for central lines. Rounds are usually carried out by the referring physician or service, who maintains primary responsibility for the patient's care. The role of the nutritional support service is to bring added expertise to a patient's care; it is not meant to usurp the attending physician's responsibility.

However, the potential effects of a team approach do not suggest that individual motivated physicians cannot provide exemplary nutritional care. I actually prefer the latter method of dealing with my patients. In teaching programs, properly supervised house staff should be able to adequately assess patients' need for nutritional support and initiate and maintain support when indicated. Alternatively, house staff may gain necessary knowledge and experience through formal rotations or on daily rounds with the nutritional support team.

Determining Nutritional Requirements

While any single patient defies accurate determination of caloric, protein, lipid, carbohydrate, fluid, electrolyte, vitamin, and mineral requirements, a "starting" point for nutritional support can be taken from the generalities that have been developed which allow calculation of all these needs from standard formulas and tables. All of these references have inherent limitations. Some are dated; others refer to unclearly defined basal states. Stresses on a patient are estimated from empirically derived data, and many references do not discuss how to begin when the basal state is clearly abnormal. Nevertheless, they serve admirably to allow one to begin, placing the obligation for subsequent alterations on the clinician who may at will overrule the standard (Table 11–3).

Fluid requirements can be calculated on a kilogram basis, an incremental kilogram basis, or based on surface area.[45] I prefer the incremental kilogram approach: 100 mL/kg for the first 10 kg, 50 mL/kg for the second 10 kg, and then 20 mL/kg for each remaining kg. Maintenance fluids are increased by

TABLE 11–3. Patient Nutritional Requirements

Fluid Requirements (FR) for 24 hours:

FR = 100 mL/kg × 10 + 50 mL/kg × 10 + 20 mL/kg for each remaining kg

Example: For a 60-kg pt.:
$$\begin{aligned}
FR &= (100\ mL \times 10) + (50\ mL \times 10) + (20\ mL \times 40) \\
&= 1{,}000\ mL + 500\ mL + 800\ mL \\
&= 2{,}300\ mL
\end{aligned}$$

Electrolyte Requirements:

Na: 3 mEq/100 mL   K: 2 mEq/100 mL   Cl: 5 mEq/100 mL

Caloric Requirements:

$$\text{kcal/day} = 665 + (9.6 \times \text{wt. [kg]}) + (1.7 \times \text{ht. [cm]}) - (4.7 \times \text{age [yr]})$$

or

$$30\ \text{kcal/kg/day} - 25\%$$

Sources of calories:

Glucose	1 g = 3.4 kcal
Protein	1 g = 4 kcal
Lipid	1 g = 9 kcal

10 mL/kg for each degree of temperature above 101° F. Urinary output and fluid assessment is performed after 8 hours, or sooner, and adjustments are made empirically. Fluid losses through nasogastric tubes, fistulas, open wounds, or other sources are not included in this approach, and needs must be estimated separately based on clinical assessment. Using the same incremental kilogram approach, electrolytes are given as 3 mEq/100 mL for sodium, 2 mEq/100 mL for potassium, and 5 mEq/100 mL for chloride.

Caloric requirements are usually calculated from modifications of the Harris-Benedict formula, which was derived from indirect calorimetry performed on normal, nonanxious, fasting adults in the semidark early morning hours. This is hardly a realistic environment or practical clinical situation. Nonetheless, caloric requirements or the basal metabolic rate (BMR) can be calculated as follows:

$$\text{BMR (kcal/d)} = 666 + [9.6 \times \text{weight (kg)}] + [1.7 \times \text{height (cm)}] - [4.7 \times \text{age (yr)}].^{1,32}$$

Although slightly different versions of this formula, which result in minor differences in final calculated BMR, appear in various texts or articles, none is clearly superior; and the BMR is, after all, only an estimate. An alternative approach is to cal-culate the caloric needs from standard nomograms, which involves determining body surface area from the patient's height and weight and basal energy expenditure from a table, and then using these two numbers to determine calorie needs by a nomogram.[45] Finally, one could simply use a formula that empirically suggests a hospitalized patient needs 30 kcal/kg/day with a correction factor for inactivity (−25%).[44] The difference between the estimates obtained by using these varied approaches is small, and the imprecision of clinical nutritional support would suggest that small differences are not clinically significant.

Clinically, it is readily apparent that the myriad clinical therapeutic or diagnostic interventions available are not of equal nutritional insult to any one patient. Further, each patient is at a given stage or phase of her disease. Consequently, some estimate of the severity of the insult or stress is needed to temper other estimates of nutritional needs, since patients with greater stress logically will need greater nutritional support. All of the measurable parameters of nutritional status can be arbitrarily or empirically quantified when abnormal into mildly, moderately, or severely abnormal. It is not clear that this is of any proven value; changes and trends are more reflective of outcome and success of intervention.

A nutritional risk index has been proposed, determined by the following formula:

$$1.519 \times \text{serum albumin (g/L)} + 0.417 \times \text{current wt./usual wt.} \times 100.^{40}$$

Values greater than 97.5 are indicative of borderline malnutrition, values of 83.5 to 97.5 indicate mild malnutrition, and values below 83.5 indicate severe malnutrition. The integral components of this formula are all subject to various confounding factors which are magnified by the formula. However, the formula does emphasize the need for assessing multiple parameters in assessing malnutrition.

Glucose solutions are the most common supplement given to patients. A gram of glucose supplies 3.4 kcal, so a liter of D5W supplies 170 kcal. One could divide the BMR by 3.4 and obtain the volume of D5W needed to provide the calculated caloric needs for a given patient. Large volumes would obviously be needed, although more concentrated solutions could be used, such as dextrose 20% or dextrose 50%.

Protein requirements, provided as amino acid solutions, should reflect the patient's age, sex, nutritional status, and current stress level. Only a fourth of the daily protein need can be expected from dietary sources; the rest comes from breakdown of serum and organ protein.[46] Roughly 50% of body protein is contained in bone and cartilage and is unavailable for mobilization to meet synthetic needs.[34,35] Hence, malnutrition or prolonged periods of inadequate oral intake rapidly lead to visceral protein breakdown. As an estimate, 1 g of nitrogen is needed for every 150 kcal of total caloric need, or 1 g/kg body wt./day.[44,45] Protein provides 4 calories per gram if metabolized.[47] Once nutritional support is in place, the adequacy of protein supplementation can be assessed by sequentially following serum protein levels, with the limitations previously discussed. Alternatively, one could determine if the desired clinical result is occurring, such as wound or fistula healing. Excellent laboratory values do not compensate for adverse clinical outcome. Another approach is to follow the patient's nitrogen balance. This is estimated from the following formula:

$$\text{Nitrogen balance} = \text{protein intake}/6.25 - (\text{urinary urea nitrogen} + 4).^{24,32}$$

The protein intake is divided by 6.25 to convert to grams of nitrogen and the urinary urea nitrogen is expressed in grams and based on a 24-hour collection. The correction factor of 4 is meant to adjust for grams of nitrogen lost in stool or nonurea nitrogen loss.

If a patient is given no fats, essential fatty acid deficiency would be expected to develop in 4 to 6 weeks.[47] Giving a liter of 10% lipids each week will prevent this problem. However, lipids are given much more frequently because they offer a means of delivering a large amount of calories in a relatively small volume. A gram of fat provides 9 kcal, while a gram of glucose yields 3.4 kcal and gram of protein 4 kcal. Many recommend that approximately 50% of nonprotein calories be given as lipids.[15]

Over 30 different amino acid solutions and at least ten different lipid preparations are available commercially. Concentrated glucose solutions can easily be obtained. The number of possible combinations one could use to provide calories as protein, lipid, and carbohydrate is mind-boggling. Common sense suggests that a hospital pharmacy, in consultation with its medical staff, should limit the solutions available to avoid ridiculously complex nutritional orders, with enormous time demands on the pharmacy. Further, all of these preparations differ slightly in electrolyte additives and the concentration of a given nutrient. To provide a semblance of order and uniformity, a standardized order form is desirable (Fig. 11–1). Selected patients may rarely require individualized preparations, but the overwhelming majority of patients can be handled by standard formulas.

Instituting, Administering, and Discontinuing TPN

The administration of TPN requires placement of a central line, which should be dedicated to TPN and not used for administering other IV fluids, blood products, or medications. A subclavian line is preferable to a jugular placement. Complications of line placement consist of pneumothorax and vessel injury but are rare when the line is placed by experienced physicians. Before solutions are infused a chest x-ray is mandatory to confirm placement into the right atrium or subclavian vein and to exclude the possibility of a pneumothorax. Considerable attention should be paid to sterile technique and to line care, but this can easily be accomplished by motivated nurses on a hospital floor, by a designated nutritional team nurse, or by home nursing services. Permanent lines are now available that may be left in place for indefinite periods of time and that have more than one lumen to allow dedication of one port for TPN and others for needed IV medications or fluids. There are data to suggest that triple-lumen catheters are more likely to become infected than single-lumen catheters (2.6% vs. 13.1%) in high-risk populations, but they also offer the great benefit of reducing the need for additional peripheral lines, which inhibit patient mobility.[48]

Before beginning TPN, the patient ideally should be in fluid and electrolyte balance. The initial infusion rate can then be that which is sufficient to provide maintenance fluids. Subsequent measurements of glucose and electrolytes can be relied on to adjust the contents of the infused solutions, with the eventual goal being to increase the infused solution to an adequate amount to provide desired calories, with stable electrolytes and glucose. Insulin can be added to TPN solutions to control glucose levels, and there is nothing to be gained by trying to avoid insulin; it is more important to provide adequate calories. With elderly patients, in whom intercurrent cardiac disease is frequent, meticulous attention to fluid balance is required. A gain of several

A. Date:

> Order solutions daily by: A. Standard Formula
> B. Individualized Formula

Instructions: Form should be completed and sent to Pharmacy by 12:00. To be written for 24 hours of parenteral nutrition.

Intravenous fat emulsion 10% _____ mL to run over _____ hours
Intravenous fat emulsion 20% _____ mL to run over _____ hours

Standard formula _____
_____ (specify by initial)

Individualized using standard formula _____ (specify by initial)
plus additives as below

Individualized using nonstandard formula plus additives as below.
Base solution _____ (see reverse of form for available solutions)
Final amino acid concentration _____
Final dextrose concentration _____

ELECTROLYTE	ADDITIVES	REQUIREMENTS/24 HOURS	AMOUNT PER LITER
Sodium	Chloride	60–125 mEq	_____ mEq
	Acetate		_____ mEq
	Phosphate	15–45 mM	_____ mEq
Potassium	Chloride	60–120 mEq	_____ mEq
	Acetate		_____ mEq
	Phosphate		_____ mmol
Calcium	Gluconate	10–20 mEq	_____ mEq
Magnesium	Sulfate	8–30 mEq	_____ mEq

ADDITIVES		DAILY REQUIREMENTS	AMOUNT PER DAY
MV$_{1-12}$	(see back)	10 mL/24 hr	_____ mL
Vitamin K	(as menadiol)	2–4 mg/wk	_____ mg
Trace elements	(see back)	5 mL/24 hr	_____ mL

MISC. ADDITIVES — AMOUNT PER LITER

Regular human insulin _____ UN

Hyperlyte® _____ ML

INFUSION RATE _____ mL/hr
MODE OF HYPERALIMENTATION ADMINISTRATION: Central ____ Peripheral ____

BASE FORMULAS—SELECT ONE
ALL FORMULAS ARE STATED AS FINAL CONCENTRATION

FORMULA A
CENTRAL PARENTERAL NUTRITION
Amino acid (Freamine 8.5% 500 mL) — 4.25% (42.5 g)
Dextrose (D50W 500 mL) — 25% (860 kcal)
Total volume — 1,000 mL

FORMULA B
CENTRAL PARENTERAL NUTRITION
Amino acid (Freamine 10% 500 mL) — 5% (50 g)
Dextrose (D70W 500 mL) — 35% (1,190 kcal)
Total volume — 1,000 mL

FORMULA C
CENTRAL RENAL FORMULATION (ESSENTIAL AMINO ACIDS)
Amino acid (Nephramine 5.4% 500 mL) — 2.7% (27 g)
Dextrose (D70W 500 mL) — 35% (1,190 kcal)
Total volume — 1,000 mL

FORMULA D
PROCALAMINE WITH ELECTROLYTES (735 mOsm/L)
Amino acid 3% — 29 g
Glycerol 3% — 130 kcal
Total volume — 1,000 mL

FORMULA E
PERIPHERAL PARENTERAL NUTRITION (1,820 mOsm/L)
Amino acid (Freamine 8.5% 500 mL) — 4.25% (42.5 g)
Dextrose (D20W 500 mL) — 10% (340 kcal)
Total volume — 1,000 mL

DAILY NUTRITIONAL GUIDELINES
Protein: 0.5 g/kg/day
Nonprotein: 10–40 kcal/kg/day
Dextrose 0–100%
Fats 0–65%

HYPERLYTE® (25 mL) CONTAINS:
Acetate	25 mEq	Sodium	25 mEq
Potassium	20 mEq	Mg^{2+}	5 mEq
Chloride	30 mEq	Ca^{3+}	5 mEq

Physician Signature: _____ *(Continued)*

FIGURE 11–1. Standard form for ordering nutritional support at Riverside Regional Medical Center. **A.** Front side of standard form. User can check off which standard formula is desired, and fill in additives and rate.

B.

AMINO ACIDS		FREAMINE 8.5% 500 mL	FREAMINE 10% 500 mL	NEPHRAMINE 5.4% 500 mL	HEPATAMINE 8% 500 mL	PROCALAMINE 3% 1,000 mL
Electrolytes (mEq)	Sodium	5	5	2.5	5	35
	Chloride	<1.5	<1.5	<1.5	<1.5	41
	Acetate	36	44	22	31	47
	Phosphate	7.3	7.3	—	7.3	7
	Potassium	—	—	—	—	24
	Magnesium	—	—	—	—	5
	Calcium	—	—	—	—	3
Protein (g)		41	48.5	10	38	29
Nitrogen (g)		7.1	8.25	1.63	6	4.6
Kcal (protein)		164	194	40	152	116
Kcal (nonprotein)		—	—	—	—	130

	CONC.	10%	20%	30%	40%	50%	70%
Dextrose	kcal/500 mL	170	340	510	680	850	1,190

VITAMINS: MV_{1-12}	(10 mL)
Ascorbic acid	100 mg
Retinol	1 mg
Ergocalciferol	5 µg
Thiamine	3 mg
Riboflavin	3.6 mg
Pyridoxine	4 mg
Niacinamide	40 mg
Dexpanthenol	15 mg
Vitamin E	10 mg
Biotin	60 µg
Folic acid	400 µg
Cyanocobalamin	5 µg

NOTE:
10 mEq calcium gluconate precipitates with more than 30 mEq potassium phosphate per liter.
15 mEq calcium gluconate precipitates with more than 20 mEq potassium phosphate per liter.
Fat emulsions separate with more than 13 mEq magnesium sulfate per liter.

FAT EMULSIONS	CALORIES	250 mL	500 mL
Intralipid 10%	1.1 kcal/mL	275 kcal	550 kcal
Intralipid 20%	2 kcal/mL	550 kcal	1,000 kcal

MULTIPLE TRACE ELEMENTS
Each 5 mL provides:

Zinc	5 mg
Copper	2 mg
Manganese	0.5 mg
Chromium	20 µg

FIGURE 11–1. (Continued) **B.** Back side of standard form. This is meant to be a brief reference for ordering physician.

pounds over the first few days or week usually indicates fluid overload, not therapeutic response.

Traditionally, TPN was administered at a constant rate over 24 hours. If the solution was unintentionally discontinued, a 5% glucose solution was immediately started to prevent rebound hypoglycemia. As home administration of TPN became more common, it was recognized that continuous infusion markedly limited a patient's mobility. As a result, stratagems were developed to allow TPN to be given over shorter periods of time, such as 8 to 12 hours, during the night. It has also been argued that cyclic administration is more natural, since it allows a postabsorption phase similar to the postpran-

dial phase after oral dietary intake.[24] There are theoretical arguments that the periods of noninfusion would allow normalization of metabolism and possibly encourage lipid utilization and improve protein metabolism. I am not convinced these advantages are real, but cyclic administration clearly simplifies both home administration and the management of patients hospitalized for long periods. Others argue there are clear advantages to cyclic administration, and a few have argued that continuous administration provides better nutritional support.[5]

When cyclic treatment is used, the solution is started and the rate increased rapidly over 1 to 2 hours; it is similarly tapered at the conclusion of the infusion. We have also discontinued continuous infusions by tapering over 1 to 2 hours and then beginning a dilute glucose infusion. Rapidly discontinuing infusions in this manner theoretically risks rebound hypoglycemia, but we have not encountered this problem with our approach. If a patient on TPN becomes able to begin oral intake, we usually do not discontinue the central feedings until the patient is ingesting more than 1,000 calories orally; then we rapidly discontinue TPN and switch to a dilute glucose solution that is discontinued after a few hours.

Home TPN is now an accepted form of treatment for patients needing long-term support. It is now possible for patients not only to live at home but also to return to their normal activities, including work. Monitoring laboratory values frequently leads to adjustments in the home formula, but major complications are rare. Most patients are readmitted to the hospital at one time or another, usually for presumed or proven line sepsis.[49] Home TPN, while orders of magnitude less expensive than in-hospital care, can still cost more than $100,000 per year.

Complications of TPN

All aspects of central TPN are fraught with potential complications, many severe. Yet the majority of patients will experience only minor problems, usually related to electrolyte imbalance.

As previously mentioned, placement of a central venous access line carries the potential risk of pneumothorax or hemothorax. The diagnosis is established from the chest radiograph obtained to confirm line placement. Proper attention to patient positioning and clinical anatomy should lessen these complications but not totally prevent them. If inserting the line on one side proves difficult, one should confirm that the lung remains inflated before switching to the second side. Bilateral pneumothoraces could be fatal. Similarly, infusion of liquids through a line without confirming the line's position could result in hydrothorax. Withdrawing the offending line and placing a chest tube should resolve these problems. Infrequently, a chest radiograph will reveal that the line is in the venous system but has crossed the midline or ascended into the neck. A technique for repositioning the line by injecting small bursts of saline through the tubing and withdrawing it has recently been described and may eliminate the need for a second puncture.[50]

Line sepsis is occasionally a difficult diagnosis

to make but must always be considered in a patient on TPN who develops fever, tachycardia, chills and sweats, leukocytosis, and a left shift in the differential. Unfortunately, these patients often have so many other concurrent problems that the source of infection is not always clear. It makes no sense to attribute infection to the central line unless pneumonia, wound infection, phlebitis, and other sources have been eliminated. Our policy is to obtain blood peripherally and through the central line for culture, to obtain urine and sputum specimens for culture, and to examine the patient in detail, searching for alternative sites of infection. We start broad-spectrum antibiotics, usually through a port in the central line. If the fever promptly lyses and subsequent WBC counts and differentials normalize over the next 24 to 48 hours, we continue the antibiotics and leave the line in place. If there is no response or if the patient is unstable, we discontinue TPN, ensure vascular access peripherally, and remove the central line. TPN is suspended until a response to the antibiotic is seen. When the patient is afebrile and improving, a new line is placed. We find replacing a line over a wire illogical but recognize that others consider this practice acceptable, and use the culture of the removed line to assess need for replacement. If fungicemia is detected, we remove all central lines and treat with systemic antifungal agents (fluconazole).

In elderly patients, particularly those with gynecologic cancer, line sepsis may manifest as mental confusion, lethargy, tachypnea, and hypotension. These markedly debilitated women do not have chills or fever. WBC counts may be deceptively low. One may be misled and begin looking for intracranial bleeding or drug toxicity. Hyperglycemia may also occur in a patient previously in good balance and in whom no formula changes have been made. A high index of suspicion is needed.

Abnormalities in serum liver function tests occur in up to 90% of patients receiving long-term TPN. The clinical significance of these abnormalities is unclear. Dextrose or lipid overload, fatty acid deficiency, amino acid toxicity, and deficiencies in various factors have been suggested as causes. Leaseburge and colleagues recently determined that the composition of TPN solutions was not associated with liver enzyme changes but that the degree of underlying malnutrition was associated with alkaline phosphatase elevations.[51] All of their patients received lipids (an average of 20% nonprotein kcal) and none were significantly overfed. They also observed that the pattern of enzyme elevations was suggestive of cholestasis. Lack of oral intake and gall hyperbilirubinemia have led us, very infrequently, to discontinue TPN. We have had one patient in the past 14 years who developed progressive liver dysfunction after many months of TPN given as treatment for a complex small bowel fistula. She ultimately died of hepatic failure, and autopsy revealed only massive fatty liver. However, if a patient becomes lethargic or somnolent, the evaluation must include determination of the serum ammonia level. Severe hepatic dysfunction of any cause may manifest in this way.

The glucose load in TPN solutions is usually handled well by the patient. However, there may occasionally be profound hyperglycemia, glucosuria with osmotic diuresis, and hyperosmolar nonketotic glycosuria, which is best managed by discontinuing TPN, treating with insulin, and hydrating with 0.5N saline while carefully correcting electrolytes. In these situations it is usually necessary to administer considerable amounts of potassium replacement. Periodic serum glucose or finger-stick determinations and periodic urine glucose and ketone determinations by dipstick should confirm the diagnosis. The onset of lethargy, stupor, or convulsions suggests that the problem has already occurred and has been missed. Special attention is needed when initiating support or when infection is present.

Stupor, confusion, and coma may also occur with marked hypoglycemia, usually attributable to accidentally discontinuing the TPN solution or overdosing the patient with insulin. Treatment involves the instillation of D50W and careful monitoring of blood sugar. If the line is disconnected, hypoglycemia may be prevented by starting a dilute glucose solution. It is wise to have standing nursing orders to cover this situation.

Electrolyte abnormalities are frequently found during the first few days of therapy. Hypokalemia may cause generalized muscle weakness, or ileus, while hyperkalemia may lead to cardiac arrhythmias. Potassium can be supplemented by increasing the amount in the solution or by utilizing a peripheral line or alternate port. Hyperkalemia is treated by administering insulin and glucose, hydration with concurrent lasix, or dialysis if necessary. Hyponatremia due to the administration of excessive free fluid or inadequate amounts of sodium in the TPN solution is corrected by restricting fluids. If untreated, it can lead to coma and seizures. Hypernatremia occurs infrequently, usually manifesting as edema. Treatment involves sodium restriction. Chloride abnormalities are uncommon.

Hypocalcemia may cause muscle cramps and aches or seizures. The free calcium levels may be normal in patients with low serum calcium values, owing to concomitant low serum albumin concentrations. Formulas and tables exist to allow calculation of free calcium from total calcium, but for most purposes it is sufficient to follow total serum calcium values. Deficiencies can be corrected with Ca^{2+} infusion. Excessive calcium administration can cause calcium deposition in soft tissues.

Muscle weakness and seizures may also result from hypomagnesemia, which is common in oncology patients who have been treated with cisplatin and have developed a magnesium-losing nephropathy. This deficiency is treated by infusing the needed element.

In the past, essential fatty acid deficiency and rare vitamin deficiencies were clinical problems. With the liberal addition of multivitamins and minerals to modern TPN solution and the use of weekly or more frequent lipid infusions, these entities are rare.

Anemia secondary to deficiencies or intercurrent blood loss is treated by ensuring adequate replacement of folate, B_{12}, and iron and transfusing as needed. Occasional patients are encountered with profound anemia who for religious or other reasons refuse transfusion. In these patients IV iron supplementation can be given using doses as large as 140 mL.[52] Hemoglobin synthesis is higher after IV administration than after oral or intramuscular injection, and anaphylactic reactions are rare.[53]

Other complications associated with TPN include cholelithiasis/cholecystitis, probably due to sludging in the inactive gallbladder; polymyopathy, possibly related to low fatty acid levels; and bone diseases related to aluminum or to the interaction of calcium, phosphate, and vitamin D.[54,55]

Peripheral Parenteral Nutrition

The risks associated with inserting and maintaining a central line have prompted efforts to develop a method of providing nutritional support using peripheral veins. Concentrated glucose solutions (D20W, D50W) cause severe phlebitis when perfused through a peripheral vein. Peripheral parenteral nutrition (PPN) solutions generally contain less concentrated amino acid solutions than TPN (3% or 8.5%), dilute glucose with approximately 100 g of glucose, or glycol solutions, and lipid solutions (10%).[56] Various PPN solutions are probably capable of reversing nutritional problems associated with mild stress in relatively well-nourished patients. This clinical situation in most instances does not require intervention. In general, PPN is not considered appropriate for use in moderately or severely malnourished patients. These peripheral solutions do not offer significant cost savings. Therefore, until further studies better define a role for PPN, at this time there is little to suggest they are of value to practicing gynecologists.

There are those who do suggest that preoperative PPN reduces surgical complications. Muller et al. randomized patients with gastrointestinal cancer to PPN or no support and found that patients who received 10 days of PPN had fewer major complications and a lower perioperative mortality than similar patients fed a hospital diet.[57] This was a well-conceived and well-executed study that should be replicated. However, one could interpret the results as showing that "starving" cancer patients in a hospital environment worsens outcome. Interestingly, in their discussion of the rationale for including patients who were not malnourished, the authors stated that "a survey of 187 patients . . . showed no difference in complications and mortality rates between those with normal nutritional status and those who were malnourished." This statement would suggest that nutritional status does not influence outcome. Their data indicate that being in a hospital 10 days preoperatively worsens outcome.

Another potential approach to using peripheral veins to provide adequate calories involves attempts to prevent protein breakdown to spare peripheral protein. This type of nutritional support is intended to be used in adequately nourished patients for short durations of treatment. The goal is "to accelerate and maximize normal adaptation to starvation."[5] It is unclear that there is any role for peripheral protein sparing in patients undergoing gynecologic surgery.

Enteral Feeding

If the gastrointestinal tract is functionally intact, enteral nutrition is more physiologic, safer, and less expensive than TPN.[58] However, for the GI tract to be intact it must be anatomically and physiologically present. Patients with multiple resections, bypassed loops, obstruction, or fistulas may lack an adequate length of functional bowel for nutritional needs. Similarly, starved patients or those with an atrophic bowel mucosa or chronic radiation enteritis do not have a physiologically intact intestine. It must be emphasized that the actual length of functional bowel necessary to maintain adequate absorption of nutrients differs in each patient.[14]

Feeding patients through nasogastric tubes has been possible for over a century, but until a few decades ago this involved the "use of large transnasal tubes . . . blenderized foods . . . and bolus feeding techniques: an unwieldy, malodorous, uncomfortable, and difficult procedure."[45] Modern techniques use commercially prepared defined solutions and slender catheters. These feeding tubes can be passed nasally or orally, or placed directly into the bowel and externalized through the skin. Enteral catheter placement is associated with fewer complications related to insertion than central lines, and although infection can occur, it is less common than with central TPN.[59] The most common problem encountered with catheters is clogging or dislodgment. Both TPN and enteral feedings through a needle jejunostomy were able to adequately support patients undergoing major gastrointestinal surgery.[60] Some studies suggest that glucose given enterally preserves the patient's ability to maintain homeostasis by utilizing endogenous pancreatic function, whereas parenteral solutions lead to hyperglycemia and require insulin administration.[61,62] Enteral therapy also maintains the integrity of the intestinal wall thickness, mucosal enzymes, and mucosal architecture; gastric feeding appears superior to direct small bowel feedings in maintaining enterointestinal hormone function.[45] Cyclic enteral feedings are possible but may not result in good nutritional support when compared to a 24-hour constant infusion.[63]

Enteral feeding covers a spectrum and includes providing the patient with a nutritious diet; adding high-calorie, high-protein supplements; tube feeding the patient with a liquid diet; or combining any enteral method with PPN or TPN. It is also feasible to use enteral diets to supplement patients in situations normally requiring TPN to situations eventually involving oral feedings.[34] A large number of diet supplements and liquid formulas exist for this purpose.

Just as with TPN, there are myriad confounding clinical variables in patients receiving enteral nutritional support, resulting in a lack of double-blind, controlled studies to support the benefit of enteral feeding in any given clinical circumstance. I have found enteral feedings of little benefit in patients with radiation enteritis, short bowel syndrome due to extensive resections for ovarian malignancy, or partial or complete bowel obstruction due to malignant disease. A major difficulty arises in providing adequate calories without using volumes that result in osmotically induced diarrhea. The long periods of time needed to gradually increase the initial dilute preparations to allow the bowel time to accommodate have been frustrating when adequate calorie support can usually be established with TPN in 48 hours. Admittedly, many describe enteral feedings to be valuable in these same patients.

Glutamine

Glutamine is a nonessential amino acid that carries ammonia from the periphery to the splanchnic bed and acts as a donor of nitrogen for the synthesis of purines and pyrimidines. It also may serve as a preferred fuel for rapidly multiplying cells such as those that line the bowel or marrow components.[64] It is possible that under conditions of severe nutritional demand, glutamine becomes an essential amino acid. There is now evidence that including glutamine in TPN or enteral solutions may increase nitrogen balance, help maintain the integrity of the intestinal mucosa, and decrease breakdown of skeletal protein.[32,58,65,66] The clinical role and potential benefit of glutamine administration are exciting and will require close observation for future use.

Future Goals

Clinical and basic research is focusing on determining the optimal combinations of lipids, proteins, and glucose to provide optimal support. In addition, different types of lipids and fatty acids are being evaluated, and alternative energy forms such as fructose, sorbitol, and ethanol are being considered. More precise determinations of mineral, vitamin, and trace element requirements are needed. Delivery catheters are being improved, as are delivery systems, particularly devices that can be implanted permanently. Computers and long-distance communications systems that allow central monitoring and adjusting of solutions while the patient remains at home are feasible.[67] And of course, medical students and house staff will continue to need exposure to the principles of clinical nutrition.

Summary

Most patients undergoing gynecologic surgery for benign conditions and many being treated for gynecologic malignancies are adequately nourished and tolerate the nutritional insult of the planned surgery without difficulty. Rarely, complications will develop after surgery for benign gynecologic or obstetric conditions and will lead to progressive nutritional deterioration; this will occur in numerous cancer patients with debilitating complications of advanced disease or treatment-related problems, or both. These malnourished patients are not always easily detected. A thorough, directed history and physical examination and pointed laboratory assessment may identify patients with significant malnutrition. When these malnourished patients are identified, the physician of record or consultants with more expertise in nutritional support must weigh the potential risks and benefits of nutritional support. If it is felt that the patient needs nutritional therapy, then the type and route of support must be decided. Once therapy is in place, vigilance is needed to prevent and identify complications. Physical assessment and laboratory evaluation can be used to assess the efficacy of treatment. Obtaining the desired patient result is the best measure of success.

Sources in the Field

There are numerous textbooks of clinical nutrition available. However, the second edition of Grant's *Handbook of Total Parenteral Nutrition* remains a superior reference for skilled clinicians, house staff, medical students, nurses, and other members of the health team. This text presents the experience gained at Duke University by a skilled nutrition team dealing with all types of patients needing nutritional support. Basic principles as well as obscure and esoteric problems are thoughtfully presented. The book is divided into chapters that stand alone, allowing the reader to refer to the text without having to read it cover to cover (which I do encourage).

The field of nutritional support is rapidly changing. Articles appear in numerous journals, but there are two sources dedicated to this topic: the *Journal of Parenteral and Enteral Nutrition* and *Nutrition in Clinical Practice*. The serious practitioner who manages a large number of patients needing nutritional support will find these journals helpful for staying abreast with current events. There is also a young but enthusiastic society, the American Society for Parenteral and Enteral Nutrition, which attempts to improve the knowledge base of health professionals involved in nutritional support, encourages exchange of information, and offers postgraduate assemblies focused on various topics in clinical nutrition.

References

1. Bessey PQ, Custer MD: Nutrition support in surgical care. Ala J Med Sci 24:158–168, 1987.
2. Dudrick SJ, Wilmore DW, Vars HM, Rhoads JE: Long-term total parenteral nutrition with growth, development and positive nitrogen balance. Surgery 64:134–142, 1968.
3. Dudrick SJ: The genesis of intravenous hyperalimentation. JPEN J Parenter Enter Nutr 1:23–29, 1977.
4. Wilkinson AW: Historical background of intravenous feeding. Nutr Dieta 5:295–297, 1963.
5. Grant JP: Handbook of Total Parenteral Nutrition, 2nd ed. Philadelphia: WB Saunders, 1992.
6. Hansen LM, Hardie WR, Hidalgo J: Fat emulsion for intravenous administration: Clinical experience with Intralipid 10%. Ann Surg 184:80–88, 1976.
7. Kokal WA: The import of anti tumor therapy on nutrition. Cancer 55:273–275, 1985.
8. Pezner R, Archambeau JO: Critical evaluation of the role of nutritional support for radiation therapy patients. Cancer 55:263–267, 1985.
9. McGreer AJ, Detsky ASg, O Rourke K: Parenteral nutrition in patients receiving cancer chemotherapy. Ann Intern Med 110:734–736, 1989.
10. Chlebowski RT: Critical evaluation of the role of nutritional support with chemotherapy. Cancer 55:268–272, 1985.
11. McIntyne PB, Ritchie JK, Hawley PR, Bartram CI, Lennard-Jones JE: Management of enterocutaneous fistulas: A review of 132 cases. Br J Surg 71:293–295, 1984.
12. Meguid MM, Campos AC, Hammond WG: Nutritional support in surgical practice: Part II. Am J Surg 159:427–443, 1990.
13. Di Costanzo J, Cano N, Martin J, et al: Treatment of external gastrointestinal fistulas by a combination of total parenteral nutrition and somatostatin. JPEN J Parenter Enter Nutr 11:465–470, 1987.
14. Dudrick SJ, Lofiti R, Fosnocht DE: Management of the short bowel syndrome. Surg Clin North Am 71:625–643, 1991.
15. Burns HJG: Nutritional support in the perioperative period. Br Med Bull 44:357–373, 1988.
16. Detsky AS, Baker JP, O Rourke K, Goel V: Perioperative parenteral nutrition: A meta-analysis. Ann Intern Med 107:195–203, 1987.
17. Fasth S, Hulten L, Magnussion O, Nordgren S, Warnold I: Postoperative complications in colorectal surgery in relation to preoperative clinical and nutritional state and postoperative nutritional treatment. Int J Colorect Dis 2:87–92, 1987.
18. Askanazi J, Hensle TW, Starker PM, et al: Effect of immediate postoperative nutritional support on length of hospitalization. Ann Surg 203:236–239, 1986.
19. Health and Public Policy Committee, American College of Physicians: Perioperative parenteral nutrition. Ann Intern Med 107:252–253, 1987.
20. Buzby GP, Knox LS, Crosby LO, et al: Study protocol: A randomized trial of total parenteral nutrition in malnourished surgical patients. Am J Clin Nutr 47:366–381, 1988.
21. Buzby GP, Williford WO, Peterson OL, et al: A randomized clinical trial of total parenteral nutrition in malnourished surgical patients: The rationale and import of previous clinical trials and pilot study on protocol design. Am J Clin Nutr 47:357–365, 1988.
22. Moley JF, August D, Norton JA, Sugarbaker PH: Home parenteral nutrition for patients with advanced intraperitoneal cancers and gastrointestinal dysfunction. J Surg Oncol 33:186–187, 1986.
23. American Society of Parenteral and Enteral Nutrition Board of Directors: Guidelines for use of total parenteral nutrition in the hospitalized adult patient. JPEN J Parenter Enter Nutr 10:441–445, 1986.
24. Martin R, Blackburn G: Nutritional support of the oncologic patient. In Knapp RC, Berkowitz RS (eds): Gynecologic Oncology, pp 553–557. New York: Macmillan, 1986.
25. Daly JM, Redmond HP, Luberman MD, Jardines L: Nutritional support of patients with cancer of the gastrointestinal tract. Surg Clin North Am 71:523–536, 1991.
26. Torosian MH, Daly JM: Nutritional support in the cancer bearing host: Effects on host and tumor. Cancer 58:1915–1929, 1986.
27. Dempsey DT, Mullen JL, Buzby GP: The link between nutritional status and clinical outcome: Can nutritional intervention modify it? Arch Surg 120:721–727, 1985.
28. Morgon DB, Hill GL, Burkinshow L: The assessment of weight loss from a single measurement of body weight: The problem and limitations. Am J Clin Nutr 33:2101–2105, 1980.
29. Heijmsfield SB, McManus OB: Tissue components of weight loss in cancer patients. Cancer 55:238–249, 1985.
30. Garn SM, Rosenberg KP, Hawthorne VM: Smoking, weight standards and "ideal" weight. Ecol Food Nutr 17:353–355, 1985.
31. Albanes D, Jones Y, Micozzi MS, Mattson ME: Associations between smoking and body weight in the US population: Analysis of NHANES II. Am J Public Health 77:439–444, 1987.
32. Blackburn GL, Bistrian BR, Moini BS, Schaum HT, Smith MF: Nutritional and metabolic assessment of the hospitalized patient. JPEN J Parenter Enter Nutr 1:11–22, 1977.
33. Smith LC, Mullen JL: Nutritional assessment and indications for nutritional support. Surg Clin North Am 71:449–457, 1991.
34. Orr JW, Shingleton HM: Importance of nutritional assessment and support in surgical and cancer patients. J Reprod Med 29:635–650, 1984.
35. Winkleer MF, Gerrior SA, Pomp A, Albina JE: Use of retinol-binding protein and prealbumin as indicators of the response to nutrition therapy. Perspect Pract 89:684–687, 1989.
36. Mullen JL, Gertner MH, Buzby GP, Goodhart GL, Rosato EF: Implications of malnutrition in the surgical patient. Arch Surg 114:121–125, 1978.
37. Detsky AS: Parenteral nutrition—Is it helpful? N Engl J Med 325:573–574, 1991.
38. Seltzer MH, Bastidas JA, Cooper DM, Engler P, Slocum B, Fletcher HS: Instant nutritional assessment. JPEN J Parenter Enter Nutr 3:157–159, 1979.
39. Verderey R: Perioperative total parenteral nutrition in surgical patients. N Engl J Med 326:273, 1991.
40. Veterans Affairs Total Parenteral Nutrition Cooperative Study Group: Perioperative total parenteral nutrition in surgical patients. N Engl J Med 325:525–532, 1991.
41. Baker JP, Detsky AS, Wesson DE, et al: Nutritional assessment: A comparison of clinical judgment and objective measurements. N Engl J Med 306:969–972, 1982.
42. Detsky AS, Baker JP, O Rourke K, et al: Predicting nutrition-associated complications for patients undergoing gastrointestinal surgery. JPEN J Parenter Enter Nutr 11:440–446, 1987.
43. Meguid MM, Campos AC, Hammond WG: Nutritional sup-

port in surgical practice: Part I. Am J Surg 159:345–357, 1990.

44. Muller JM, Keller HW, Brenner V, Walter M, Holgmuller W: Indications and effects of preoperative parenteral nutrition. World J Surg 10:53–63, 1986.

45. Page CP, Hardin TC: Nutritional Assessment and Support: A Primer. Baltimore: Williams & Wilkins, 1989.

46. Dudrick PS, Souba WW: Amino acids in surgical nutrition. Surg Clin North Am 71:459–476, 1991.

47. Heber D, Byerley LO, Chi J, et al: Pathophysiology of malnutrition in the adult cancer patient. Cancer 58:1867–1873, 1986.

48. Clark-Christoff N, Watters IA, Sparks W, Snyder P: Use of triple-lumen catheters for administration of total parenteral nutrition. JPEN J Parenter Enter Nutr 16:403–407, 1992.

49. Burns JV, O Keefe SJU, Fleming CR, Devine RM, Berkner S, Herrick L: Home parenteral nutrition: A 3-year analysis of clinical and laboratory monitoring. JPEN J Parenter Enter Nutr 16:327–332, 1992.

50. Warner BW, Ryckman FC: A simple technique to redirect malpositioned Silastic central venous catheters. JPEN J Parenter Enter Nutr 16:473–476, 1992.

51. Leaseburge LA, Winns NJ, Schloerb PR: Liver test alterations with total parenteral nutrition and nutritional status. JPEN J Parenter Enter Nutr 16:348–352, 1992.

52. Dudrick SJ, O Donnell JJ, Raleigh DP, Matheny RG, Unkel SP: Rapid restoration of red blood cell mass in severely anemic surgical patients who refuse transfusion. Arch Surg 120:721–727, 1985.

53. Hamstra RD, Block MH, Schochet AL: Intravenous iron dextran in clinical medicine. JAMA 243:1726–1731, 1980.

54. Klein GL, Rivera D: Adverse metabolic consequences of total parenteral nutrition. Cancer 55:305–308, 1985.

55. Koo WWK: Parenteral nutrition-related bone disease. JPEN J Parenter Enter Nutr 16:386–397, 1992.

56. Waxman K, Day AT, Stellin GP, Tominaga CT, Gazzangia AB, Bradford RR: Safety and efficacy of glycerol and amino acids in combination with lipid emulsion for peripheral parenteral nutrition support. JPEN J Parenter Enter Nutr 16:374–378, 1992.

57. Muller JM, Dienst C, Brenner U, Pichlmaier H: Preoperative parenteral feeding in patients with gastrointestinal carcinoma. Lancet 1:68–71, 1982.

58. Ellis LM, Copeland EM, Soriba WW: Perioperative nutritional support. Surg Clin North Am 71:493–507, 1991.

59. Payne-Jones JJ, Rana SK, Bray MJ, McSwigger DA, Silk DBA: Retrograde (ascending) bacterial contamination of enteral diet administration systems. JPEN J Parenter Enter Nutr 16:369–373, 1992.

60. Bower RH, Talamini MA, Sax HC, Hamilton F, Fischer JE: Postoperative enteral vs parenteral nutrition. Arch Surg 121:1040–1045, 1986.

61. Magnusson J, Tranberg KG, Jeppsson B, Lunderquist A: Enteral versus parenteral glucose as the sole nutritional support after colorectal resection. Scand J Gastroenterol 24:539–549, 1989.

62. Zielger F, Ollivier JM, Cynober L, et al: Efficiency of enteral nitrogen support in surgical patients: Small peptides v non-degraded proteins. Gut 31:1277–1253, 1990.

63. Campbell IT, Morton RP, Macdonald IA, Judd S, Shapiro L, Stell PM: Comparison of the metabolic effects of continuous post operative enteral feeding and feeding at night only. Am J Clin Nutr 52:1107–1112, 1990.

64. Hammerquist F, Wemeiman J, Ali R, Von Der Decker A, Vinna E: Addition of glutamine to total parenteral nutrition after elective abdominal surgery spares free glutamine in muscle, counteracts the fall in muscle protein synthesis, and improves nitrogen balance. Ann Surg 209:455–461, 1989.

65. Furst P, Albers S, Stehle P: Glutamine-containing dipeptides in parenteral nutrition. JPEN J Parenter Enter Nutr 14:118S–124S, 1990.

66. Ziegler TR, Benfell K, Smith RJ, et al: Safety and metabolic effects of L-glutamine administration in humans. JPEN J Parenter Enter Nutr 14:137S–146S, 1990.

67. Dudrick SJ: Past, present, and future of nutritional support. Surg Clin North Am 71:439–448, 1991.

Index

Page numbers followed by *t* and *f* indicate tables and figures, respectively.

ISBN 0-397-51269-4

90000